ACUTE CARE CASEBOOK

ACUTE CARE CASEBOOK

Edited by Bret P. Nelson

PROFESSOR, EMERGENCY MEDICINE CHIEF
ULTRASOUND DIVISION DEPARTMENT OF EMERGENCY MEDICINE
ICAHN SCHOOL OF MEDICINE AT MOUNT SINAI
NEW YORK, NY

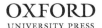
OXFORD
UNIVERSITY PRESS

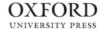

OXFORD
UNIVERSITY PRESS

Oxford University Press is a department of the University of Oxford. It furthers
the University's objective of excellence in research, scholarship, and education
by publishing worldwide. Oxford is a registered trade mark of Oxford University
Press in the UK and certain other countries.

Published in the United States of America by Oxford University Press
198 Madison Avenue, New York, NY 10016, United States of America.

Library of Congress Cataloging-in-Publication Data
Names: Nelson, Bret, 1973-, editor.
Title: Acute care casebook / edited by Bret P. Nelson.
Description: New York, NY : Oxford University Press, [2019] |
Includes bibliographical references.
Identifiers: LCCN 2018035754 | ISBN 9780190865412 (pbk.)
Subjects: | MESH: Critical Care—methods | Emergency Medical
Services—methods | Case Reports
Classification: LCC RC86.7 | NLM WX 218 | DDC 616.02/8—dc23
LC record available at https://lccn.loc.gov/2018035754

This material is not intended to be, and should not be considered, a substitute for medical or other professional
advice. Treatment for the conditions described in this material is highly dependent on the individual
circumstances. And, while this material is designed to offer accurate information with respect to the subject
matter covered and to be current as of the time it was written, research and knowledge about medical and health
issues is constantly evolving and dose schedules for medications are being revised continually, with new side
effects recognized and accounted for regularly. Readers must therefore always check the product information
and clinical procedures with the most up-to-date published product information and data sheets provided by
the manufacturers and the most recent codes of conduct and safety regulation. The publisher and the authors
make no representations or warranties to readers, express or implied, as to the accuracy or completeness of this
material. Without limiting the foregoing, the publisher and the authors make no representations or warranties as
to the accuracy or efficacy of the drug dosages mentioned in the material. The authors and the publisher do not
accept, and expressly disclaim, any responsibility for any liability, loss or risk that may be claimed or incurred as
a consequence of the use and/ or application of any of the contents of this material.

1 3 5 7 9 8 6 4 2

Printed by Webcom, Inc., Canada

CONTENTS

SECTION V
MEDICINE FLOOR
Allen Tran

SECTION VI
PEDIATRIC CLINIC
Jennifer Sanders

PREFACE

This book was inspired by countless discussions over the years with the teams who brought patients in to my emergency department and the teams who cared for them after me. As medics, nurses, doctors, students, and physician's assistants caring for patients in and out of the hospital, we see the same pathology through different lenses. We can learn a tremendous amount from each other by sharing our stories.

We have over 70 cases written by experts who care for patients in many different environments. In every case, something goes acutely wrong. Snakes bite hikers, ward patients become hypotensive, and hypoxic patients need emergent transport. The cases highlight common pathologies and the approach to care, including images and a debrief of key learning points. We hope you enjoy the journey; in the end, we all learn medicine one patient at a time.

I am grateful to all our editors for their commitment to excellent clinical care and education. Thank you for your incredible contributions and for teaching me so much! To Susan, Holden, and Austin, I thank you for your patience and inspiring me to be better.

Bret P. Nelson

CONTRIBUTORS

Andrea Austin, MD
Emergency Medicine Instructor
Assistant Professor
Uniformed Services University
Naval Medical Center
San Diego, CA

Marko Balan, MD, FRCPC
Department of Critical Care
Dalhousie University
Halifax, Nova Scotia, Canada

Jennifer Bellis, MD, MPH
Instructor, Department of Pediatrics
Section of Emergency Medicine
University of Colorado
Aurora, CO

Alexander Berk, MD
Assistant Clinical Professor of Medicine
Education Director, Hawaii Emergency
  Physicians Associated
The John H. Burns School of Medicine
University of Hawaii
Honolulu, HI

Katherine Biggs, DO, LT, MC, USN
Emergency Medicine PGY-4, Chief Resident
Naval Medical Center Portsmouth
United States Navy
Portsmouth, VA

Caroline Black, MD
Pediatric Emergency Medicine
Department of Emergency Medicine
Ichan School of Medicine
Mount Sinai Hospital
New York, NY

Rachelle Blackman, MD
Department of Medicine
Dalhousie Internal Medicine
Queen Elizabeth II Health Sciences
  Centre
Halifax, Nova Scotia, Canada

Andrew Caddell, MD
Department of Medicine
Division of Cardiology
Dalhousie University
Halifax, Nova Scotia, Canada

Carlo Canepa, MD
Emergency Medicine Physician
Commonwealth Healthcare
  Corporation
Saipan, Northern Mariana Islands

Martin Casey, MD, MPH
Department of Emergency Medicine
Icahn School of Medicine
Mount Sinai
New York, NY

Rittik Chaudhuri, MD, PhD
Department of Emergency Medicine
Massachusetts General Hospital
Brigham and Women's Hospital
Harvard Medical School
Boston, MA

Drew Clare, MD
Resident, Department of Emergency
    Medicine
Virginia Commonwealth University
    Health System
Richmond, VA

Kara Cockrum, DO
Resident, Department of Pediatrics
Medical University of South Carolina
Charleston, SC

Heidi Cordi, MD, MPH, MS, EMTP, FACEP
Assistant Professor of Clinical
    Medicine
Associate Medical Director of Emergency
    Medical Services
The New York Presbyterian Hospital
New York, NY
Associate Professor of Emergency Medicine
Core Faculty, Division of Emergency Medical
    Services
Albany Medical Center
Albany, NY

Angela Creditt, DO
Assistant Professor and Clinical Faculty
Department of Emergency Medicine
Virginia Commonwealth University
    Medical Center
Richmond, VA

Jeremy T. Cushman, MD, MS
Associate Professor of Emergency Medicine
Chief of the Division of Prehospital Medicine
University of Rochester
School of Medicine and Dentistry
Rochester, NY

Elizabeth DeVos, MD, MPH, FACEP
Associate Professor, Emergency Medicine
University of Florida College of Medicine
Jacksonville, FL

Sean Donovan, MB, BCh, BAO
Assistant Professor of Emergency
    Medicine
Division of Emergency Ultrasound
Division of Prehospital & Operational
    Medicine
Albany Medical Centre
Rochester, NY

Maia Dorsett, MD, PhD
Clinical Instructor of Emergency Medicine
Division of Prehospital Medicine
University of Rochester Medical Center
Rochester, NY

Shannon Drohan, MD
Pediatrician
Eastern Carolina Pediatrics
Wilson, NC

Patrick Engelbert, MD
Department of Emergency Medicine
Naval Medical Center
San Diego, CA

Aaron Farney, MD
Department of Emergency Medicine
University of Rochester Medical Center
Rochester, NY

Christopher J. Fullagar, MD, EMT-P, FACEP
Assistant Professor of Emergency
    Medicine
State University of New York Upstate
    Medical University
Syracuse, NY

Christopher Galton, MD
Assistant Professor
Departments of Anesthesiology and
    Emergency Medicine
University of Rochester Medical Center
Chief Medical Director, Mercy Flight Central
Deputy EMS Medical Director
Monroe County, NY

Sylvia E. Garcia, MD
Assistant Professor of Emergency Medicine
Assistant Professor of Pediatrics
Icahn School of Medicine at Mount Sinai
New York, NY

Harman S. Gill, MD
Assistant Professor of Medicine
Emergency Medicine and Critical Care
    Medicine
Dartmouth Hitchcock Medical Center
Lebanon, NH

Christopher J.M. Green, MD
Physician Fellow
Division of General Internal Medicine
Department of Medicine
Dalhousie University
Halifax, Nova Scotia, Canada

Peter Gutierrez, MD
Fellow of Pediatric Emergency Medicine
Emory University School of Medicine
Atlanta, GA

N. Stuart Harris, MD
Chief, Division of Wilderness Medicine
Department of Emergency Medicine
Massachusetts General Hospital
Boston, MA

John Haggerty, DO
Resident Physician, Emergency Medicine
Naval Medical Center
San Diego, CA

Douglas Hofstetter, MD
Department of Emergency Medicine
Uniformed Services University
Naval Medical Center
San Diego, CA

Oliver Hulland, MD
Resident, Emergency Medicine
Yale School of Medicine
New Haven, CT

Michael Joyce, MD
Virginia Commonwealth University School
    of Medicine
Richmond, VA

Ali Kamran, MD
Resident, Emergency Medicine
Yale School of Medicine
New Haven, CT

Aamer Khan, MD
Resident, Emergency Medicine
Yale School of Medicine
New Haven, CT

Olga Kovalerchik, MD
Instructor of Emergency Medicine
Yale University School of Medicine
New Haven, CT

Benjamin J. Lawner, DO, MS
Department of Emergency Medicine
Allegheny General Hospital
Department of Emergency Medicine
Temple University School of Medicine
Pittsburgh, PA

Jaclyn LeBlanc, PharmD, MD
Internal Medicine Resident
Saint John Regional Hospital
Saint John, New Brunswick, Canada

Eric Lee, MD
Department of Emergency Medicine
Maimonides Medical Center
Brooklyn, NY

Scott Lee, MD
Dalhousie University
Halifax, Nova Scotia, Canada

Kathleen Li, MD
Resident, Department of Emergency
    Medicine
Icahn School of Medicine at
    Mount Sinai
New York, NY

S. Terez Malka, MD
Physician, Emergency Medicine and Pediatric
    Emergency Medicine
Department of Emergency Medicine
University of Colorado School of Medicine
Carepoint Healthcare
Aurora, CO

Nathaniel R. Mann, MD
Department of Emergency Medicine
Massachusetts General Hospital
Boston, MA

Evie Marcolini, MD, FACEP, FAAEM, FCCM
Assistant Professor of Surgery
   and Neurology
Director of Critical Care Education
Emergency Medicine Fellowship Director
University of Vermont Medical Center
Burlington, VA

Michelle N. Marin, MD
Assistant Professor of Pediatric Emergency
   Medicine
Department of Emergency Medicine
Icahn School of Medicine at Mount Sinai
New York, NY

Ryan Maves, MD
Department of Emergency Medicine
Uniformed Services University
Naval Medical Center
San Diego, CA

Julie Mayglothling Winkle, MD
Assistant Professor, Emergency Medicine
Virginia Commonwealth University
Medical College of Virginia School of
   Medicine
Richmond, VA

Jeff Meyer, MD
Assistant Professor
Division of General Pediatrics
Department of Pediatrics
University of Louisville
Louisville, KY

Stephen Miller, DO
Assistant Professor of Emergency Medicine
Residency Assistant Program Director
Virginia Commonwealth University
Richmond, VA

David Mills, MD
Assistant Professor
Department of Pediatrics
Medical University of South Carolina
Charleston, SC

Michael Mohseni, MD
Assistant Professor of Emergency Medicine
Mayo Clinic
Jacksonville, FL

Sarah Morgan, MD
Resident of Internal Medicine
Virginia Commonwealth University
   Health System
Rochester, VA

Philip Nawrocki, MD
Department of Emergency Medicine
Allegheny General Hospital
Pittsburgh, PA

Jillian Nickerson, MD, MS
Department of Emergency Medicine
Icahn School of Medicine at Mount Sinai
New York, NY

Cynthia Oliva, MD
Resuscitation/Ultrasound Fellow
Virginia Commonwealth University
Richmond, VA

Glenn Patriquin, MSc, MD, FRCPC
Resident Physician, Infectious Diseases and
   Medical Microbiology
Dalhousie University
Halifax, Nova Scotia, Canada

Jacqueline Paulis, MD
Clinical Instructor and Ultrasound Fellow
Department of Emergency Medicine
New York University School of Medicine
Bellevue Hospital Center
New York, NY

Christopher M. Perry, DO, LCDR, MC
Emergency Medicine Resident
Portsmouth Naval Hospital
Portsmouth, VA

Elysha Pifko, MD
Division of Pediatric Emergency Medicine
Nemours/Alfred I. DuPont Hospital for
   Children
Wilmington, DE

Justin T. Pitman, MD
Physician
Department of Emergency Medicine
Mount Auburn Hospital
Cambridge, MA

David Poliner, DO
Department of Emergency Medicine
Allegheny General Hospital
Pittsburgh, PA

Steven Portouw, MD
Staff Emergency Physician
Naval Medical Center
San Diego, CA

Usama Qadri, MD
Resident, Emergency Medicine
Yale New Haven Hospital
New Haven, CT

Megha Rajpal, MD
Resident
Icahn School of Medicine at Mount Sinai
New York, NY

Megan Rashid, MD
Assistant Professor of Anesthesiology
Virginia Commonwealth University
    Health System
Richmond, VA

Essie Reed-Schrader, MD
Fellow in EMS Medicine
University at Buffalo
Erie County Medical Center
Buffalo, NY

Jennifer Repanshek, MD
Associate Professor, Emergency Medicine
Lewis Katz School of Medicine
Temple University
Philadelphia, PA

William T. Rivers, MD
Department of Emergency Medicine
Jacobs School of Medicine and Biomedical
    Sciences
University at Buffalo
Buffalo, NY

Alison Rodger, MD, FRCPC
Department of Medicine
Division of Geriatric Medicine
Dalhousie University
Halifax, Nova Scotia, Canada

Erik Rueckmann, MPH, MD, FACEP
Assistant Professor of Emergency
    Medicine
University of Rochester Medical Center
Medical Director, American Medical
    Response
Rochester, NY

Abbie Saccary, MD
Resident
Department of Emergency Medicine
Yale University School of Medicine
New Haven, CT

Renee N. Salas, MD, MPH, MS
Assistant Wilderness Medicine Fellowship
    Director
Division of Wilderness Medicine
Department of Emergency Medicine
Massachusetts General Hospital; Instructor
    in Emergency Medicine
Harvard Medical School
Boston, MA

Jennifer Sanders, MD
Assistant Professor, Emergency Medicine
Assistant Professor, Pediatrics
Icahn School of Medicine at Mount Sinai
New York, NY

Aman Shah, MD
Instructor of Emergency Medicine
Department of Emergency Medicine
Yale School of Medicine
New Haven, CT

Daniel Shocket, MD
Emergency Physician
Carson Tahoe Emergency Physicians
Carson City, NV

Leslie V. Simon, DO
Assistant Professor of Emergency Medicine
Mayo Clinic
Jacksonville, FL

Ashley Sutherland, MSc, MD
Dalhousie Medical School
Halifax, Nova Scotia, Canada

Todd W. Thomsen, MD
Attending Physician
Department of Emergency Medicine
Mount Auburn Hospital
Cambridge, MA
Instructor in Medicine
Harvard Medical School
Boston, MA

Anthony Tomassoni, MD, MS, FACEP, FACMT, FAACT
Associate Professor
Department of Emergency Medicine
Yale School of Medicine
Medical Director
Yale New Haven Center for Emergency
    Preparedness and Disaster Response
New Haven, CT

Jordan Tozer, MD, MS
Assistant Professor of Emergency Medicine
Virginia Commonwealth University School
    of Medicine
Richmond, VA

Allen Tran, MD
Assistant Professor
Division of General Internal Medicine
Department of Medicine
Dalhousie University
Halifax, Nova Scotia, Canada

Colin Turner, MD
Resident
Dalhousie University Department of
    Medicine
Halifax, Nova Scotia, Canada

Temima Waltuch, MD
Resident, Emergency Medicine
Icahn School of Medicine at Mount Sinai
New York, NY

Denise Whitfield, MD
Adjunct Faculty
Department of Emergency Medicine
Assistant Professor of Clinical
    Medicine
David Geffen School of Medicine
Harbor-UCLA Medical Center
University of California, Los Angeles
Los Angeles, CA

Thomas Williams, MD
Department of Emergency Medicine
Glens Falls Hospital
Glens Falls, NY

Sarah Yale, MD
Resident, Department of Pediatrics
The Medical University of
    South Carolina
Charleston, SC

ACUTE CARE CASEBOOK

SECTION I

WILDERNESS/EXPEDITION MEDICINE

N. STUART HARRIS

CHAPTER 1

HEADACHE AT HIGH ALTITUDE

RENEE N. SALAS

SETTING

Wilderness, Everest Base Camp, Nepal

CHIEF COMPLAINT

Headache

HISTORY

A 45-year-old female presents to an expedition physician at Mount Everest Base Camp (5,380 m/17,650 ft) in Nepal (Figure 1.1) with a complaint of headache. The headache has been present for 12 hours, was gradual in onset, was worse this morning, and described as a bitemporal and throbbing. She currently rates it as a 7/10. She denies preceding trauma, fever, photophobia, or neck stiffness. She reports mild nausea, anorexia, moderate fatigue, generalized weakness, mild dizziness, and poor sleep last night. She denies vomiting, focal weakness or speech disturbances, gait instability, confusion, cough, dyspnea on exertion or at rest, or decreased exercise tolerance. She denies being around a gas stove in closed quarters. No one else on her team has had similar symptoms. She arrived to camp late yesterday after ascending from Gorak Shep (5,140 m/16,863 ft) after following a gradual ascent schedule.

She endorses a past medical history of acute mountain sickness (AMS) when summiting Mount Kilimanjaro (5,895 m/19,341 ft).

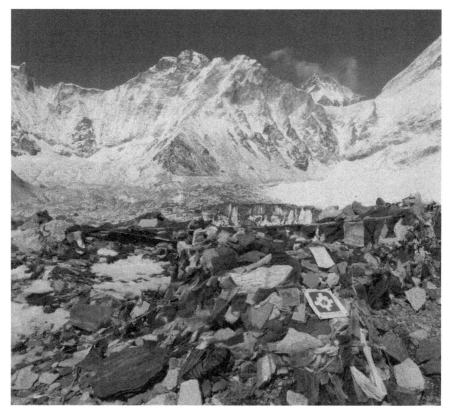

FIGURE 1.1 Everest Base Camp (5,380 m/17,650 ft) in Nepal.
Photograph by Dr. Renee N. Salas and used with permission.

She has been taking acetazolamide and acetaminophen and denies allergies.
She denies smoking, recent alcohol use, or the use of other illicit drugs.
She denies any family history of cerebral aneurysms.

PHYSICAL EXAMINATION

Vital signs: HR 115, BP 110/85, RR 26, SpO_2 81%, on room air, temp 36.5°C.

Examination reveals a muscular female in no acute distress. Examination of head and neck is normal with no jugular venous distension. She exhibits tachypnea but lungs are clear bilaterally with good air movement. She is tachycardic but regular with normal S1/S2 and no murmurs, rubs, or gallops appreciated. Her abdomen is soft, nontender, and nondistended. She has no lower extremity edema. Her extremities are warm and well-perfused. Neurologic examination reveals she is alert and orientated × 4. Cranial nerves 2 to 12 and motor/sensory function are intact throughout. She completes finger to nose and heel to shin without past pointing. Bicep and patellar reflexes are 2+ equal and symmetric. Gait and tandem gait are fully intact with no ataxia.

DIFFERENTIAL DIAGNOSIS

1. AMS
2. High altitude headache
3. High altitude cerebral edema (HACE)
4. High altitude pulmonary edema (HAPE)
5. Viral syndrome
6. Dehydration
7. Carbon monoxide poisoning
8. Intracranial hemorrhage
9. Meningitis/central nervous system infection

TESTS

Ambulatory saturation with warm fingers were 79% to 82% without notable dyspnea on exertion. Orthostatic vital signs are normal. No laboratory or radiographic tests are available.

CLINICAL COURSE

The patient was given an analgesia and antiemetic. Oral fluid intake was encouraged and tolerated. She was given a treatment dose of acetazolamide. She was directed to not ascend to higher sleeping elevations until her symptoms resolved. She came for a recheck the following day and felt significantly improved. She was symptom free at 48 hours other than continued mild sleep disturbances.

KEY MANAGEMENT STEPS

1. In austere environments, radiographic or laboratory testing are not typically available. Providers must rely on careful history and physical exam to make a diagnosis.
2. Awareness that "normal" vital signs at high altitude are markedly different from standard sea level values. Following a graded ascent, for patients newly at 5,300 meters, a pulse oximeter reading of approximately 80% is "normal." In addition, one should recognize that normal physiologic acclimatization to high altitude includes tachycardia and tachypnea.
3. It is critical to differentiate AMS from HACE and/or HAPE. The presence of altered mental status or ataxia suggests cerebral edema, and the presence of resting dyspnea, crackles, cough productive of frothy sputum, or hypoxia out of proportion to altitude suggests pulmonary edema. HACE and HAPE are immediate life threats that cannot be missed.
4. Acclimatization and symptom management are the mainstay of AMS treatment. Do not advance to a higher sleeping altitude until the symptoms resolve. Pharmacological interventions include symptom management with analgesics (nonsteroidal

anti-inflammatory drugs or acetaminophen) and antiemetic (Ondansetron) as indicated. If symptoms do not improve, consider oral steroids (dexamethasone) and descent.

DEBRIEF

The first step in caring for a patient with a headache at high altitude is to assess for life-threatening pathology. This patient's "abnormal" tachycardia, tachypnea, and hypoxia are all consistent with normal acclimatization following acute exposure to high altitude. Overall, her presentation is most consistent with AMS. Generally, AMS can occur when an individual ascends from lower elevations to an altitude above 2,500 meters. While objective criteria would be ideal, currently AMS is defined by subjective self-reported criteria called the Lake Louise Score. Using this scoring system, in which each category is rated mild (1) to severe (3), AMS is defined as a headache plus 1 or more of the following: gastrointestinal symptoms (anorexia/nausea/vomiting), fatigue/weakness, dizziness/lightheadedness, and/or sleep difficulty. Other than potential vital sign changes (when compared with sea-level "normal"), physical examination in AMS is unremarkable. Abnormal physical examination or fever suggests other concurrent pathology. This patient's benign headache with associated symptoms following recent ascent to high altitude are sufficient to diagnose AMS. Even though she followed the ascent guidelines, she is still at risk for AMS. The patient should be advised not to ascend to a higher sleeping altitude while symptoms remain. Pharmacological interventions include symptom management: antiemetics to assist with maintaining appropriate hydration, nonsteroidal anti-inflammatory drugs, or acetaminophen for headache treatment. Acetazolamide, a carbonic anhydrase inhibitor, can assist in acclimatization and may be used for treatment. If the symptoms worsen or continue for more than 24 hours, then descent to a lower altitude is recommended. In patients with severe or continued symptoms without other findings, oral steroids may be considered—but only in patients who will not resume ascent until they are off of steroids and asymptomatic. In austere environments, it is critical that the patient be closely monitored by friends for progression of symptoms and have short-term follow-up with strict return precautions provided to the patient and teammates.

In the patient with an isolated headache at altitude without other features of AMS, a diagnosis of high altitude headache may be made. Two common life-threatening pathologies at high altitude that cannot be missed are HACE and HAPE. HACE is typically associated with preceding moderate to severe AMS symptoms and has exam findings that may include ataxia, altered mental status, or papilledema (though fundoscopy is often unavailable). To rule out HACE, all patients at altitude with headache need to be assessed for altered mental status and ataxia. Tandem gait testing to assess for ataxia is the test of choice. HAPE can occur with both AMS and/or HACE. HAPE patients typically have dyspnea at rest and/or dyspnea on exertion, a change in exercise tolerance, and/or cough. Physical exam features can include hypoxia out of proportion to altitude and crackles on pulmonary exam. Both HACE and HAPE are best treated with supplemental oxygen and immediate descent. In addition, HACE may be treated with dexamethasone, and HAPE, with nifedipine.

FURTHER READING

Bartsch P, Swenson ER. Acute high-altitude illnesses. *N Engl J Med*. 2013;368:2294–2302.

Grissom CK, Roach RC, Sarnquist FH, Hackett PH. Acetazolamide in the treatment of acute mountain sickness: clinical efficacy and effect on gas exchange. *Ann Intern Med*. 1992; 116:461–465.

Hackett PH, Luks AM, Lawley JS, Roach RC. High-altitude medicine and pathophysiology. In Auerbach PS, Cushing TA, Harris NS, eds. *Auerbach's Wilderness Medicine*. 7th ed. Philadelphia, PA: Elsevier; 2017: 8–28.

Luks AM, McIntosh SE, Grissom CK, et al. Wilderness medical society practice guidelines for the prevention and treatment of acute altitude illness: 2014 update. *Wild Environ Med*. 2014;25(4):S4–S14.

HEAD TRAUMA

TODD W. THOMSEN

SETTING

Wilderness, Utah

CHIEF COMPLAINT

Blunt head injury with loss of consciousness

HISTORY

A 67-year-old male patient is backcountry skiing with a group of friends. On the final descent of the day, while skiing through a glade, he loses control and strikes a large pine tree at a moderate rate of speed. Witnesses describe a complete loss of consciousness lasting about 3 minutes. No seizure activity or abnormal posturing are noted. He is not wearing a helmet. After regaining consciousness, the patient is confused and disoriented and is noted to repetitively question his companions about where he is and what has happened. He is also noted to be slightly dyspneic. Despite the group's wishes to help him ski back down to the base of the mountain, he is unable to continue. He vomits multiple times and gradually becomes more lethargic. The search-and-rescue team is summoned to the scene to provide assistance and evacuation.

He has no chronic medical problems.

He does not take any medications and has no known drug allergies.

PHYSICAL EXAMINATION

Vital signs: HR 110, BP 92/60, RR 24, SpO₂ 91% on room air, temp. 37.1°C.

   Examination reveals an athletic man who appears much younger than his stated age. He is lethargic but opens his eyes on command. He is confused, does not remember what happened to him, and is occasionally uttering inappropriate words. He inconsistently follows commands and localizes light painful stimuli. Motor strength, sensation, and reflexes are normal in all extremities. There is a 3 cm laceration on the right forehead with a surrounding hematoma. His pupils are 3 mm and reactive bilaterally. The cervical spine is nontender and without step-offs. There is tenderness to palpation to the right anterior chest wall; however, no crepitus or flail segments are noted. The lungs are clear bilaterally. His heart is regular rhythm with limited tachycardia. Radial pulses are normal. The abdomen is soft and nontender. No tenderness, deformities, or other trauma are noted in the extremities. His skin is warm and well-perfused.

DIFFERENTIAL DIAGNOSIS

1. Epidural hematoma
2. Subdural hematoma
3. Subarachnoid hemorrhage
4. Cerebral parenchymal contusion
5. Concussion

TESTS

Detailed serial neurologic examinations were performed to document any changes in the patient's clinical status. A noncontrast computed tomography (CT) scan of the brain revealed a traumatic subarachnoid hemorrhage (Figure 2.1A).

CLINICAL COURSE

Members of the ski party realized that they would be unable to evacuate the patient without assistance. A wilderness search-and-rescue team was summoned to the scene. Oxygen was applied to maintain saturations >90%, and intravenous fluids were started to maintain systolic pressures >90 mm Hg. Given high mechanism injury, C-spine precautions and immobilization were applied. The patient was evacuated from the mountainside and transferred to a regional trauma center. He was admitted to the trauma intensive care unit for close monitoring. He was given a gram of Keppra. His laceration was sutured. His neurological exam remained nonfocal, and his confusion gradually improved. No other serious injuries were discovered, and he was discharged home after a relatively uneventful 4-day hospital stay.

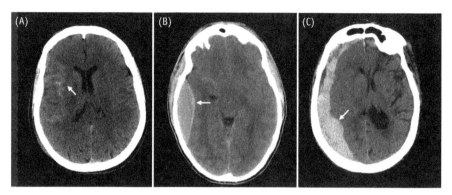

FIGURE 2.1 (A) Traumatic subarachnoid hemorrhage. Note the presence of hyper-dense blood layering in the subarachnoid space along the right sylvian fissure. (B) Epidural hematoma (EDH). EDH's are lenticular collections, usually found in the temporal regions. The lenticular morphology is due to the hemorrhage being contained by dural reflections. These injuries are usually arterial in nature. (C) Acute subdural hematoma (SDH). The crescentic shape of this lesion is characteristic of SDH, and the hyper-density of the hematoma indicates this is an acute injury. SDHs can occur anywhere in the cranium, however they do not cross the midline as they are contained by the falx cerebri.

KEY MANAGEMENT STEPS

1. Recognizing that this patient had a significant mechanism of injury, displayed signs of potentially serious intracranial injury, and required emergent neuroimaging to rule out intracranial hemorrhage.
2. Recognizing that hypoxia and hypotension can lead to secondary brain injury and treating these conditions appropriately.
3. Arranging for expedient transfer to a trauma center for definitive diagnostic and therapeutic intervention.

DEBRIEF

This patient sustained a high-energy deceleration injury and was at risk for multisystems trauma. Given the severity of injury, the backcountry location of the incident, and the logistical difficulties of an evacuation, the prompt and appropriate decision to evacuate the patient to a trauma center was correct.

The Canadian CT Head Rule is a validated clinical decision rule that can be utilized to determine which head injury patients require neuroimaging. The rule dictates that a patient with any 1 of the following high-risk criteria require an imaging study: Glasgow Coma Scale (GCS) <15 at 2 hours post injury; suspected open or depressed skull fracture; signs of basilar skull fracture (e.g., hemotympanum, raccoon eyes, Battle's sign, central serous retinopathy, otorrhea, or rhinorrhea); 2 or more episodes of vomiting; age ≥65; retrograde amnesia >30 minutes; or "dangerous" mechanism of injury (e.g., pedestrian struck by motor vehicle, occupant ejected from motor vehicle, fall from >3 feet or >5 stairs). Our patient "failed" the rule by 5 measures—age, GCS, amnesia, vomiting, and dangerous mechanism—and thus required urgent brain imaging.

The ultimate goal of wilderness and prehospital management of the severely head-injured patient is timely delivery to a trauma center. Maintenance of oxygen saturations >90% and systolic pressures >90 mm Hg is important to prevent secondary brain injury. Appropriate cervical spine immobilization and treatment of concomitant injuries should be undertaken during transport. If feasible, the patient should be positioned with the head of the bed raised to 30° to mitigate increases in intracranial pressures.

Definitive management of intracranial trauma depends on the type of injury present. Patients with traumatic subarachnoid hemorrhage (see Figure 2.1A) rarely require neurosurgical intervention; however, they may need treatment for complications such as hydrocephalus and cerebral vasospasm (similar to aneurysmal subarachnoid patients.) Treatment with Keppra intravenously to decrease risk of complicating seizure is recommended. Patients with epidural hematomas (see Figure 2.1B) often require emergent surgery, although select patients with smaller hemorrhages can be observed clinically. General indications for operative intervention of epidural hematomas include hematoma volume >30 cm^3, hematoma width >15 mm, and midline shift >5 mm. Patients with acute subdural hematomas (see Figure 2.1C) may also require operative interventions. General indications for surgery on these lesions include hematoma thickness >10 mm, midline shift >5 mm, decreasing GCS, and asymmetric or fixed and dilated pupils.

FURTHER READING

Borczuk P, Penn J, Peak D, Chang Y. Patients with traumatic subarachnoid hemorrhage are at low risk for deterioration or neurosurgical intervention. *J Trauma Acute Care Surg*. 2013; 74:1504–1509.

Bullock MR, Chesnut R, Ghajar J, et al. Surgical management of acute epidural hematomas. *Neurosurgery*. 2006;58(Suppl 3):S7–S15.

Bullock MR, Chesnut R, Ghajar J, et al. Surgical management of acute subdural hematomas. *Neurosurgery*. 2006;58 (Suppl 3):S16–S24.

Nassiri F, Badhiwala JH, Witiw CD, et al. The clinical significance of isolated traumatic subarachnoid hemorrhage in mild traumatic brain injury: a meta-analysis. *J Trauma Acute Care Surg*. 2017;83:725–731.

Papa L, Stiell IG, Clement CM, et al. Performance of the Canadian CT Head Rule and the New Orleans Criteria for predicting any traumatic intracranial injury on computed tomography in a United States Level I trauma center. *Acad Emerg Med*. 2012 Jan;12(1):2–10.

CHAPTER 3

DIZZINESS WHILE TRAVELING

JACQUELINE PAULIS

SETTING

Wilderness, Nepal

CHIEF COMPLAINT

Dizziness

HISTORY

A healthy 28-year-old male traveling in rural Nepal presents with a complaint of 2 days of progressively worsening dizziness. He describes it as lightheadedness that is exacerbated upon standing or sitting up. It is better with lying flat. He denies room spinning or syncope. Over a similar period of time, he has also experienced 8 to 10 episodes of watery bowel movements daily, with no blood or mucous. Due to intermittent, diffuse, crampy abdominal pain, and nausea, he has had decreased oral intake. He notes decreased frequency and increased concentration of his urine. He denies fever, chills, vomiting, chest pain, cough, headache, vision changes, and shortness of breath.

He denies past medical or surgical history.

He denies smoking, drinking, or illicit drug use.

Family history is without notable findings.

PHYSICAL EXAMINATION

Vital signs: HR 92, BP 115/75, RR 17, SpO$_2$ 97% on room air, temp. 36.1°C.

Examination reveals a well-developed young man with dry mucous membranes and sunken eyes. When seated, his cardiac rate and rhythm are regular without murmurs, rubs, or gallops. On standing his heart rate increases to 116 bpm, and his presenting complaint of dizziness occurs. His lungs are clear to auscultation bilaterally. His abdomen is soft, nontender, and nondistended. His skin exhibits decreased turgor. His extremities are warm and well-perfused. Capillary refill is intact. On neurologic exam, his cranial nerves and sensation are intact, and motor is 5/5 in all extremities. His coordination and gait are normal. He has no pronator drift; Romberg is negative. While initially unsteady on first standing, his tandem gait testing is intact.

DIFFERENTIAL DIAGNOSIS

1. Dehydration
2. Acute central nervous system pathology (ischemia or hemorrhage)
3. Increased vasovagal tone
4. Hypoglycemia
5. Cardiac arrhythmia
6. Anemia
7. Benign paroxysmal positional vertigo

TESTS

Finger-stick glucose: 87 mg/dL

CLINICAL COURSE

Based on the history and physical exam, orthostatic vital signs were obtained. After standing for 3 minutes, the patient was noted to have an increase in heart rate to 116 bpm and a decrease in blood pressure to 90/60 mm Hg. A blood glucose level was obtained, which was within normal limits. Due to limited resources, access to an electrocardiogram (ECG) was unavailable. On examination, the patient was clinically dehydrated. Oral rehydration therapy was initiated. After 2 days, his diarrhea abated, oral intake increased, and dizziness resolved. His neurologic examination remained nonfocal. He was able to complete the rest of his expedition.

KEY MANAGEMENT STEPS

1. Perform a detailed history and a thorough neurologic exam in patients with dizziness. In the appropriate clinical context with a reassuring neurologic exam, consider dehydration as a cause of postural dizziness.

2. Obtain a blood glucose level and an ECG (resource permitting) in all patients presenting with dizziness. Patients with concerning features on history or physical exam warrant a more thorough workup. This may require evacuation to an established medical facility.
3. In both well-resourced hospitals and austere conditions, the use of oral rehydration therapy (ORT) for treatment of mild to moderate dehydration is safe, cost-effective, and convenient.

DEBRIEF

This patient experienced postural hypotension due to dehydration in the setting of an acute diarrheal illness and decreased oral intake. He was young and otherwise healthy, endorsed orthostatic symptoms, and had a normal neurologic exam with postural dizziness that followed shortly after the onset of his gastrointestinal (GI) complaints. The diarrhea itself is not concerning for an acute bacterial or parasitic infection requiring specific therapy given lack of fever, blood or mucous in stool, and a benign abdominal examination. A blood glucose level was normal. On exam, his dizziness was reproduced with postural change, and his orthostatic testing was consistent with dehydration. Despite not having access to an ECG to rule out unlikely acute cardiac pathology, the rest of his evaluation was reassuring and supported the diagnosis of acute dehydration.

When evaluating patients who present with dizziness, first determine if they are experiencing lightheadedness (presyncope) or vertigo (room-spinning). Determine exacerbating and relieving factors. Isolated postural dizziness suggests global central nervous system hypoperfusion. A detailed history should include questions about syncope, headache or trauma, focal neurologic deficits, and any cardiac, thrombotic, or infectious symptoms. A comprehensive neurologic exam should always be performed.

An ECG can be used to screen for an underlying cardiac arrhythmia, and a finger-stick glucose can alert the clinician to a reversible etiology. Patients with advanced age, comorbidities, or any neurologic abnormalities on exam warrant a more thorough workup, including consideration of labs and neuroimaging. If a patient presents with vertigo, the Head Impulse, Nystagmus, and Test of Skew (HINTS) exam can help elucidate whether the vertigo is of peripheral or central origin. Concern for focal cerebellar involvement should prompt emergent transfer of the patient to an appropriate care facility for appropriate imaging.

ORT for mild to moderate dehydration from gastroenteritis is a reasonable and cost-effective therapy in advanced facilities and may be the only option in low-resource environments. The World Health Organization recommends that oral rehydration salts (ORS) be a balanced glucose-electrolyte mixture with a specific osmolality. ORS solutions are effective because glucose aids the absorption of sodium, and so water; sodium, and potassium repletion are required to replace GI losses from diarrhea and emesis; citrate counters the acidosis caused by dehydration. Figure 3.1 is an example of a commercially available ORS packet.

According to the Centers for Disease Control and Prevention, ORS should be immediately provided to dehydrated patients capable of sitting up and drinking, even if they are vomiting. Multiplying the patient's weight in kilograms by 75 and adding in additional volume to compensate for GI losses can estimate the milliliters of ORS required. For adults, roughly 100 mL of ORS is required every 5 minutes until the patient improves. Reassessment of hydration status should be performed hourly, and a normal diet should be resumed as soon as tolerated. ORT is not appropriate for patients with altered mental status, ileus, underlying intestinal malabsorption,

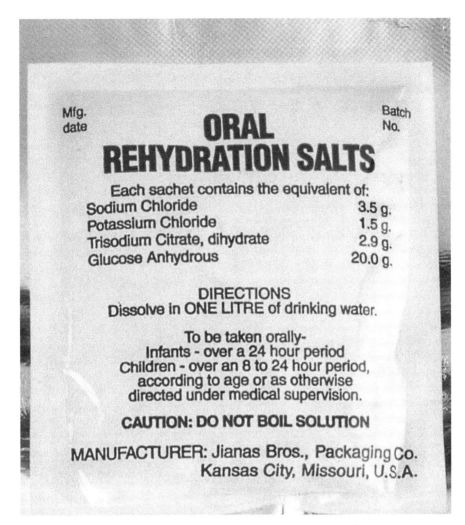

FIGURE 3.1 Example of a commercially available packet of oral rehydration salts.

or severe dehydration. Intravenous fluid rehydration should be initiated if ORT cannot keep up with GI losses.

FURTHER READING

Centers for Disease Control and Prevention. Cholera—vibrio cholera infection: rehydration therapy. May 15, 2018. https://www.cdc.gov/cholera/treatment/rehydration-therapy.html

Chang AK. Dizziness and vertigo. In: Walls RM, Hockberger RS, Gausche-Hill M, eds. *Rosen's Emergency Medicine: Concepts and Clinical Practice*. 9th ed. Philadelphia, PA: Elsevier; 2018: 145–152.

Newman-Toker DE, Kerber KA, Hsieh YH, et al. HINTS outperforms ABCD2 to screen for stroke in acute continuous vertigo and dizziness. *Acad Emerg Med*. 2013;20(10):986–996.

World Health Organization. Oral rehydration salts: production of the new ORS. 2006. http://www.who.int/maternal_child_adolescent/documents/fch_cah_06_1/en/

DIZZINESS ON AIRPLANE

JUSTIN T. PITMAN

SETTING

Emergency Department

CHIEF COMPLAINT

Ear Pain

HISTORY

A 32-year-old female presents to the emergency department with a complaint of left-sided ear pain and dizziness. The patient was returning from a trip to Italy, and pain began during aircraft descent 2 hours ago. The pain is associated with dizziness, mild nausea, and a sense of mild hearing loss in the affected ear. She denies ear drainage, tinnitus, vomiting, gait disturbance, numbness, or weakness. She is recovering from an upper respiratory tract infection that she acquired during her travels. Symptoms are worsened with manipulation of ear and head movement. Pain has somewhat improved since her plane landed but are still persistent.

She has a past medical history of seasonal allergies and no history of surgery.

She has never smoked and consumes approximately 3 to 4 drinks per week. She uses marijuana infrequently.

She denies family history of stroke or cardiac disease.

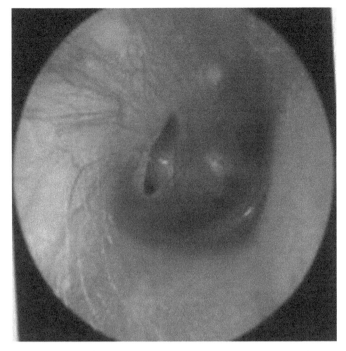

FIGURE 4.1 Otoscopic visualization of tympanic membrane hemorrhage and perforation.
Courtesy of GoFlightMedicine.com

PHYSICAL EXAMINATION

Vital signs: HR 62, BP 118/62, RR 18, SpO_2 99% on room air, temp. 36.7°C.

Patient is a well-developed female in no acute distress. Examination of her head and neck reveals normal oropharyngeal examination. Face is without tap tenderness. Otoscopic evaluation of the left ear reveals a retracted tympanic membrane and evidence of limited tympanic membrane hemorrhage (Figure 4.1). There is no mastoid tenderness or external canal findings. Her lungs are clear without respiratory distress. Cardiac evaluation reveals regular rate and rhythm without murmurs, rubs, or gallops. Her abdomen is soft without focal tenderness. Neurological examination reveals normal extraocular movement with left-beating nystagmus (fatiguable) and preserved facial symmetry and sensation. There is mild to moderate conductive hearing loss in the left ear. There is a negative Dix-Hallpike maneuver bilaterally. Strength and sensation are grossly symmetrical. She is normal gait and coordination.

DIFFERENTIAL DIAGNOSIS

1. Ear barotrauma
2. Sinus barotrauma
3. Acute otitis media/acute otitis externa
4. Mastoiditis
5. Acute cerebrovascular accident

TESTS

Based on history and physical examination findings, no testing is indicated.

CLINICAL COURSE

Frenzel maneuver was attempted (simultaneous oral and nasal cavity occlusion with positive pressure introduced into posterior oropharynx) with significant pain reduction and immediate improvement in hearing. Patient was recommended to use NSAIDS for pain reduction, oral and nasal decongestants, gentle Frenzel maneuver and physical activity reduction. Outpatient otolaryngology consultation was requested given associated vertiginous symptoms. Patient improved significantly over the next several days. During ENT evaluation, she was not exhibiting any symptoms of vertigo and audiology testing had returned to normal.

KEY MANAGEMENT STEPS

1. The diagnosis of acute ear barotrauma can be made by history and physical examination alone.
2. Treatment is largely supportive. Nonsteroidal anti-inflammatory drugs and Tylenol may be used for pain. Antihistamines and decongestants (oxymetazoline 0.05% nasal spray) may have a role in treatment of eustachian tube dysfunction, but studies have not reliably demonstrated reduction of ear barotrauma when used prophylactically.
3. Antibiotics are not required unless there is evidence of tympanic perforation present with gross contamination.
4. Appropriate early consultation with otolaryngology in cases where patient has unrelieved pain (and may require decompressive myringotomy) or persistent/severe tinnitus, hearing loss, or vertigo concerning for perilymphatic fistula requiring potential surgical intervention.

DEBRIEF

This patient was experiencing discomfort from acute ear barotrauma, caused by a pressure gradient between the middle ear and outer ear. The most common presenting symptom of acute ear barotrauma is acute onset of progressive pain of the middle ear during rapid pressure changes (e.g., on take-off or landing in an airplane or on ascent or descent during diving). It can be associated with hearing loss, tympanic membrane perforation, round or oval window perforation, perilymphatic fistula, disequilibrium, and tinnitus.

During changes in atmospheric pressure, a patent eustachian tube allows equalization of the inner ear external pressure gradient and so preserves hearing at a wide range of altitudes. If external pressure change is rapid or if there is an abnormality of the eustachian tube (eustachian tube dysfunction), the pressure within the middle ear cannot equalize, causing either bulging or retraction of the tympanic membrane and associated pain and potential injury to inner ear structures.

The degree of ear barotrauma can be quantified by the TEED grading system:

- Grade 0: Symptoms without otologic findings
- Grade 1: Erythema and mild retraction of the tympanic membrane
- Grade 2: Erythema of the tympanic membrane with mild or spotty hemorrhage within the membrane
- Grade 3: Gross hemorrhage throughout the tympanic membrane
- Grade 4: Grade 3 changes plus gross hemorrhage within the middle ear (hemotympanum)
- Grade 5: Free blood in the middle ear plus perforation of the tympanic membrane

Treatment of ear barotrauma is typically supportive. In addition to analgesic therapy, decongestants may also provide ancillary relief. Typically, oral decongestants (such as phenylephrine or pseudoephedrine) are combined with nasal decongestants (such as oxymetazole or phenylephrine) and accompanied by repeated gentle Frenzel maneuvers for the first 3 to 5 days following insult. Antihistamines may be used if allergic eustachian tube dysfunction is suspected. Antibiotic otic drops should only be provided if tympanic membrane perforation present and accompanied by gross contamination (e.g., occurs while diving).

Pain accompanied by tinnitus, vertigo, and hearing loss is strongly suggestive of inner ear barotrauma and could be accompanied by a perilymphatic fistula due to rupture of either the round or oval windows. Treatment remains generally conservative although recovery usually is more gradual than an isolated middle ear injury. In addition to standard treatments, bed rest with head elevation (30°) and cessation of strenuous activities are also recommended. As there is no consensus regarding need or timing of surgical repair of a perilymphatic fistula, urgent otolaryngology referral should be considered.

FURTHER READING

Byyny RL Shockley LW. Scuba diving and dysbarism. In Marx JA, Hockberger RS, Walls RM, eds. *Rosen's Emergency Medicine: Concepts and Clinical Practice*. 7th ed. Philadelphia, PA: Elsevier; 2010: 1915–1927.

Van Hoesen KB, Lang MA. Diving medicine. In: Cushing TA, Harris NS, Auerbach PS. *Auerbach's Wilderness Medicine*. 7th ed. Philadelphia, PA: Elsevier; 2017: 1583–1618.

Veronica DM. Ear barotrauma. In: Deschler DG, Sullivan DJ, eds. *UpToDate*. July 18, 2016. https://www.uptodate.com/contents/ear-barotrauma

ENVENOMATION

JILLIAN NICKERSON

SETTING

Emergency Department

CHIEF COMPLAINT

Abdominal Pain

HISTORY

A 34-year-old male presents to the emergency department complaining of severe diffuse crampy abdominal pain for the last 2 hours. The pain was abrupt in onset, is severe, and without radiation. He has had nausea and vomiting as well as crampy muscular pain in both legs. He denies fevers, diarrhea, sick contacts, recent travel, or antibiotic use. The pain started about 30 minutes after he suffered a spider bite on the posterior aspect of this right thigh while removing a pile of wood from his garage. He has brought the spider into the emergency department in a jar. A picture of the spider is shown in Figure 5.1. He is unsure of when he last received a tetanus vaccine.

He has no past medical or surgical history. He denies allergies to medications or environmental allergies.

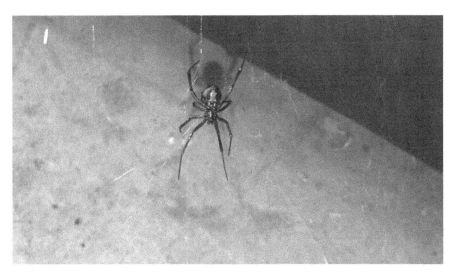

FIGURE 5.1 Lactrodectus specimen.
Courtesy of the author.

PHYSICAL EXAMINATION

Vital signs: HR 106, BP 170/80, RR 16, SpO$_2$ 99% on room air, temp. 37.0°C.

- General: well-developed, well-nourished male screaming in pain.
- Head and neck: moist mucous membranes, no abnormalities.
- Cardiovascular: tachycardia, regular rhythm.
- Respiratory: clear bilaterally to auscultation.
- Abdomen: stiff, board-like diffusely with rectus spasm noted. Diffusely tender to palpation in all 4 quadrants. No distention. Normal bowel sounds.
- Lower extremities: 3 cm area of erythema to the posterior right thigh with 2 central puncta, no erythema, induration, fluctuance.
- No edema, strong peripheral pulses, warm and well perfused
- Neurologic: normal strength, normal gait

DIFFERENTIAL DIAGNOSIS

1. Latrodectism
2. Acute abdomen secondary to appendicitis versus perforated viscus
3. Pancreatitis
4. Peptic ulcer disease

TESTS

Complete blood count: normal hemoglobin, hematocrit, white blood cell count and platelets.

Chemistry panel: normal sodium, potassium, chloride, bicarbonate, blood urea nitrogen, creatinine, and glucose

Lipase: normal

Upright abdominal and chest X-ray: normal cardiac silhouette, clear lungs; no free air; unremarkable bowel gas pattern

CLINICAL COURSE

Based on history, exam, and evaluation of spider consistent with a black widow (*Latrodectus*), the patient was suspected to have latrodectism. An intravenous (IV) line was placed, and IV opiates were given for pain and IV benzodiazepines for muscle cramping. An upright abdominal and chest X-ray was obtained given peritoneal findings on exam, raising concern for possible perforated viscus to rule out free air. Results were reassuring as noted. The wound was cleaned, and ice was applied to reduce swelling and pain. The patient's tetanus vaccine was updated. Given ongoing severe abdominal discomfort and hypertension, patient was given antivenom. Symptoms improved, and patient was admitted to the observation unit for pain control and 6 to 24 hours of monitoring.

KEY MANAGEMENT STEPS

1. Recognize that an examination consistent with an "acute abdomen" can result from envenomation and may not be an indication for surgical exploration.
2. Pain control may require high doses of IV opiates for pain and benzodiazepines for cramping.
3. Wound management directly to bite site.
4. Tetanus update if indicated.
5. Antivenom should be reserved for patients failing initial symptom management and to treat high-risk populations (children, elderly and pregnant women).

DEBRIEF

The patient was experiencing severe abdominal pain, nausea, vomiting, muscle cramping, tachycardia, and hypertension after a spider bite. Examination of the patient's arachnid specimen was consistent with a black widow spider. Together, the components of the patient's presentation are strongly suggestive of acute latrodectism and not of an intra-abdominal catastrophe, despite the worrisome abdominal exam and hemodynamic instability. Latrodectism should be considered in patients with peritoneal signs in the right clinical context (e.g., after black widow spider envenomation). Failure to appropriately consider latrodectism as a reason for a patient's abdominal wall rigidity can lead to an unnecessary exploratory laparotomy.

Black widow spiders (*Latrodectus* genus) have a classic red hourglass on the abdomen. They are found throughout the continental United States, commonly in woodpiles and other dark, protected areas. The venom contains a neurotoxin that stimulates release of acetylcholine in the neuromuscular junction. This causes muscle cramping, abdominal distress, nausea, vomiting, and, in severe cases, seizures and respiratory depression.

The only other venomous spider in the United States is the brown recluse (*Loxosceles reclusa*). It is identified by its tan color and violin-shaped marking on the cephalothorax. *Loxosceles* species are found most commonly in the south-central United States, especially Kansas, Missouri, Arkansas, Oklahoma, Louisiana, and Texas. The brown recluse venom causes vasoconstriction, which can result in local tissue necrosis. In rare cases, patients can develop systemic symptoms including shock, multiorgan failure, and disseminated intravascular coagulation.

Treatment for latrodectism consists of local wound care, appropriate tetanus prophylaxis, and aggressive symptom management. Pain control may require high doses of IV opiates, and muscle cramps may require significant doses of benzodiazepines. Lactrodectism is unlikely to be life-threatening, but in cases of severe symptoms recalcitrant to initial symptom management— or in high risk populations (i.e., children, the elderly, or pregnant patients)—providers may consider using antivenom. Rarely, patients can develop an anaphylactic reaction to the antivenom. If hypertension is severe, it may be treated with anti-hypertensive medications.

FURTHER READING

Isbister GK, Graudins A, White J, Warrell D. Antivenom treatment in arachnidism. *J Toxicol Clin Toxicol*. 2003;41(3):291–300.

Isbister G, Fan HW. Spider bite. *Lancet*, 2011;378(9808):2039–2047.

Monte AA, et al. A US perspective of symptomatic latrodectus spp. envenomation and treatment: a National Poison Data System review. *Ann Pharmacother*. 2011;45(12):1491–1498.

Swansen DL, Vetter RS, White J. Clinical manifestations and diagnosis of widow spider bites. In: Deschler DG, Sullivan DJ, eds. *UpToDate*. March 20, 2018. https://www.uptodate.com/contents/clinical-manifestations-and-diagnosis-of-widow-spider-bites

Venomous animal injuries. In: Walls RM, Hockberger RS, Gausche-Hill M, eds. *Rosen's Emergency Medicine: Concepts and Clinical Practice*. 9th ed. Philadelphia, PA: Elsevier; 2018: 698–714.

CHAPTER 6

WRIST PAIN

ERIC LEE

SETTING

Wilderness

CHIEF COMPLAINT

Wrist Pain

HISTORY

A 35-year-old male hiker presents with a swollen and painful right wrist after a fall. He states he tripped on a branch while descending a steep hill and fell forward onto his outstretched arm. He reports "landing hard on my right hand." He noted immediate pain and worsening swelling in his right wrist since then. After walking to the trailhead, emergency medical services was called and noted the patient to have a wrist deformity consistent with acute fracture. He was neurovascularly intact. His right wrist and forearm was placed in a volar splint for immobilization. He was given oral ibuprofen and transported to an emergency department for further care. He denies any head injury, loss of consciousness, numbness, tingling, or other injuries. He is right-hand dominant. He has no unusual dexterity requirements.

He has no past medical or surgical history.

PHYSICAL EXAMINATION

Vital signs: HR 80, BP 135/90, RR 18, SpO$_2$ 98% on room air, temp. 36.8°C.

Examination reveals a well-developed, well-nourished male in no acute distress. His right wrist has a mild dorsally displaced deformity with no open wounds or lacerations. There is diffuse swelling and tenderness throughout the right wrist, most prominently over the radial aspect. He has a +2 radial pulse and normal capillary refill. His sensation is grossly intact, and he can wiggle all his fingers. His range of motion of the right wrist is limited by pain but intact. He has no snuffbox tenderness or pain with axial loading of the thumb. He exhibits no elbow or radial head tenderness. Light touch sensation is intact. He is fully ambulatory and without other physical or neurologic exam findings.

DIFFERENTIAL DIAGNOSIS

1. Distal radial fracture
2. Scaphoid fracture
3. Distal ulnar fracture
4. Wrist dislocation
5. Wrist sprain

TESTS

X-ray right wrist: mildly displaced distal radius fracture; ultrasound forearm; visibly displaced distal radius fracture

No blood tests are indicated unless the patient requires preoperative labs for possible operative intervention at the hospital.

CLINICAL COURSE

A bedside ultrasound revealed a displaced distal radius fracture. An X-ray confirmed a mildly displaced distal radius fracture. There was no articular surface involvement. A hematoma block and a closed reduction were performed. He was placed in a reverse sugar tong splint without complication. Post-reduction X-ray showed an improvement in alignment. He was discharged with orthopedic follow-up.

KEY MANAGEMENT STEPS

1. Consider an acute fracture in the differential diagnosis of a patient with wrist pain after a fall.
2. Perform a comprehensive physical exam that includes assessment of circulation, sensation, and motor function to evaluate for neurovascular compromise.

3. Utilize appropriate imaging modalities to confirm and characterize fracture. Point-of-care ultrasound can be used initially to help confirm a fracture. X-ray radiography provides definitive imaging to help guide diagnosis and treatment of an uncomplicated acute wrist fracture.
4. Use appropriate immobilization and splinting techniques,

DEBRIEF

A distal radial fracture is the most common type of wrist fracture seen in adults. It is commonly caused by a hard fall on an outstretched hand. This mechanism is consistent with the patient's history of falling down a steep hill and landing on his right wrist. Swelling, tenderness, and visible deformity on physical exam are all suggestive of an acute fracture. Immobilization in the field is indicated based on these findings.

A careful physical exam to assess circulation, sensation, and motor function of the affected limb is required. Confirm that the patient has a palpable pulse, normal capillary refill, and normal sensation and motor function within the injured extremity. If there is any evidence of neurovascular compromise, a closed reduction—whether in the field or in the emergency room—is indicated. Following this, prompt immobilization with a splint will help prevent further neurovascular injury, avoid the conversion of a closed fracture into an open fracture, and reduce pain.

Assess for potential scaphoid fracture by palpating for snuffbox tenderness. Definitive diagnosis of a distal radial fracture can be made on imaging. Historically, X-ray radiography of the wrist is the most common modality for diagnosis (Figure 6.1). With the advent of mobile point-of-care ultrasound, ultrasound can be used (in the field or the emergency department) to help confirm a fracture. On ultrasound, the fracture will appear as an interruption of the linear bony cortex (Figure 6.2). Ultrasound may also aid in the treatment of a distal radial fracture to

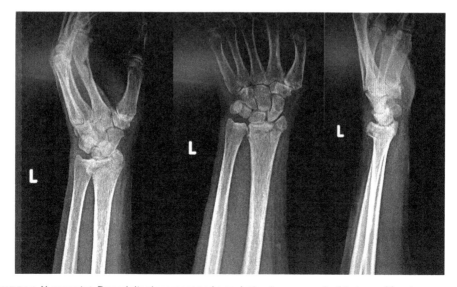

FIGURE 6.1 X-ray wrist. Dorsal displacement and angulation is common in this type of fracture.
Courtesy of Dr. Melissa Leber, Icahn School of Medicine at Mount Sinai.

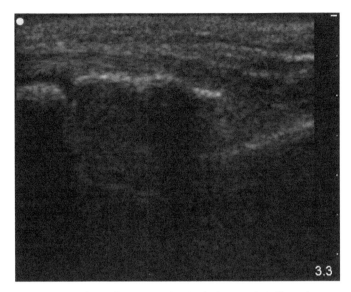

FIGURE 6.2 Ultrasound forearm. Note the interruption in the hyperechoic linear bony cortex.
Courtesy of the author.

guide injection of a hematoma block (for analgesia prior to a closed reduction) and to confirm its alignment after a closed reduction.

A closed reduction involves the external manipulation of the fractured bone to recreate normal anatomic alignment. Following a reduction, a splint is required. A temporary splint may be applied in the prehospital setting, and a more definitive splint may be applied after a successful reduction to maintain alignment. When creating a splint, it is critical to (i) use adequate padding over bony prominences and high-pressure areas, (ii) keep the extremity in anatomic alignment throughout the entire procedure, and (iii) perform a neurovascular exam before and after splinting. A splint should immobilize the joint above and below the site of injury. A sugar tong or reverse sugar tong splint is ideal for a distal radial fracture, as it immobilizes the wrist and elbow. Even if initial imaging is reassuring, if examination raises concern for potential scaphoid fracture (i.e., snuffbox tenderness), the patient should be placed in a thumb spica splint and instructed to follow up with orthopedics. With a distal radius fracture, the patient may be discharged to home with appropriate orthopedic follow-up after successful reduction and splinting.

FURTHER READING

Chinnock B, Khaletskiy A, Kuo K, Hendey GW. Ultrasound-guided reduction of distal radius fractures. *J Emerg Med*. 2011;40(3):308–312.

Geiderman JM, Katz D. General principles of orthopedic injuries. In: Marx J, Rosen P. *Rosen's Emergency Medicine: Concepts and Clinical Practice*. 9th ed. Philadelphia, PA: Elsevier/Saunders; 2017: 445–463.

Gottlieb M, Cosby K. Ultrasound-guided hematoma block for distal radial and ulnar fractures. *J Emerg Med*. 2015;48(3):310–312.

Lin, M. Trick of the trade: reverse sugar tong splint (blog post). *Academic Life in Emergency Medicine Medical Blog*. August 26, 2009. https://www.aliem.com/2009/08/trick-of-trade-reverse-sugar-tong/

Williams DT, Kim HT. Wrist and forearm. In: Marx JA, Rosen P, eds. *Rosen's Emergency Medicine: Concepts and Clinical Practice*. 9th ed. Philadelphia, PA: Elsevier/Saunders; 2017: 508–529.

ABDOMINAL PAIN

CARLO CANEPA

SETTING

Emergency Department

CHIEF COMPLAINT

Abdominal Pain

HISTORY

A 20-year-old male presents with crampy abdominal pain. He reports have enjoyed a white-water rafting trip in the southwest United States 3 weeks ago. A couple of weeks after his trip, he developed crampy, intermittent abdominal pain accompanied by nonbloody, foul-smelling, and watery stools and flatulence. He also feels bloated and nauseous but does not vomit. He has had no fever or chills. His symptoms have been ongoing for several days and are not improved with changes in diet or with over-the-counter medications. No sick contacts. No international travel. During his trip, he used chlorine tablets to treat his water.

He has no past medical or surgical history.

He is an occasional, limited alcohol drinker and cigarette smoker.

He has no pertinent family history.

PHYSICAL EXAMINATION

Vital signs: HR 85, BP 110/70, RR 14, SpO$_2$ 100% on room air, temp. 37.2°C.

Examination reveals a well-developed, well-nourished male in no acute distress. Minimally dry mucus membranes are noted. Examination of his head and neck is normal. His lungs are clear bilaterally with good air movement, and his cardiac rate and rhythm are normal; no murmurs, rubs, or gallops are appreciated. His abdomen is soft, nontender, and hyperactive bowel sounds. There is no rebound or guarding. He has a negative Murphy's sign and no tenderness at McBurney's point. His extremities are warm, well-perfused, and without edema. He has no rashes. Neurologic examination is grossly normal.

DIFFERENTIAL DIAGNOSIS

1. Giardia infection
2. Enteritis
3. Colitis
4. Appendicitis
5. Cholecystitis
6. Diverticulitis

TESTS

Complete blood count: normal hemoglobin, hematocrit, white blood cell count, and platelets
Chemistry panel: normal sodium, potassium, chloride, bicarbonate, blood urea nitrogen, creatinine, and glucose
Stool ova and parasites: giardia trophozoites and cysts visualized.

CLINICAL COURSE

The patient was well-appearing and comfortable with a nontender abdomen. His blood work was normal, and he was orally rehydrated. He was treated empirically for Giardia based on his symptoms and recent potential exposure to contaminated and insufficiently treated drinking water while rafting. He was discharged home. Following his discharge, his stool samples revealed Giardia cysts and parasites, which confirmed the diagnosis. The patient's symptoms quickly resolved after treatment.

KEY MANAGEMENT STEPS

1. Consider Giardia infection in someone recently returned from a wilderness trip with abdominal pain, bloating, and nonbloody diarrhea.
2. Recognize and treat dehydration in this patient with ongoing symptoms. Oral replacement therapy is typically sufficient.

3. Treat empirically for suspected Giardia infection with appropriate antibiotics.
4. Obtain stool samples to confirm the diagnosis.

DEBRIEF

This patient was experiencing abdominal symptoms due to a Giardia infection. Typical symptoms of this protozoal infection include abdominal cramping, bloating, and foul-smelling loose stools that are nonbloody. No fever is expected. Patients may complain that their stools are mushy and greasy. The typical patient has been exposed to poorly or untreated drinking water and poor hand hygiene. Symptoms typically present 1 to 3 weeks after the initial exposure. Giardia cysts can be resistant to chlorine-treated water.

Giardiasis can often be diagnosed clinically based on careful history and examination. It is confirmed by testing stool testing for ova and parasites. Because cysts can be excreted irregularly, multiple stool samples should be sent (3 samples will increase sensitivity to >90%). Newer tests (e.g., fecal immunoassays and polymerase chain reaction) are more sensitive but may not be available at many hospitals and clinics.

When Giardia infection is suspected, the patient should be assessed for dehydration. This is particularly important in children, pregnant women, the immunosuppressed, and the elderly. Giardial protozoa can adhere to the intestinal wall and cause villous flattening, secretion of fluids, and result in malabsorption. The vast majority of patients do not require intravenous hydration and can be safely treated with oral rehydration and oral antibiotics. Unless alternative diagnoses are being actively entertained, blood work (i.e., complete blood count and electrolytes) are unlikely to help make the diagnosis. Imaging is not necessary.

Giardia intestinalis is an anaerobic, flagellated protozoan parasite with a life cycle alternating between trophozoite and the infective cyst. Giardia is found throughout the United States and the world. All age groups are affected. Giardia lives in intestines and is spread via oral–fecal contamination by ingesting cysts in untreated drinking water, on uncooked food, or by direct contact with contaminated surfaces (e.g., unwashed hands). The incubation period is 1 to 2 weeks. Symptoms typically last 2 to 6 weeks in the untreated patient. Antibiotics (metronidazole, albendazole, tinidazole, or nitazoxanide) can decrease the duration of symptoms. In the absence of treatment, some patients will become asymptomatic carriers, while others will develop long-term irritable bowel syndrome-like symptoms.

As in most cases, this patient's symptoms and history were sufficient to make a provisional diagnosis and start empiric antibiotic treatment for giardia infection. Subsequent stool ova and parasite results confirmed the clinical diagnosis. No further testing was necessary.

FURTHER READING

Adachi JA, Backer HD, Dupont HL. Infectious diarrhea from wilderness and foreign travel. In: Auerbach PS, Cushing TF, Harris NS, eds. *Auerbach's Wilderness Medicine.* 7th ed. Philadelphia, PA: Elsevier; 2017: 1859–1870.

Centers for Disease Prevention and Control. Parasites—Giardia. July 22, 2015. https://www.cdc.gov/parasites/giardia/index.html

Minetti C, Chalmers RM, Beeching NJ, Probert C, Lamden K. Giardiasis. *Brit Med J.* 2016;355:i5369.

FEVER

RITTIK CHAUDHURI

SETTING

Emergency Department

CHIEF COMPLAINT

Fever

HISTORY

A 45-year-old male presents to the emergency department with a chief complaint of fever. The patient states that 2 weeks ago he traveled to Cape Cod, Massachusetts, where 3 days after hiking in the woods, he reports discovering a tick attached to the back of his neck. His wife promptly removed the tick with forceps. The patient denies any rash associated with the tick bite. He states that he was in his usual state of health until 4 days ago, when he developed intermittent cyclic fevers as high as 103.4°F and chills. He has noted progressive fatigue and malaise. He endorses a mild headache when he has the high fevers. He denies any neck stiffness, photophobia, phonophobia, or confusion. The patient further denies any rhinorrhea, sore throat, cough, abdominal pain, dysuria, or diarrhea. He does not have any sick contacts. He reports recent travel only to New England.

He has a past medical history of hypertension. He denies any prior surgeries.

He denies any intravenous drug use, tobacco, or alcohol use.

PHYSICAL EXAMINATION

Vital signs: HR 110, BP 143/86, RR 18, SpO$_2$ 98% on room air, temp. 39.5°C.

Examination reveals a well-developed and well-nourished male in no acute distress. Oropharynx is clear, with no erythema, edema, or exudate. His neck is supple. There is no cervical, supraclavicular, or axillary lymphadenopathy. Auscultation reveals tachycardia with a regular rhythm and no appreciable murmurs; his lungs are clear bilaterally with no wheezing and no focal decreased breath sounds. Abdominal exam reveals mild hepatomegaly and splenomegaly; the abdomen itself is nontender with no guarding or rebound tenderness. He has no tenderness at the costovertebral angle. His extremities are warm and well perfused. Careful examination of his skin reveals no jaundice or rash.

DIFFERENTIAL DIAGNOSIS

1. Babesiosis
2. Anaplasma
3. Lyme disease
4. Ehrlichiosis
5. Rocky Mountain Spotted Fever
6. Influenza
7. Malaria

TESTS

Abnormal lab values: hematocrit: 31.5% (36.0-46.0), platelets 130,000 per mm^3 (150,000-450,000), creatinine 1.4 mg/dL (0.6-1.2), indirect bilirubin 2.5 mg/dL (0.2-0.7), direct bilirubin 0.3 mg/dL (0-0.3), aspartate aminotransferase 135 U/liter (9-32), ALT 124 U/liter (7–33)

Normal lab values: white blood cell count, sodium, potassium, chloride, bicarbonate, blood urea nitrogen, total protein, and albumin

CLINICAL COURSE

This patient's history and physical exam raised concern for a tick-borne disease. Based on his recent travel to the Northeast, babesiosis and anaplasmosis were highest on the differential. In the setting of only domestic travel, the patient's cyclic fevers and hepatosplenomegaly further increased the likelihood of acute babesiosis. Lyme disease was considered as well, but it was thought to be less likely as the patient denied any history of rash associated with the tick bite.

In the emergency department, intravenous access was established and the following laboratory studies were sent: complete blood count and comprehensive metabolic panel, thick/ thin smear, *Babesia* polymerase chain reaction (PCR), *Anaplasma* PCR, and Lyme antibody with reflex to western blot. The patient was initially treated with acetaminophen and intravenous fluids with resolution of his fever and tachycardia. One hour later, his laboratory studies revealed anemia, thrombocytopenia, elevated creatinine, elevated bilirubin, and a mild transaminitis. The thin smear was positive for *Babesia* parasitemia. The patient was started on atovaquone and azithromycin and observed overnight. He remained nontoxic. In the morning, his complete blood count and comprehensive metabolic panel were checked again and found to be unchanged. *Anaplasma* PCR and Lyme testing sent the previous day were negative. His diagnosis of babesiosis was confirmed by PCR. The patient was discharged on a 7-day course of atovaquone and azithromycin. His fever resolved after 2 days, and he had no relapses.

KEY MANAGEMENT STEPS

1. Obtain a detailed history in a patient with fever, including recent travel and possible tick exposures.
2. Perform a careful physical exam to evaluate for other causes of fever.
3. Pursue appropriate diagnostic testing for tick-borne diseases.
4. Consider empiric treatment with appropriate antibiotics pending results of final testing.

DEBRIEF

Babesiosis is a disease caused by protozoa of the *Babesia* genus. A number of species within the *Babesia* genus have been identified. In the United States, *Babesia microti* is most common, is endemic to the Northeast and upper Midwest, and is transmitted to humans by the tick *Ixodes scapularis* (more commonly known as the deer tick). Rare cases of tickborne babesiosis have been reported in the western United States and Europe, which are believed to be caused by other *Babesia* species transmitted by ticks native to those regions. *Babesia* infections have also been found in patients who received blood products from infected donors. Congenital transmission, though exceedingly rare, has been documented as well.

Babesia infects red blood cells, causing hemolytic anemia. Individuals infected with *Babesia* can have varying degrees of illness, ranging in severity from an asymptomatic parasitemia to fulminant sepsis and even death. Patients at greatest risk for developing severe disease are those with a high parasite load, impaired or absent splenic function, or other immunocompromise. Individuals with asymptomatic babesiosis may progress to severe disease after splenectomy or administration of immunosuppressive medications.

Most patients with babesiosis will develop symptoms 1 to 6 weeks after being bitten by an infected tick. The most common symptoms are fever (38–40°C), chills, and fatigue. Patients may also experience headache, sore throat, myalgias, athralgias, anorexia, and nausea. Dark-colored urine and shortness of breath are rare and concerning for more severe infection. The majority of patients will have a nonfocal exam, although mild hepatomegaly and splenomegaly may be noted. Jaundice is an uncommon finding and suggestive of advanced disease.

Laboratory workup is often notable for classic signs of hemolytic anemia: decreased hematocrit, elevated bilirubin and lactate dehydrogenase, and decreased haptoglobin. Free hemoglobin and hemosiderin, produced by hemolysis, can cause renal injury and result in an elevated creatinine. Thrombocytopenia and mild transaminitis are common as well. Diagnosis of babesiosis is most easily made by thick/thin smear (Wright or Giemsa staining under oil immersion), which can be performed rapidly and is of low cost. Under light microscopy, *Babesia* parasites appear within erythrocytes as round or oval-shaped and form rings or tetrads. In cases where there is a low parasite burden, multiple thin slides may need to be examined. PCR, while more expensive, can also be used to diagnose babesiosis and is particularly helpful for detecting low-level parasitemia.

Patients who are asymptomatic may be observed without intervention. However, if the parasitemia persists for greater than 3 months, they should be treated with antibiotics. All symptomatic patients should be treated as well. For patients who are asymptomatic or have mild to moderate disease, the Infectious Disease Society of America recommends a combination of atovoquone and azithromycin. For patients with severe disease (which may result in renal failure, congestive heart failure, acute respiratory distress syndrome, and disseminated intravascular coagulation), quinine and clindamycin should be used. These patients may require exchange transfusion and substantial supportive care.

It is important to consider possible co-infections when treating a patient for babesiosis. The deer tick is the vector for several other zoonotic diseases, including Lyme disease and anaplasmosis. Recent studies have shown that up to two thirds of patients with babesiosis have concurrent Lyme disease and one third have anaplasmosis. Early Lyme disease is often marked by a distinctive rash (erythema migrans), but this may not be a prominent feature, and the rash may have resolved by the time a patient presents with babesiosis. Anaplasmosis, which does not cause a rash, produces symptoms similar to babesiosis and can be very difficult to exclude by history and physical exam alone. Additional testing (e.g., Lyme antibody with reflex to western blot and *Anaplasma* PCR) may be helpful. If there is strong suspicion for these diseases, particularly anaplasmosis, treatment should be initiated while confirmatory tests are pending. The recommended treatment for both Lyme disease and anaplasmosis is doxycycline.

FURTHER READING

Bolgiano EB, Sexton J. Tick-borne illnesses. In: Marx JA, ed. *Rosen's Emergency Medicine: Concepts and Clinical Practice*. 8th ed. Philadelphia, PA: Elsevier/Saunders; 2014: 1785–1808.

Diuk-Wasser MA, Vannier E, Krause PJ. Coinfection by Ixodes tick-borne pathogens: ecological, epidemiological, and clinical consequences. *Trends Parasitol*. 32;2016:30–42.

Edlow JA. Tick-borne diseases. In: Adams JG, ed. *Emergency Medicine: Clinical Essentials*. 2nd ed. Philadelphia, PA: Elservier/Saunders; 2013: 1518–1525.

Manian FA, Barshak MB, Lowry KP, Basnet KM, Stowell CP. Case 27-2016: a 71-year-old woman with Mullerian carcinoma, fever, fatigue, and myalgias. *New Engl J Med*. 375;2016:981–991.

Sanchez E, Vannier E, Wosmer GP, Hu LT. Diagnosis, treatment, and prevention of Lyme disease, human granulocytic anaplasmosis, and babesiosis: a review. *JAMA-J Am Med Assoc*. 315(2016):1767–1777.

Vannier E, Krause PJ. Human babesiosis. *New Engl J Med*. 366(2012):2397–2407.

C H A P T E R 9

ACUTE MOUNTAIN SICKNESS

NATHANIEL R. MANN

SETTING

Himalayan Rescue Association Clinic. Pheriche, Nepal. 4500 meters

CHIEF COMPLAINT

Acute Mountain Sickness

HISTORY

A 24-year-old male is brought into your clinic by his friend who is concerned that "he may have mountain sickness." He reports they both live in San Diego, California and are in Nepal to hike. They arrived in the area from Kathmandu (1400 meters) three days ago. Yesterday at about 4500 meters, the patient had complained of a headache, some general malaise, and fatigue. Despite this, they decided to continue on, believing his symptoms to be the result of a mild ongoing diarrheal illness. Today, they hiked up to 5600 meters. There the patient was noted to be frequently stumbling and having a difficult time staying on the trail. They were able to slowly descend on foot to the clinic. The patient reports a diffuse, global headache that has been present over 2 days. He notes limited nausea, and reports his diarrhea has resolved. He denies numbness, weakness, speech or vision changes, and fever or chills. He has moderate dyspnea on exertion, but none at rest. He has no abdominal or chest pain.

He has no past medical history, and currently takes no medications
He is a social drinker, though has not had any alcohol since leaving Kathmandu
He has no significant family history

PHYSICAL EXAMINATION

Vital Signs: HR 110, BP 165/95, RR 22, SpO_2 88%, Temp 37.2 C

The patient's exam shows a well-developed male who appears to be healthy at baseline. He has no signs of trauma. His neck is supple. His lungs are clear bilaterally. His heart rate is elevated, but he has no murmurs. His abdomen is soft, non-tender, and non-distended. Other than bilaterally-symmetric trace non-pitting edema of the ankles, has no abnormalities of the extremities. A neurologic examination reveals intact cranial nerves and negative pronator drift. He demonstrates repetitive questioning, confusion to his situation and location, an unsteady ataxic gait, and dysmetria.

DIFFERENTIAL DIAGNOSIS

1. High altitude cerebral edema (HACE)
2. Acute cerebral vascular accident
3. Carbon monoxide (CO) poisoning
4. Meningitis
5. Acute mountain sickness (AMS)
6. High altitude pulmonary edema (HAPE)

TESTS

No testing is available in the given setting

CLINICAL COURSE

With the patient's history of rapid ascent to high altitude, exam findings of ataxia, and confusion without evidence of other focal neurologic deficits, a clinical diagnosis of high altitude cerebral edema (HACE) was made. He had no signs of pulmonary edema on exam, and his SpO2 was normal for the altitude (Table 9.1). Given the potential lethality of a HACE diagnosis, the patient required urgent descent and evacuation. Poor weather made evacuation by foot or helicopter (the only two options) unsafe until the following day. The clinic's oxygen supply was exhausted, and so the patient was administered 8 mg of IM dexamethasone and was placed in the portable hyperbaric chamber. The chamber's internal pressure provided a barometric pressure equivalent to an altitude of 2500 meters—effectively "descending" him by 2000 meters. A personnel rotation was created to continue to pump air into the chamber throughout the night. The following morning, the patient was significantly improved, and he was removed from the hyperbaric chamber. His headache had improved, he was fully oriented, and showed only trace residual ataxia without signs of other neurologic dysfunction. He was given an additional 4 mg PO of dexamethasone, and arrangements were made for an assisted descent with trusted colleagues to a low-altitude clinic.

Table 9.1. Expected Arterial Saturation by Altitude. Oxygen Saturation Drops with Decreasing Barometric Pressure

Altitude in Meters	Expected SpO_2
0	100%
1500	95%
3000	93%
4500	88%
5500	82%
6500	75%
8000	68%

KEY MANAGEMENT STEPS

1. Obtaining a thorough history and ascent profile to establish likelihood of HACE and to rule out other potentially lethal diagnoses.
2. Performing a careful physical exam (with oxygen saturation if available), paying close attention to neurologic and pulmonary findings.
3. In an otherwise healthy young man newly at high altitude, recognizing that acute ataxia and confusion are overwhelmingly likely to be due to HACE.
4. Arranging for definitive HACE therapy (descent and oxygen) as soon as safely possible.
5. Providing supplemental HACE treatment (a portable hyperbaric chamber and steroids) as able.

DEBRIEF

Patients with acute focal neurologic deficits—whether at sea level or high altitude—should be considered to have a life-threatening condition until proven otherwise. For patients newly at high altitude, with acute ataxia or altered mental status, HACE should be the first consideration. HACE is a potentially life-threatening condition that tends to strike those who ascend too quickly to high altitude. To mitigate against the risk of acute altitude illnesses, it is recommended that above 3000 meters, climbers should not increase their sleeping elevation more than 300-500 meters per day.

It is believed that HACE exists on a spectrum of acute cerebral dysfunction due to acute high-altitude exposure. The more common AMS is on one end of this spectrum; rare, but potentially-lethal HACE exists on the other. The risk for developing AMS or HACE is higher among younger patients. In AMS, headaches are typical, but the subject will have a normal neurologic examination. In HACE, the patient will display either ataxia and/or confusion. HACE patients should have no other focal neurologic deficits, fever, or neck stiffness.

In HACE, hypobaric hypoxia is thought to lead to dysregulation of cerebral blood flow and cause vasogenic edema, which later leads to cytotoxic edema and neurologic dysfunction. HACE can be fatal if not promptly recognized and treated. The treatment of choice is rapid descent in altitude, typically at least 1,000 meters, or until the patient's systems improve. When HACE is diagnosed early and and treatment rapidly initiated, descent may be completely curative. If available, supplemental oxygen and dexamethasone (8 mg initially, then 4 mg every 6 hours) are excellent adjunctive therapy—but should never replace immediate descent. If descent is not immediately possible, portable altitude chamber therapy can be utilized until arrangements can be made for the patient descent.

Patients with HACE can often suffer concomitant HAPE. If a patient is suffering significant respiratory symptoms, has pulmonary exam findings (crackles, frothy sputum), or oxygen saturation below the expected "normal" for the altitude (Table 9.1), the diagnosis of HAPE should be made. Again, oxygen and descent are the key interventions. In addition, nifedipine can be employed.

If the patient may have been exposed to combustion products (e.g., heating or cooking devices) within a closed space, CO poisoning should be on the differential. Symptoms of CO poisoning (e.g., headache, confusion, nausea/vomiting) can overlap with those of AMS and HACE. For patients with mild to moderate CO symptoms, treatment with oxygen (or potentially hyperbaric therapy) and removal from the environment will generally have improvement of their symptoms, even while staying at the same altitude. Conversely, HACE patients who stay at the same altitude will not improve. If available, co-oximetry (measuring CO levels) can be diagnostic. In a mountain environment, if there is any clinical concern or diagnostic uncertainty, the patient should descend.

Additionally, acute cerebral events (ischemic and hemorrhagic) may mimic HACE. This is an unlikely occurrence in an otherwise fit young individual at high altitude, but can be easy to overlook in this setting. Altitude has also been known to occasionally cause focal neurologic deficits, usually reversible with descent or oxygen administration. Findings of fever or meningismus would raise concern for an acute infectious etiology. Acute alcohol intoxication may also mimic HACE. A careful history can be telling.

If there is any suspicion for acute severe altitude diseases (HACE or HAPE), descent is advised.

FURTHER READING

Hackett PH, Roach RC. "High-Altitude Medicine and Physiology." *Auerbach's Wilderness Medicine, 7e. Ed.* Paul S Auerbach, Tracy C Cushing, N Stuart Harris. Philadelphia: Elsevier, 2016. 2–119. Print.

Forgey WW. "High-Altitude Illness." *Wilderness Medical Society Practice Guidelines for Wilderness Emergency Care, 5e.* Guilford: Falcon Guide, 2006. 46–53. Print.

Houston CS, Zafren K, Grissom CK. "Disorders Caused by Altitude." *Medicine for Mountaineering & Other Wilderness Activities,* 6e. Ed. James A Wilkerson. Ed. Ernest E Moore, Ken Zafren. Seattle: The Mountaineers Books, 2010. 238–255. Print.

HYPOTHERMIA

S. TEREZ MALKA

SETTING

Outdoors

CHIEF COMPLAINT

Cold Water Immersion

HISTORY

The patient is a 28-year-old male who presents by emergency medical services in cardiac arrest. Cardiopulmonary resuscitation (CPR) has been in progress for 25 minutes. He is accompanied by his girlfriend and a park ranger.

   The patient and his girlfriend were a running alongside an icy creek on a winding snowy trail earlier in the day. While running, the patient appeared to lose his footing and slip down an embankment before breaking through thin ice over a deep pool. He was immersed to the chest in water and was unable to pull himself onto the bank. After approximately 10 minutes, his girlfriend was successful in pulling him to shore. He was noted to be shivering while lying in the snow and was unable to stand or walk. She removed his wet jacket and gave him her own and then ran out to the trailhead to call for help. By the time she returned with a park ranger 2 hours later, the patient was barely responsive. He had removed the coat, and his lips were blue. He was minimally verbal, mumbling "I'm Keith" in response to all questions. The ranger removed Keith's wet pants and socks and wrapped him in a wool blanket. He arranged for an ambulance and evacuation to a nearby access road. While waiting for the ambulance to arrive, Keith became unresponsive and his pulse was no longer palpable. The ranger began CPR and continued it while he was being transported by ambulance to your hospital.

The patient has no known medical problems, takes no medications, and has no known drug allergies. He neither smokes nor drinks alcohol.

PHYSICAL EXAMINATION

Vital signs: HR 0. BP is unmeasurable. Good carotid pulses with chest compressions. RR 0. SpO_2 has no wave form without chest compressions. Temperature 18°C.

Examination reveals a cool, pale, unresponsive male.

Head and neck are normal without evidence of acute trauma.

No respirations are noted.

Cardiac exam reveals no heart sounds. He has no palpable pulses.

Extremities are cool to the touch, pale, and atraumatic with normal passive range of motion.

Neurologic exam: pupils 4 mm and fixed, no response to external stimuli, and Glasgow Coma Scale 3.

DIFFERENTIAL DIAGNOSIS

1. Acute hypothermia
2. Closed head injury
3. Acute coronary syndrome/ischemic arrhythmia
4. Toxic ingestion
5. Dehydration
6. Electrolyte abnormality

TESTS

Chest X-ray with clear lungs, and endotracheal tube 2 cm above the carina. Head CT shows normal grey–white border and no evidence of hemorrhage or trauma. C-spine computed tomography is negative.

Unremarkable complete blood count, chem 7, urinalysis, and creatine kinase. Negative troponin. Electrocardiogram (ECG) on rewarming is as noted in the following discussion.

CLINICAL COURSE

Medics placed a cervical collar and immobilized the patient as traumatic injury could not be excluded, obtained intravenous access, and began warm normal saline infusion as well as heated oxygen by bag-valve-mask while continuing CPR. Warm packs were placed behind the neck, in the axillae, and the groin. No cardiac activity was noted on the monitor.

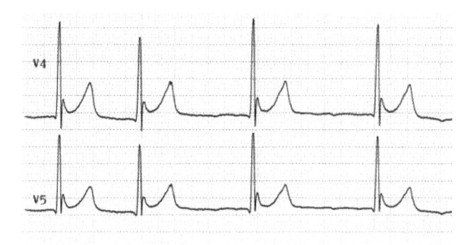

FIGURE 10.1 Electrocardiogram. Osborne J waves, seen as the positive defection at the J point, as seen here in leads V_4 and V_5.

Photo used with permission of Dr. Malka.

On arrival to your emergency department, CPR was continued, and the patient was intubated observing C-spine precautions. Two large-bore chest tubes were placed, and warm saline was infiltrated into the thoracic cavity. A nasogastric tube and Foley catheter were placed and irrigated with warm fluids. After an hour of rewarming and CPR, electrical activity was seen on the cardiac monitor, and an ECG was obtained (Figure 10.1), demonstrating J waves. Twenty minutes later, the patient regained pulses. He was admitted to the intensive care unit and made a full recovery.

KEY MANAGEMENT STEPS

1. Assuming complicating traumatic injury or medical illness until rewarming is complete.
2. Initiating active core rewarming prior to external warming measures.
3. Continuing CPR until a normal core temperature is achieved.
4. Recognizing that in hypothermia complete neurologic recovery can occur after even prolonged CPR.
5. Recognizing of Osborne J waves on ECG.

DEBRIEF

This patient was experiencing hypothermia due to cold water immersion. Hypothermia occurs when the core temperature drops below 35°C (95°F). Acute hypothermia often occurs following an environmental exposure, such as hiking on a windy day or falling into cold water. If a person gets wet or is improperly dressed, hypothermia can occur even in relatively warm ambient conditions. Windy conditions can further increase heat loss. Once the body becomes significantly hypothermic, central processes of thermoregulation fail, and the body will continue to cool to ambient temperature if external warming is not initiated.

Hypothermia is classified into 4 categories. Mild hypothermia occurs with a core body temperature of between 33.3 and 37.6°C. Victims will shiver and develop decreases in muscle tone and blood pressure. Mental processes will slow and patients may demonstrate slurred speech, an unsteady gait, poor judgement, unusual behaviors, and amnesia. The peripheral blood vessels will constrict, increasing blood return to the heart and brain, and leading to increased urine output, known as cold diuresis. ECG changes can be noted in this stage with the characteristic Osborne J Wave appearing (Figure 10.1).

Moderate hypothermia occurs at 29 to 32°C. Shivering ceases and level of consciousness decreases until patients become unresponsive. Cardiac arrhythmias or significant bradycardia may occur. Acid-base abnormalities and coagulopathies are common.

In severe hypothermia (22–28°C), the heart becomes predisposed to ventricular dysrhythmias, and the victim will become comatose and areflexic with no response to pain.

The final stage, profound hypothermia, occurs at less than 22°C. In this stage, the victim will appear to be "dead" and have no discernible heart beat and a flat electroencephalogram. Survival has been reported even in cases of profound hypothermia following hours of CPR. Resuscitative efforts should not be abandoned until the victim's core temperature has be restored to normal. In hypothermic cardiac arrest, patients are not dead until "they are warm and dead."

Treatment efforts should focus on increasing core temperature as quickly as possible. Passive external warming (e.g., applying a blanket or a coat) will work only in mild cases. In all other cases, active rewarming is required.

Outside of the hospital, wet clothing should be removed and replaced with dry layers, making sure to cover the head. The patient should be kept as still as possible, and in a horizontal position—minimize movement as cardiac irritability can lead to arrhythmias. Warm intravenous fluids should be started. If the patient is conscious, warm, sugar-containing oral liquids can be helpful. Warm packs may be placed in the axillae and groin. The patients should then be wrapped in several insulating and wind-resistant layers and gently evacuated. Avoid massaging or rubbing the extremities. These maneuvers can lead to a sudden vasodilation that causes "afterdrop," a phenomenon in which the rush of cool blood returning from the periphery causes the core temperature to suddenly drop further. This can lead to dysrhythmias and death.

In the hospital, rewarming methods should be continued using warm intravenous fluids, warm humidified oxygen, and warm packs to the axillae and groin. If cardiac instability is present, more aggressive core rewarming using thoracic lavage, peritoneal lavage, bladder lavage, or gastric lavage may be considered. In severe cases, where patients have significant metabolic abnormalities or are in cardiac arrest, extracorporeal warming devices may be life-saving. Continuous veno-venous hemofiltration, extracorporeal membrane oxygenation, and cardiac bypass techniques may be considered in addition to standard airway management and CPR. The use of antiarrhythmic drugs is controversial. Many arrhythmias will spontaneously improve once the core temperature begins to normalize. Resuscitative efforts should be continued until a normal core temperature is present.

FURTHER READING

Alhaddad IA, Khalil M, Brown EJ Jr. Osborn waves of hypothermia. *Circulation* 2000;101(25):E233–E244.

Danzl DF, Huecker, MR. Accidental hypothermia. In: Auerbach PS, Cushing TF, Harris NS, eds. *Wilderness Medicine*. 7th ed. Philadelphia, PA: Elsevier; 2017: 135-161.

Giesbrecht GG, Steinman, AM. Immersion into cold water. In: Auerbach PS, Cushing TF, Harris NS, *Wilderness Medicine*. 7th ed. Editors: Philadelphia, PA: Elsevier; 2017:162–196.

Zafren K, Giesbrecht GG, Danzl DF, et al. Wilderness Medical Society practice guidelines for the out-of-hospital evaluation and treatment of accidental hypothermia: 2014 update. *Wilderness Environ Med* 2014;25(Suppl 4):S66–85.

SECTION II

PREHOSPITAL

JEREMY T. CUSHMAN

VOMITING

MAIA DORSETT

SETTING

Rural Farm Area

CHIEF COMPLAINT

Vomiting

HISTORY

Emergency medical services is dispatched to a peach orchard where a 45-year-old male farmer complains of vomiting, difficulty breathing, and blurred vision. The symptoms started 30 minutes prior to emergency medical services arrival. Earlier in the day, the patient was cleaning out the tool shed and inadvertently spilled pesticide that had been stored on a top shelf. Soon after, he developed sweating, blurry vision, and watery eyes. The farmer's wife called 911 when he began to vomit and have difficulty breathing, both of which have gotten progressively worse. He also had a single episode of diarrhea. He denies chest pain or headache.

He has no significant past medical history.

He is a current smoker with a 15 pack-year history.

He denies any family history of cardiac, endocrine, or lung disease.

PHYSICAL EXAMINATION

Vital signs: HR 40, BP 88/60, RR 26, SpO_2 86% on room air, temp. 37.0°C.

Examination reveals a well-developed, well-nourished male in severe distress. His clothing is damp, and he is confused. His head is without trauma, and his pupils are 2 mm and reactive bilaterally. The patient has excessive tearing. Mucous membranes are excessively moist, and he is drooling. Cardiac rate is regular, and bradycardic without murmurs, gallops, or rubs. Radial pulses are palpable. There is no jugular venous distension. He is tachypneic with subcostal retractions. There are expiratory wheezes bilaterally. Abdomen is soft and nontender. He has no lower extremity edema. Skin is warm and diaphoretic. He is oriented to self and place. He has grossly normal strength and sensation in all extremities with intermittent muscle fasciculations.

DIFFERENTIAL DIAGNOSIS

1. Cholinergic toxidrome
2. Hypoglycemia
3. Heart block with cardiogenic shock
4. Viral syndrome/gastroenteritis

TESTS

Finger-stick blood glucose: 135 mg/dL
Electrocardiogram (ECG): sinus bradycardia

CLINICAL COURSE

After double-gloving with nitrile gloves and applying a particulate mask, the paramedic initiates a nebulizer treatment with bronchodilators and supplemental oxygen. Because the provider is suspicious of cholinergic toxicity due to organophosphate pesticide, an intravenous line is established, and 2 mg of atropine is administered intravenously. The patient has mild improvement in his heart rate but persistent hypotension and respiratory distress.

The patient is decontaminated by removing and bagging his clothing in such a way to minimize contamination. He is then copiously washed with soap and water. The patient is placed on a cardiac monitor, and an ECG is performed, demonstrating sinus bradycardia. A finger-stick blood glucose is obtained and found to be within normal limits. A 1 L normal saline bolus is initiated for hypotension. Pralidoxime chloride 2 g is administered intravenously. Given persistent respiratory distress, an additional 2 mg of intravenous atropine is administered, and the patient is placed on continuous positive airway pressure. En route to the hospital, paramedics notify the emergency department of the likely organophosphate exposure, treatment so far, and measures taken to decontaminate the patient. Local fire/hazmat is also notified of the pesticide spill.

In the hospital, the patient is intubated for persistent respiratory distress and hypoxia despite noninvasive positive pressure ventilation. An atropine drip is started, and the patient is admitted to the intensive care unit.

KEY MANAGEMENT STEPS

1. Recognition of cholinergic toxidrome in a patient with miosis, lacrimation, vomiting, diarrhea, bradycardia, bronchospasm, and muscle fasciculations.
2. Rapid initiation of treatment for immediate life threats.
3. Administration of correct antidote.
4. Recognizing the need for patient decontamination.
5. Notification of appropriate agencies (hospital, hazmat) of probable organophosphate exposure.

DEBRIEF

A toxidrome is a clinical syndrome that results from poisoning by a specific class of substances. When a patient presents with a diverse set of physical findings and/or history of exposure to a poisonous substance (e.g., a pesticide spill), identification of a specific toxidrome is critical in guiding diagnosis and treatment. This patient presented with a constellation of findings consistent with a cholinergic toxidrome. As implied by the name, the cholinergic toxidrome results from an excess of the neurotransmitter acetylcholine (ACh) at nerve endings. ACh binds to and activates nicotinic and muscarinic receptors present in the autonomic nervous system, central nervous system, and neuromuscular junction. In general, overstimulation of the parasympathetic nervous system dominates the clinical presentation of cholinergic excess. The symptoms of parasympathetic excess have been described by the pneumonic DUMBELS:

Defecation
Urination
Miosis
Bradycardia, bronchorrhea, bronchospasm ("Killer Bs")
Emesis
Lacrimation
Salivation

Nicotinic-receptor activation at the neuromuscular junction can lead to muscle fasciculations and/or muscle weakness. Cholinergic excess in the central nervous system can cause delirium, confusion, and seizures in severe cases.

Organophosphates are a common component of insecticides and are used in agriculture to protect food crops. Organophosphate exposure can occur by ingestion, inhalation, or skin absorption. This patient's exposure to pesticides was therefore a significant clue to the diagnosis. Organophosphates cause toxicity by increasing the concentration of ACh primarily by phosphorylation of acetylcholinesterase found at nerve endings. Normally, synaptic acetylcholinesterase inhibits neurotransmission by hydrolyzing acetylcholine to acetic acid and choline. In the absence of functional acetylcholinesterase, ACh accumulates leading to symptoms of cholinergic excess. Chemical warfare nerve agents (e.g., tabun, sarin, soman, VX) are acetylcholinesterase inhibitors that have been weaponized to cause more severe symptoms at lower concentrations.

When a toxic exposure is suspected, it is important that medical providers protect themselves so that they are not poisoned as well. In this case, double nitrile gloves are sufficient protection and should be worn at all times when treating the patient and handling his clothes. Initial care should focus on immediate life threats, in this case breathing and circulation. These are treated by the rapid administration of oxygen and antidote. In cases of refractory hypoxia, respiratory muscle weakness, or severe alteration of mental status, patients should be emergently intubated. Succinylcholine, a depolarizing muscle relaxant that is metabolized by acetylcholinesterase, should be avoided. Once initial measures are initiated, the patient warrants rapid decontamination to prevent further toxin absorption and to minimize contamination of care providers. This should be done in a manner that avoids increasing toxin absorption by exposing the mouth, airway, or eyes (Figure 11.1). Removal of clothing alone will reduce the exposure by more than half.

Treatment of organophosphate toxicity focuses on competitive inhibition of ACh at nerve endings and restoration of acetylcholinesterase function. Atropine antagonizes the effects of ACh at muscarinic receptors and blocks parasympathetic excess. It may be administered by the intravenous or intramuscular routes. Atropine dosing should be increased until bronchial secretions are cleared and the patient can be adequately oxygenated—this may require very large doses of atropine. Additionally, pralidoxime restores acetylcholinesterase activity by reactivating acetylcholinesterase and should be initiated early in severe poisonings. In addition to antidotes,

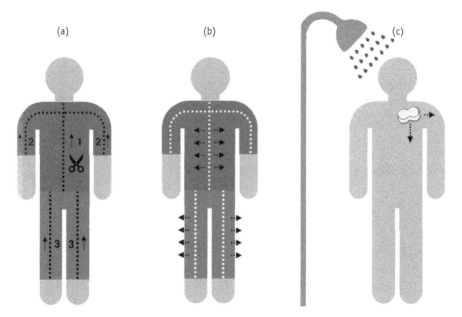

FIGURE 11.1 Decontamination procedure. (A and B) Cut the patient's clothing down the middle and roll down the sides to avoid contaminating the eyes, nose, and mouth. The clothing should be placed in a double plastic bag and tagged appropriately. (C) If the patient is ambulatory, they should wash from head to toe with soapy water. If the patient is nonambulatory, wash using a sideways motion from head to toe and then roll them to repeat on their backside. Ideally, runoff should be collected for appropriate disposal.

severe toxicity is managed with supportive care including oxygen, frequent suctioning, mechanical ventilation, and benzodiazepines should the patient begin seizing.

FURTHER READING

Beuhler MC. Treatment and evaluation of specific toxins. In: Cone D, Brice JH, Delbridge TR, Myers JB, eds. *Emergency Medical Services: Clinical Practice and Systems Oversight*, Vol. 1. *Clinical Aspects of EMS*. West Sussex, United Kingdom. Wiley; 2015: 341–350.

King AM, Aaron CK. Organophosphate and carbamate poisoning. *Emerg Med Clin N Am.* 2015;28;33(1):133–151.

Robey WC, Meggs WJ. Pesticides. In: Tintinalli JE, Stapczynski JS, Ma OJ, Cline DM, Cydulka RK, Meckler GD, eds. *Tintinalli's Emergency Medicine: A Comprehensive Study Guide*. 7th ed. New York, NY: McGraw-Hill Education; 2011: 1297–1305.

FALL WITH SYNCOPE

CHRISTOPHER J. FULLAGAR

SETTING

Outdoor Skate Park

CHIEF COMPLAINT

Fall and Syncope

HISTORY

A 23-year-old male is found at an outdoor skate park after calling 911 because he was concerned that he broke his arm after falling on an outstretched hand while inline skating. The patient complains of severe pain of the wrist with visible deformity of the distal right forearm. He was wearing a helmet but no wrist guards. He denies striking his head and has no neck nor back pain. He denies previous injury and explains that a pebble on the sidewalk caused him to fall. Subsequent to the fall, the patient states that he became very lightheaded and nauseated. His vision became fuzzy, which he described as "tunnel vision," and states that his ears began to ring before he passed out. He thinks he lost consciousness because of the severe pain. The feeling of lightheadedness and "fainting" has happened to him before, even with minor injuries and once when donating blood. Bystanders state that the patient's whole body shook about 4 or 5 times when he passed out, and he was unconscious for only a few seconds. He was not confused upon awakening.

He has no significant past medical history.

He does not smoke.

There is no significant family history.

PHYSICAL EXAMINATION

Vital signs: HR 65, BP 90/72, RR 16, SpO$_2$ 99% on room air.

Examination reveals a young, age-appropriate male in significant distress. He is awake and alert, without confusion. He appears pale and mildly diaphoretic. Examination of the head reveals no abrasions, lacerations, edema, or ecchymosis. A bicycle helmet is still in place and appears undamaged. The pupils are equal and 4 mm. There is no ear or nasal discharge, no loose or missing teeth, and no bite marks on the tongue. Neck reveals no cervical spinal tenderness, step-off, or deformity. The patient has no apparent range of motion limitation of the neck. Lungs are clear. Cardiac exam reveals a regular rate and rhythm. Abdomen is soft, nontender, and without ecchymosis. His back reveals no midline tenderness, step-off, or deformity. There is no ecchymosis of the flank. Pelvis is not tender. Examination of the right arm reveals a dorsal deformity of the distal forearm with associated tenderness. Distal pulses are full and capillary refill is brisk. Sensory function is grossly intact. The remainder of his extremities have full range of motion and are without evidence of injury.

DIFFERENTIAL DIAGNOSIS

1. Fractured arm with subsequent vasovagal syncope
2. Cardiac arrhythmia causing a syncopal episode leading to fall and subsequent fractured arm
3. Mechanical fall with closed head injury leading to a brief loss of consciousness
4. Seizure leading to fall and subsequent fracture

TESTS

No tests were administered.

CLINICAL COURSE

The patient's right forearm was immobilized in a commercial splint. Voids were padded, and the hand was placed in a position of function. Neurovascular integrity was assessed both before and after splint placement and was intact. An ice pack was placed. The patient reported significant pain relief at that point. No other injury was identified on examination. The patient was placed in a supine position and reported significant improvement of his lightheadedness. His pallor and diaphoresis resolved. His vital signs were reassessed, and his blood pressure was 122/76 with a heart rate of 82 and respirations of 16. Advanced life support (ALS) was initially considered for pain management and for syncope; however, the patient reported adequate pain control after immobilization and the syncope was felt to be vasovagal in nature. The patient was transported to the emergency department without incident where his fracture was subsequently reduced and splinted, and he was discharged for outpatient orthopedic follow-up.

KEY MANAGEMENT STEPS

1. Assess for neurovascular integrity before and after splint placement.
2. Maximize basic life support (BLS) pain management with optimal immobilization and cold packs.
3. Look for evidence of other trauma, not just what is initially obvious.
4. Consider all causes of syncope and do not prematurely assume a vasovagal etiology.

DEBRIEF

The importance of prehospital BLS is often minimized or completely overlooked, but these interventions may have a significant effect on the patient's course. Knowing the basics and implementing them well is applicable whether you are a first responder in the field or an attending physician in a tertiary care center. In this case, the patient had a very painful angulated forearm fracture.

Often, a cursory splint is applied, and the patient is given opioid pain medication. In this case, the responding ambulance crew was trained and equipped at the BLS level. Calling an ALS unit for a rendezvous is a valid consideration for patients with uncontrolled severe pain. Even in cases of relatively short transport times, there can be a significant delay before the patient receives analgesia after arrival in the emergency department. Pain medication administered by emergency medical services can greatly reduce time to adequate analgesia even if the medication is given in close proximity to the hospital. Adequate pain management, however, does not necessarily require parenteral opioids. Proper immobilization and the placement of a cold pack can have a significant effect on the level of pain. Even small movements of the sharp bone fragments can be excruciating. Don't overlook these simple steps, especially in the field environment or any other time when it is necessary to move the patient.

In this case, this BLS crew utilized a commercial splint. Depending on the particular splint used, one may presume that the splint simply has to be applied and secured without any other intervention. Figure 12.1 depicts a simulated angulated fracture with a commercial splint. If the device was simply secured with the hook and loop fasteners, optimal immobilization would not be achieved. Figure 12.2 illustrates that sufficient padding and placing the hand in the position of function is necessary to provide the proper support to achieve maximal effect of the splint. Note that the hook and loop fasteners in this case had to be reinforced with tape because the padding rendered the native fasteners too short (Figure 12.3).

The patient also presented with a brief episode of unconsciousness. Syncope has many worrisome etiologies, and in any acute care situation, it is always crucial to consider the worrisome potential causes of the patients' presentation rather than hastily settling on what might be the most likely cause. It is a common pitfall in acute care to misinterpret the patient's findings as something benign when there is a more serious underlying process. Like uncontrolled severe pain, syncope is also a valid reason for a BLS crew to consider calling an ALS unit. Excluding

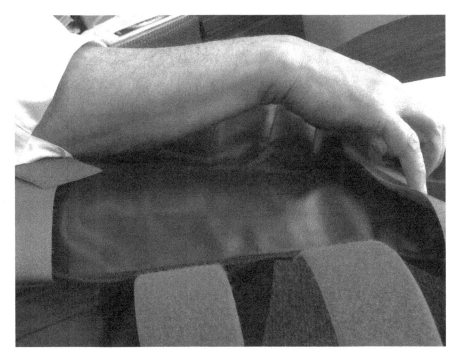

FIGURE 12.1 Simulated angulated forearm fracture with a commercial splint. If the hook and loop closure is secured without any other provisions, the limb will be improperly immobilized. This can lead to unnecessary pain and, possibly, vascular compromise with movement.

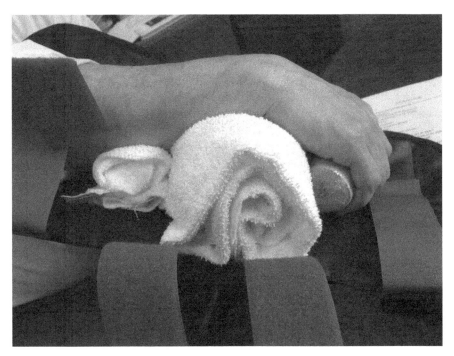

FIGURE 12.2 Commercial splint with voids padded and the hand placed in the position of function. This allows for maximal support of the injury which minimizes movement. Sharp bone fragments can cause immense pain with even small movements. Unnecessary movement of the limb may even lead to vascular compromise. Basic interventions, such as immobilization and cold packs, can significantly reduce the patient's pain and need for opiate medications while reducing complications.

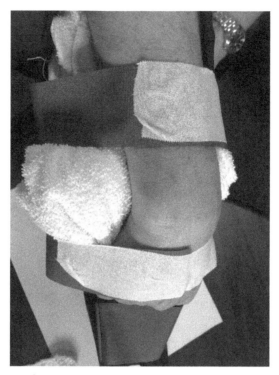

FIGURE 12.3 Reinforcement of splint straps with tape. It is possible that the native securing device may require reinforcement if padding is utilized. In this case, tape is used to secure the splint because the hook and loop closure is too short to encompass the additional padding.

worrisome etiologies does not always require advanced tests, but it does require careful history taking and decision-making.

In this case, the patient is a young, healthy male without a significant past medical history, such as an arrhythmia (like Wolf-Parkinson-White syndrome) or diabetes (suggesting the possibility of hypoglycemia). Furthermore, the symptoms followed the classic pattern of vasovagal syncope: a severe pain trigger with a prodrome of lightheadedness, nausea, "tunnel vision," and tinnitus prior to losing consciousness. There was no evidence of head trauma on examination, and the history clearly indicates a mechanical etiology of the fall that is spontaneously recalled by the patient.

As vasovagal syncope is mediated by inappropriate vagal or autonomic tone, it is often associated with bradycardia and hypotension (secondary to vasodilation). Even though the patient appeared to be in significant pain, his initial heart rate was not tachycardic. This is consistent with his persistent vagal signs of mild hypotension, pallor, and diaphoresis. As with any instance of hypotension, the patient should be positioned appropriately. Simply having the patient lie flat will facilitate cerebral blood flow and decrease symptoms of presyncope. In this case, on reassessment after positioning the patient supine, his heart rate and blood pressure improved and his vagal symptoms resolved. If a patient is unresponsive, placing the patient in the recovery (lateral recumbent) position has the added benefits of reducing the potential of aspiration of fluid into the lungs and keeping the airway open. In at least 1 study, the simple act of placing an unresponsive child in the recovery position was associated with a reduced rate of hospital admission.[1]

Besides syncope, other etiologies such as seizure must be considered. Bystanders noted that the patient's whole body shook 4 or 5 times after he passed out. These myoclonic jerks are common with syncope and are often misinterpreted as seizure activity, especially by laypersons.[2] Other clues of generalized seizure activity, such as tongue biting and a postictal period of confusion, are also absent.

REFERENCES

1. Julliand S, Desmarest M, Gonzalez L, et al. Recovery position significantly associated with a reduced admission rate of children with loss of consciousness. *Arch Dis Child*. 2016;101:521–526.
2. Josephson Syncope Convulsions (web video). *YouTube*. December 30, 2014. https://youtu.be/YaktxCXiUyY

FURTHER READING

Costantino G, Sun BC, Barbic F, et al. Syncope Clinical Management in the Emergency Department: A Consensus From the First International Workshop on Syncope Risk Stratification in the Emergency Department. *Eur Heart J*. 2016;37(19):1493–1498.

Limmer D, O'Keefe MF. Musculoskeletal injuries. In: Limmer D, O'Keefe MF, eds. *Emergency Care*. 11th ed. Upper Saddle River, NJ: Pearson Education; 2009: 700–713.

Qiunn J. Syncope. In: Tintinalli JE, ed. *Tintinalli's Emergency Medicine: A Comprehensive Study Guide*. 7th ed. New York, NY: McGraw-Hill; 2011: 360–365.

CHAPTER 13

EXCITED DELIRIUM

THOMAS WILLIAMS

SETTING

Urban College Campus

CHIEF COMPLAINT

Agitation

HISTORY

911 is called for an altercation at a party on a college campus. On arrival, police and emergency medical services find a 22-year-old male agitated and expressing aggressive language and behavior. The initial physical altercation between the patient and 2 other men resolved on arrival of police; however, the patient is now pacing, speaking loudly, and appears to be interacting with unseen figures and voices. He becomes more agitated and angry with each interaction with police and emergency medical services and threatens them with violence when they attempt to question him or approach to evaluate him. Friends say the patient has been drinking alcohol and may have been using recreational drugs but aren't sure what he may have taken.

His roommate indicates he has attention deficit hyperactivity disorder for which he takes Adderall but does not know of any other medical problems. No additional information is available.

PHYSICAL EXAMINATION

Vital signs are unable to be obtained due to his agitation.

A visual exam from a distance is all that can be obtained due to his aggressiveness. His exam is limited but reveals an agitated patient who is pacing, diaphoretic, and verbally aggressive and abusive. He has evidence of a contusion and swelling to the left side of his face with a laceration and bleeding over his left eye. He appears to be breathing rapidly but without distress. His skin is diaphoretic, and he is shirtless. There are abrasions noted to his forearms, and he is purposeful in his movements, although at times nonsensical in his speech.

DIFFERENTIAL DIAGNOSIS

1. Intoxication
2. Excited delirium
3. Acute psychosis
4. Acute mania
5. Head injury

CLINICAL COURSE

Verbal de-escalation and show-of-force fails to calm the patient. He becomes increasingly agitated and aggressive. When approached by law enforcement, he lashes out again, and there is increasing concern that the patient may hurt himself or others. After discussion among responders, five police officers swarm the patient and physically restrain him on the ground while the paramedic administers 250 mg ketamine intramuscularly (IM) to the anterolateral thigh.

Within minutes, the patient begins to calm. He is transferred to the ambulance gurney and physically restrained. Once in the ambulance, vital signs and a physical exam can be completed. They reveal: HR 132, BP 146/85, RR 24, SpO$_2$ 98% on room air.

The patient is diaphoretic and warm to the touch. His head has evidence of a laceration to the left superior orbital rim with mild bleeding controlled with gauze and direct pressure. He has contusions to bilateral periorbital regions with swelling and ecchymosis. Pupils are 6 mm, equal and reactive. There is no intraoral trauma, and although sedated, the patient is maintaining his own airway. His cardiac exam is notable for tachycardia, and his lung sounds are clear bilaterally. His abdomen is soft and without tenderness. His extremities have abrasions to the forearms and hands but no obvious lacerations or deformities. His skin is warm and diaphoretic.

The patient is placed on a cardiac monitor and waveform capnography is monitored while an intravenous (IV) line is established and crystalloids are begun. The patient is transported to the nearest emergency department with a police officer on board. In the emergency room, the patient is provided with IV fluids, receives blood work, a head computed tomography, and is closely monitored. After 6 hours in the emergency department, the patient is reevaluated and appears sober and no longer agitated or aggressive. He reports drinking heavily at the party and using cocaine for the first time; however, he denies any history of psychiatric illness. He denies any suicidal or homicidal thoughts, and after discussion with social work regarding substance abuse and outpatient resources, he was discharged home.

TESTS

Head computer tomography: normal
Complete blood count: normal
Complete metabolic panel: normal
Ethanol level: 168 mg/dL
Urine tox screen: (+) cocaine, (–) benzodiazepines, (–) amphetamines, (–) opiates
Serum drug screen: (–) Salicylate, (–) Acetaminophen, (–)Tricyclic
Creatinine kinase: 450 IU/L (30–225 IU/L)
Troponin: 0.01 ng/mL (0–0.04 ng/mL)
Electrocardiogram: sinus tachycardia, no arrhythmias, no ST elevation.

KEY MANAGEMENT STEPS

1. Recognize excited delirium and take appropriate personal safety precautions.
2. Attempt verbal de-escalation.
3. Consider chemical restraint for extremely agitated or combative patients.
4. Do not allow physical restraints to restrict the patient's ability to breathe.
5. Treat for hyperthermia, acidosis, and rhabdomyolysis until proven otherwise.
6. Consider all causes of agitation and acute delirium.

DEBRIEF

In this scenario, the patient exhibited behavior consistent with that of excited delirium, which is described as a triad of delirium, psychomotor agitation, and physiologic excitation. Delirium is a state in which the patient has an altered level of consciousness where he or she may experience delusions, hallucinations, and disorganized thought as well as a decreased ability to maintain or shift his or her attention and focus. Psychomotor agitation coupled with emotional and physical excitation or aggression make these patients highly volatile and dangerous. They are prone to explosive outbursts that can result in violent behavior toward providers and those perceived as authority figures. They may also exhibit extraordinary strength and pain tolerance, making them very difficult to restrain.

Common precipitants for excited delirium include psychiatric disturbances, alcohol intoxication, and ingestion of recreational drugs, such as cocaine, methamphetamines, or phencyclidine (PCP). Although infrequent, it's important to recognize that infections, metabolic disturbances, and hypoglycemia may also present similarly. While the exact mechanism by which these precipitants cause excited delirium is not yet clear, the common pathway appears to be excessive dopamine stimulation in the brain.

With an overly aggressive, agitated patient, such as one in a state of excited delirium, standard de-escalation techniques often fail, and providers may be put in harm's way. Therefore, one must be vigilant to maintain personal safety at all times. Careful and clear coordination with law enforcement personnel can help in physically restraining an agitated patient and thereby allowing medical providers to safely approach and administer a sedative agent. The most common sedatives used in the prehospital setting are benzodiazepines and ketamine, and both can be given IM into large muscles such as the thigh, gluteus, or deltoid.

Ketamine is often dosed at 4 to 5 mg/kg IM for excited delirium, while doses ≤200 mg have been associated with higher risk of treatment failure. Ketamine is advantageous as it has a short onset of action, generally achieving sedation in as little as 2 to 5 minutes and does not reduce the patient's respiratory drive. Additionally, it has been found safe in the setting of head trauma with no significant increase in intracranial pressure. There are 2 adverse reactions that are particularly relevant: laryngospasm and hypersalivation. The incidence of hypersalivation is low, and in the event it develops, atropine 0.5 mg and suction are the initial treatments of choice. Laryngospasm is rare, but when it occurs, it can be difficult to manage. The initial approach starts with providing supplemental oxygen and performing a modified jaw thrust with pressure at the laryngospasm notch, a procedure called the Larson maneuver. This maneuver may help relax the vocal cords and involves a jaw thrust with the addition of pressure to the space above the superior aspect of mandibular ramus, called the laryngospasm notch. Noninvasive positive pressure ventilation can then be used for persistent laryngospasm or hypoxemia. If this fails or the patient has refractory or recurrent laryngospasm, paralysis and intubation may be required.

Benzodiazepines have a long history in the management of agitated patients and have predictable respiratory depression with minimal effects on hemodynamics. Midazolam is the preferred agent in the prehospital setting as it has a fast time of onset relative to other benzodiazepines and when given IM has a reliable onset of action and a rapid time until clinical effect compared to other benzodiazepines such as lorazepam. The initial starting dose of midazolam is often 5 to 10 mg with repeat doses of 2.5 to 10 mg IM as needed with careful attention to respiratory status.

Once adequately chemically sedated, care must be taken to ensure no further injury comes to the patient. The patient should be physically restrained in such a way that his or her ability to breathe is not compromised and he or she is transported in a supine position. End-tidal capnography should be initiated to monitor for adequate ventilation, and treatment for hyperthermia, rhabdomyolysis, and acidemia should be considered. This begins with establishing IV access and starting IV fluids as well as cooling patients as needed. Sodium bicarbonate may be considered in a patient at risk for rhabdomyolysis or acidosis following adequate fluid resuscitation. Once sedated and restrained, a more complete physical exam should then be performed and consideration given to other causes of agitation and delirium.

These patients pose a management challenge to providers as they are prone to aggressive outbursts and incredible strength, making a proper evaluation incredibly hard, if not impossible. It is important to work closely with law enforcement personnel to safely physically and, if necessary, chemically restrain the patient. The choice of sedative agent is often either ketamine or midazolam, but the route of administration in an agitated, aggressive patient should be intramuscularly, in either the deltoid, thigh, or gluteus, as attempting to place in IV catheter in these patients can be dangerous for both the patient and provider. Once sedated and restrained, one should complete a thorough physical exam and consider the causes of the patient's delirium, which may include many life-threatening conditions including intoxication, head injury, hypoglycemia, metabolic derangement, infection, or excited delirium. Importantly, never assume the behavior is due to primarily psychiatric or intoxicant causes until other life-threatening causes are excluded. In this manner, a dangerous patient can be safely assessed and treated with as little risk to the patient and providers as possible.

FURTHER READING

Bellolio MF, Gilani WI, Barrionuevo J, et al. Incidence of adverse events in adults undergoing procedural sedation in the emergency department: a systematic review and meta-analysis. *Acad Emerg Med.* 2016;23(2):119–134.

Cohen L, Athaide V, Wickham ME, et al. The effect of ketamine on intracranial and cerebral perfusion pressure and health outcomes: a systematic review. *Ann Emerg Med.* 2015;65(1):43–51.

Cole J, Moore J, Nystrom PC, et al. A prospective study of ketamine versus haloperidol for severe prehospital agitation. *Clin Tox.* 2016;54(7): 556–562.

Hopper A, Vilke G, Castillo EM, et al. Ketamine use for acute agitation in the emergency department. *J Emerg Med.* 2015;48(6):712–719.

Isbister G, Calver L, Downes MA, et al. Ketamine as rescue treatment for difficult-to-sedate severe acute behavioral disturbance in the emergency department. *Ann Emerg Med.* 2016;76(5):581–587.

Larson, CP. Laryngospasm—the best treatment. *Anesthesiology.* 1998;89(5):1293–1294.

Nobay F, Simon BC, Levitt MA, et al. A prospective, double-blind, randomized trial of midazolam versus haloperidol versus lorazepam in the chemical restraint of violent and severely agitated patients. *Acad Emerg Med.* 2004;11(7):744–749.

Reich J, Stinton A. Behavioral health emergencies. In: Cone D, Brice JH, Delbridge TR, Myers JB, eds. *Emergency Medical Services Clinical Practice and Systems Oversight:* Vol. 1, *Clinical Aspects of EMS.* 2nd ed. West Sussex, United Kingdom: Wiley; 2015: 412–420.

Scheppke K, Braghiroli J, Shalaby M, et al. Prehospital use of IM ketamine for sedation of violent and agitated patients. *West J Emerg Med.* 2014;15(7):736–741.

Stoelting R. Hemodynamic effects of barbiturates and benzodiazepines. *Clev Clin J Med.* 1981;48(1):9–13.

Vilke GM, DeBard ML, Chan TC, et al. Excited delirium syndrome: defining based on a review of the lLiterature. *J Emerg Med.* 2012;43(5):897–905.

CHAPTER 14

STRIDOR

SEAN DONOVAN AND HEIDI CORDI

SETTING

Private Residence

CHIEF COMPLAINT

Respiratory Distress

HISTORY

911 is activated by the mother of a 1-year-old male. For the last 24 hours her son has had a runny nose, low-grade fever, and a harsh cough. Aside from some mild fussiness, he has been acting himself and eating/drinking normally. Shortly after going to sleep tonight, the patient awoke in distress, working to breath and making an abnormal high-pitched sound with inspiration. Mom administered an albuterol nebulizer with no improvement. The patients' older sister was recently sick with an upper respiratory tract infection.

Past medical history includes reactive airway disease for which he uses albuterol on an as-needed basis. No surgical history. Vaccinations are up to date, and there is no recent foreign travel.

The patient attends playgroup during daytime hours and has no exposure to secondhand cigarette smoke.

PHYSICAL EXAMINATION

Vital signs: HR 130, BP 80/40, RR 32, SpO_2 93% on room air, temp. 37.9°C, weight 12 kg.

Examination reveals a well-developed 1-year-old male sitting in mom's arms. He is in moderate respiratory distress, with a harsh seal-like cough and intermittent stridor when crying. His trachea is midline with tugging visible at his sternal notch. In addition, he has intercostal and subcostal retractions. He does not have any nasal flaring. On auscultation, inspiratory stridor is evident at his neck but no expiratory wheeze is present in his lung fields. Normal but tachycardic heart sounds are auscultated without murmur or rub, and he is warm and well perfused. His abdomen is soft, but it is difficult to assess with his intermittent crying. Neurologically, he is alert, moving all extremities, and has normal muscle tone.

DIFFERENTIAL DIAGNOSIS

1. Croup (acute laryngotracheobronchitis)
2. Bacterial tracheitis
3. Epiglottitis
4. Inhaled foreign body
5. Angioedema
6. Congenital airway malformation

TESTS

No tests were administered.

CLINICAL COURSE

After initial assessment, the patient receives blow-by oxygen due to increased work of breathing and mild hypoxia. Given his moderate to severe distress with the presence of stridor, the decision is made to administer nebulized epinephrine (5 mls of 1mg/1ml L-epinephrine) over 10 minutes. After starting the nebulizer, the patient was noted to become increasingly agitated, with more prominent stridor. To comfort him, he was provided his favorite teddy bear, kept in his mother's arms, and further medical interventions were limited. With these adjustments, he began calming, and his work of breathing and stridor began to resolve. During transport to the nearby emergency department, the patient remained calm and a dose of dexamethasone (0.6 mg/kg) was administered orally per local emergency medical services protocol.

Transport to the emergency department was uneventful without recurrence of agitation, stridor, or respiratory distress. In the emergency department, the patient was observed for several hours to ensure no deterioration. He did not require repeat dosing of nebulized epinephrine or supplemental oxygen administration and was subsequently discharged from the emergency department with primary care follow up in 2 to 3 days.

KEY MANAGEMENT STEPS

1. Recognizing respiratory distress with development of stridor.
2. Limiting stressful/painful interventions, which could worsen respiratory distress.
3. Administering supplemental oxygen for respiratory distress or significant hypoxia.
4. Administering nebulized epinephrine for respiratory distress with stridor.
5. Considering prehospital steroid therapy if local protocol and patient stability allows.

DEBRIEF

The patient was diagnosed with croup, otherwise known as acute laryngotracheobronchitis. This is a common upper airway infection typically affecting children ages 6 months to 3 years, most frequently occurring in the late fall to winter. This infection is viral in nature, most commonly caused by the parainfluenza virus, but can also occur secondary to influenza, adenovirus, respiratory syncytial virus, or human metapneumovirus infections.

Classically, patients develop cough and runny nose 1 to 2 days before the development of airway symptoms. Edema leads to marked narrowing of the upper airway, which manifests itself as acute stridor and the harsh "seal-like" cough that is most commonly associated with acute croup. Stridor is most notable during periods of agitation and increased work of breathing. If continuous stridor is present in a nonagitated child, this is worrisome for severe airway compromise. When stridor or increased work of breathing is present, treatment with nebulized epinephrine causes vasoconstriction and reduction of airway edema. It is important to note that edema, not bronchospasm, is the main cause of the patient's symptoms and the reason inhalers such as albuterol do not have any significant effect.

While children with croup sometimes require nebulized epinephrine, all children with symptoms of acute croup should typically receive steroid therapy. Once administered, steroids typically decrease airway edema and inflammation over the following 4 to 6 hours. Dexamethasone is the most commonly utilized steroid given its prolonged duration of action. As such, most children require only 1 dose during the course of infection.

While croup is common and mainly a self-limited disease, there are a few notable alternative pathologies that present with stridor. Bacterial tracheitis is associated with an acute deterioration, toxic appearance, and copious secretions. Often, these patients will have had upper airway surgery or tracheostomy. Similarly, epiglottis will also present with a toxic, unwell appearance as well as drooling, absence of cough, and tripod self-positioning. Both of these life-threatening pathologies will not respond to nebulized epinephrine. Occasionally, deep space neck infections such as peritonsillar or retropharyngeal abscess can also cause stridor. With any signs of upper airway obstructive pathology, one should also consider inhaled foreign body, often presenting after a choking episode, or angioedema, which may have associated allergic skin findings or hereditary familial association.

FURTHER READING

Bjornson C, Johnson D. Croup in children. *Can Med Assoc J.* 2013;185(5):1317–1223.

Ortiz-Alvarez O. Acute management of croup in the emergency department. *Pediatr Child Health.* 2017;22(3):166–169.

Zoorob R, Sidani M, Murray J. Croup: an overview. *Am Fam Physician.* 2011;83(9):1067–1073.

CHAPTER 15

INTERFACILITY VENTILATOR MANAGEMENT

CHRISTOPHER GALTON

SETTING

Community Hospital ICU

CHIEF COMPLAINT

Hypoxemia

HISTORY

A 35-year-old female initially presented to a community hospital for an abdominal component separation and mesh repair secondary to an infected implant. During the 12-hour surgery, the mesh was removed and noted to be purulent. The abdominal components were separated and a new piece of mesh was reimplanted. Postoperatively, she was unable to be extubated and was transferred to the intensive care unit (ICU). After 3 days in the ICU, the community hospital contacted the aeromedical provider and a quaternary academic center for transfer to a higher level of care for persistent hypoxemia. Her current infusions include norepinephrine at 2 mcg/min, midazolam at 15 mg/hr, and fentanyl at 250 mcg/hr.

She has a past medical history of moderate chronic obstructive pulmonary disease, moderate persistent asthma, hypertension, type 2 diabetes, super morbid obesity, previous tracheostomy with successful wean and decannulation, and a pulmonary embolism.

She currently smokes approximately 1 pack/day and has been smoking for 20 years. She has a family history of hypertension and diabetes.

PHYSICAL EXAMINATION

Vital signs: HR 114, BP 88/52, RR 10 assisted, SpO_2 87% on ventilator, temp. 38.6°C, height 150 cm, weight 148 kg.

Ventilator: Assist control, rate = 10 bpm, tidal volume = 650 mL, positive end-expiratory pressure (PEEP) = 10 cm H_2O, FiO_2 = 100%.

Examination reveals an obese female, who is under the care of the ICU staff. Her head exam is normal with a 7.0 mm oral endotracheal tube at 21 cm to the teeth and feeding tube in the left nare at 55 cm. Lung sounds are very distant with no adventitious sounds noted. Cardiac exam reveals normal S_1S_2 without any murmurs, rubs, or gallops. The abdomen is very obese with a midline incision site that extends from the subxyphoid space to 5 cm above the symphysis pubis. It also extends laterally 10 cm from the inferior border to the left. The staple line is intact with no purulent drainage or erythema noted. Moderate to severe peripheral edema is appreciated in all 4 extremities, but they are all warm and well perfused. Neurologic exam reveals a patient that is interactive and able to follow commands.

DIFFERENTIAL DIAGNOSIS

1. Acute respiratory distress syndrome (ARDS)
2. Acute lung injury
3. Pleural effusion
4. Right heart failure
5. Chronic obstructive pulmonary disease exacerbation
6. Asthma exacerbation
7. Pulmonary embolism
8. Aspiration pneumonia

TESTS

Complete blood count

White blood cell count of 13,000/uL (4–10)
Hemoglobin of 12.4 g/dL (12–16)
Platelet count of 63,000/mL (150,000–450,000)

Chemistry panel

Sodium	148 mEq/L (136–144)
Potassium	5.4 mEq/L (3.7–5.2)
Chloride	99 mmol/L (92–108)

CO$_2$	14 mmol/L (22–26)
Blood urea nitrogen	73 mg/dL (7–20)
Creatinine	3.2 mg/dL (0.8–1.2)
Glucose	212 mg/dL (70–100)
D-dimer	Mildly elevated
Fibrinogen	102 mg/dL (150–400)

Arterial blood gas

pH	7.14
PaCO$_2$	41 mmHg (35–45)
PaO$_2$	52 mmHg (80–100)
Base excess	–12

Chest radiograph (Figure 15.1).

CLINICAL COURSE

The patient was moved to the transport aircraft and secured to the airframe. Prior to moving her, the PaO$_2$/FiO$_2$ ratio was calculated (52/100% or 52/1.0 = 52) and noted to be consistent with severe ARDS. She is transitioned to appropriate ventilator settings that included 5 mL/kg of ideal body weight, which placed her tidal volumes at 250 mL. Since her PaCO$_2$ was within normal limits, it was appropriate to maintain similar minute volumes, which were 6.5 L/min. Her respiratory rate was set at 26 breaths/min. Her PEEP was gradually increased during transport

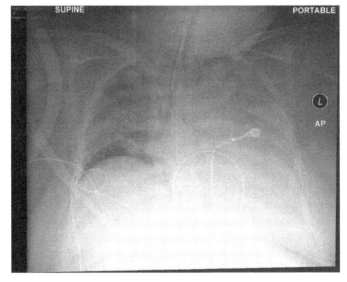

FIGURE 15.1 Chest x-ray. Endotracheal tube is 3 cm off carina, normal sized heart situated in the left chest, heart border is clear, bilateral patchy white infiltrates, mild right sided effusion, and right subclavian central venous catheter noted with tip in the superior vena cava.

until her SpO_2 improved, which was at 18 cm H_2O. The plateau pressures were 35 cm H_2O once the PEEP was finalized. Her FiO_2 was weaned down to 60% once she arrived at the destination facility to maintain PaO_2 of >60 mm Hg. Adequate sedation and analgesia was achieved with ketamine and dexmedetomidine infusions, and the high doses of midazolam and fentanyl were weaned down at appropriate rates to prevent withdrawal symptoms. Given the high PEEP needed to achieve adequate oxygenation, she was started on an atracurium infusion to maintain neuromuscular blockade. Her blood pressure was maintained with increased intravenous fluids and the norepinephrine infusion was titrated to maintain a MAP of >60 mm Hg.

After a prolonged hospital course that required another tracheostomy and multiple episodes of intraabdominal sepsis, the patient was weaned from the ventilator, decannulated, and was discharged to an acute rehabilitation facility.

KEY MANAGEMENT STEPS

1. Recognizing that ventilator settings should be based on ideal body weight, not total body weight.
2. By calculating the PaO_2/FiO_2 ratio, the level of lung injury is known and can assist with determining the proper tidal volume calculation.
3. Maintaining oxygenation is paramount and the PEEP and FiO_2 should be adjusted accordingly.
4. High PEEPs require ventilator synchrony and neuromuscular blockade is frequently necessary.
5. When neuromuscular blocker infusions are required, sedation at amnestic levels is required.

DEBRIEF

The sending facility wanted to transfer this patient because of the persistent hypoxemia despite their best efforts to ensure adequate oxygenation. This was likely related to a combination of persistent intra-abdominal sepsis and a ventilation strategy that was suboptimal. Determining proper ventilator settings in the morbidly obese and super morbidly obese populations can be challenging and when done poorly, can lead to significant parenchymal lung injuries. Using an air medical transport provider allowed for both rapid interfacility transport as well as a critical care nurse and paramedic with extensive experience managing ventilated patients with multiple vasoactive and other drips that may be beyond the scope of a ground-based emergency medical services provider in some areas.

When attempting to determine proper ventilator settings, it is important to consider both the patient's pathology as well as his or her body habitus. In patients who are having difficulty oxygenating with relatively standard ventilator settings, the first step is to calculate the $PaO_2:FiO_2$ ratio. Ratios of <300 are indicative of acute lung injury. If that ratio drops below 200, then a diagnosis of ARDS is considered. Severe ARDS occurs when those ratios drop below 100, and mortality can rise to close to 50%. This information, when combined with the chest X-ray finding of bilateral patchy white infiltrates makes the diagnosis of ARDS.

Early recognition and adjustment of ventilator settings may help to avoid severe ARDS. In this case, the patient had a tidal volume in the ICU based on total body weight (650 mL) rather than ideal body weight (250 mL), which likely transitioned an acute lung injury into severe ARDS. Understanding that patients are at risk for parenchymal stretch injuries provides us with the opportunity to reduce tidal volumes earlier in the disease process. Tidal volume reduction, when combined with aggressive treatment of the underlying etiology, can reduce mortality and morbidity.

Sedation for these patients is also very important and should not be overlooked. Many ventilator setting changes are very uncomfortable for the patient. This leads to ventilator dyssynchrony and continued injury potentiation. Typically, medications that depress the respiratory drive such as opiates or propofol are desirable for ventilator synchrony. Unfortunately, those medications have side effects and may not be appropriate for all ARDS patients. In fact, this frequently results in using alternative agents such as in this case where ketamine and dexmedetomidine provided the opportunity to safely sedate without incurring additional hypotension.

If standard ventilator adjustments do not safely reverse the process of worsening lung injury, then frequently more advanced therapies need pursuing. Some of these options include neuromuscular blockade, prone positioning, pulmonary vasodilators such as epoprostenol or nitric oxide, high-frequency oscillation ventilation, and extracorporeal membrane oxygenation. There is still considerable debate on the indications and ideal therapies for this complex condition with a high mortality.

FURTHER READING

The Acute Respiratory Distress Syndrome Network. Ventilation with lower tidal volumes as compared with traditional tidal volumes for acute lung injury and the acute respiratory distress syndrome. *New Engl J Med*. 2000;342(18):1301–1308.

Ferguson ND, Fan E, Camporota L, Antonelli M. The Berlin definition of ARDS: an expanded rationale, justification, and supplementary material. *Intens Care Med*. 2012;38(10):1573–1582.

Marino, Paul L. Acute respiratory distress syndrome. In: Marino P, ed. *Marino's The ICU Book*. 4th ed. Philadelphia, PA. Lippincott, Williams, & Wilkins; 2014: 447–463.

Petrucci N, De Feo C. Lung protective ventilation strategy for the acute respiratory distress syndrome. *Cochrane Db Syst Rev*. 2013;2:CD003844.

CHAPTER 16

DIFFICULTY BREATHING

ESSIE REED-SCHRADER AND WILLIAM T. RIVERS

SETTING

Park

CHIEF COMPLAINT

Difficulty Breathing

HISTORY

911 receives a call for a 6-year-old boy in a park who is experiencing difficulty breathing. On arrival, emergency medical services crews note a child in acute respiratory distress. Family reports the onset was 5 minutes ago, and it began suddenly. They believe they saw a bee nearby just prior to the incident. The child has never been stung nor has any food allergies. Additional history is limited due to the child being unable to speak.

No medical or surgical history.
Immunizations are up to date.
No known allergies.

PHYSICAL EXAMINATION

Vital signs: HR 135, BP 88/42, RR 32, SpO$_2$ 93%.

A well-developed pediatric male is found in significant respiratory distress and stridor. His head is normocephalic and atraumatic. His tongue is enlarged, but there is no lip swelling. Cardiac exam is tachycardic with a regular rhythm and no murmurs. Lung sounds are diminished bilaterally with significant wheezing and tachypnea. His abdomen is soft and nontender. Extremities demonstrate full range of motion, and the skin is notable for a diffuse urticarial rash and is cool to the touch.

DIFFERENTIAL DIAGNOSIS

1. Allergic reaction with anaphylaxis
2. Foreign body airway obstruction
3. Status asthmaticus

TESTS

No tests were administered.

CLINICAL COURSE

After assessing the scene and seeing that it is safe, the paramedic notes that the child is gasping for air. While her partner sets up oxygen and a nebulizer treatment, the paramedic draws up 0.15 mg of epinephrine. This is given intramuscularly in the anterolateral thigh. The child is also started on an oxygen-powered nebulizer treatment via face mask. While intravenous (IV) access is established, the child's breathing becomes less labored. Using a length-based resuscitation tape that estimates the child's weight at 20 kg, the paramedic administers 20 mg of diphenhydramine and 10 mg of dexamethasone IV. The patient is placed on the cardiac monitor ,and his vital signs are improving, heart rate is normalizing, and his breathing is becoming less labored. A 20 ml/kg fluid bolus is initiated while the child is loaded onto the stretcher and secured appropriately. The patient as well as 1 of the parents are then transported to the nearest pediatric hospital.

At the hospital, the patient's rash is improving. Breathing remains nonlabored. The patient is observed for approximately 4 hours on a cardiac monitor. He continues to improve and is playful at the end of the emergency department stay. The patient and family are discharged with primary care follow-up, careful discharge instructions, and a prescription for an epinephrine autoinjector.

KEY MANAGEMENT STEPS

1. Recognize anaphylaxis.
2. Provide epinephrine and do not delay this while performing other interventions.
3. Administer oxygen and early airway intervention if necessary.
4. Perform frequent reassessments.
5. Transport to the closest appropriate facility as soon as feasible.

DEBRIEF

Allergic reactions are commonly encountered in both the hospital and prehospital settings. Allergic reactions are hypersensitivity reactions resulting from exposure to an allergen, and may be triggered by many agents, including foods, medications, topical products, and environmental exposures such as stinging insects, as in this case. Mild reactions may result in localized edema, pruritus, or urticaria. Systemic reactions can vary from a diffuse rash to anaphylaxis. Classically, symptoms will begin within 60 minutes of exposure to an allergen, often sooner. More rapid symptom onset correlates with increased severity of the reaction. Due to the varied presentations of anaphylaxis, it is important to maintain a high index of suspicion. Even in the emergency department setting, up to 57% of patients presenting with anaphylaxis are misdiagnosed.

Anaphylaxis is a clinical diagnosis defined as the involvement of 2 or more body systems (skin, respiratory, gastrointestinal, or cardiovascular) with or without the presence of hypotension or respiratory compromise. Critical to note is that shock or hypotension will not necessarily be present in every case of anaphylaxis. Anaphylaxis is a complex process and is the most severe manifestation of hypersensitivity. The initial mechanism is through the activation of immunoglobulins, which then stimulates mast cells and basophils to release a host of inflammatory mediators. This includes the release of histamine stimulating vasodilation, increased vascular permeability, and increased heart rate and cardiac contractility; prostaglandins, which cause bronchoconstriction, pulmonary and coronary vasoconstriction, and peripheral vasodilation; and leukotrienes, which cause bronchoconstriction and peripheral vasodilation. As these inflammatory mediators have overlapping function, the cumulative effects of these substances can lead to severe respiratory distress and profound shock due to circulatory collapse.

The diagnosis of anaphylaxis may be made by meeting either of the following criteria:

1. Acute onset of an illness with involvement of the skin and/or mucosa (hives, urticaria, or oropharyngeal edema) associated with at least one of the following:
   - Respiratory compromise (wheezing/dyspnea)
   - Reduced blood pressure
   - Associated symptoms of organ dysfunction (syncope, incontinence, etc.)
2. Two or more of the following that occur rapidly after allergen exposure:
   - Involvement of the skin and/or mucosa
   - Respiratory compromise
   - Reduced blood pressure or associated symptoms
   - Persistent gastrointestinal symptoms

As with all care in the prehospital environment, scene safety is critical. If providers are exposed to the same hazard, they may be unable to render aid and may themselves be harmed (particularly in the case of stinging insects). The provider should attempt to determine what type of exposure the patient experienced if not immediately obvious, while evacuating the patient from the scene as soon as possible to prevent further exposure. Preparation should be made for potentially life-threatening airway compromise, respiratory failure, and profound shock. Up to one half of anaphylactic fatalities occur within the first hour.

The highest priority actions are those taken to stabilize the patient, and these should not be delayed by attempting to complete a detailed assessment that is focused on the patient's respiratory effort and should note if hoarseness, stridor, or wheezing is present. Facial and tongue swelling should also be assessed. Although the presence of skin findings are a significant aid to diagnosis, anaphylaxis can occur without skin findings, and one must consider anaphylaxis in any patient exposed to a known allergen that presents with signs of shock.

Treatment for anaphylaxis can divided into first- and second-line therapies. First-line therapies include airway management, epinephrine, and IV fluids. Second-line therapies include corticosteroids, antihistamines, nebulizers, and glucagon. Epinephrine is the treatment of choice for anaphylaxis. Through both alpha and beta receptor actions, it counters the inflammatory mediators responsible for pathophysiology of anaphylaxis. Alpha-1 receptor activation reduces mucosal edema and causes peripheral vasoconstriction. Beta-1 receptor stimulation increases heart rate and contractility while beta-2 receptor stimulation provides bronchodilation. There are no absolute contraindications to epinephrine in the setting of anaphylaxis. Intramuscular (IM) epinephrine has superior absorption, resulting in higher and more consistent blood levels than subcutaneous administration. IM epinephrine may redosed every 5 to 10 minutes if there is no response or symptom relapse occurs. IV epinephrine is reserved for patients with refractory hypotension despite IM epinephrine, and one must be aware that there is a risk of cardiovascular complications, most notably arrhythmias or chest pain.

Fluid resuscitation is critical to combat the distributive shock related to increased vascular permeability and is often given as 1 to 2 L fluid bolus (20 mL/kg in pediatric patients) concurrently with epinephrine. Additionally, corticosteroids are given to prevent prolonged reactions as well as to reduce the risk of biphasic reactions. Methylprednisolone and dexamethasone are commonly used corticosteroids for allergic reactions and anaphylaxis.

Most patients with anaphylaxis will benefit from antihistamine medication, specifically H_1 blockers, most commonly diphenhydramine. Often in severe anaphylaxis, providers may add an H_2 antihistamine such as ranitidine. Albuterol may be initiated if wheezing is present, while one can consider the use of glucagon in patients on beta blockers that are anaphylactic. As beta blockers can increase the risk of prolonged anaphylaxis, glucagon can be used as an adjunctive treatment, in addition to epinephrine (which remains first line even in case of concurrent beta blocker use), if hypotension is refractory.

Even if treated appropriately, biphasic reactions occur in approximately 5% of cases of anaphylaxis. Though the reaction is often less severe, the patient may still require additional treatment including epinephrine, fluid resuscitation, and airway monitoring. Transport after epinephrine administration in the field is critical, as even patients with resolving symptoms are at risk of biphasic reactions.

After arrival in the emergency department, patients are often observed 4 to 6 hours, although this duration is derived from expert consensus. Physicians should consider admission if the patient has severe anaphylaxis, slow or insufficient response to first dose of epinephrine, the need for second dose of epinephrine, or the need for repeated fluid boluses. In addition to continued monitoring, these patients will require primary care follow-up. All patients should obtain and may benefit from referral to an Allergy and Immunology specialist as well as a prescription for an epinephrine auto-injector on discharge.

FURTHER READING

Campbell RL, Hagan JB, Manivannan V, et al. Evaluation of National Institute of Allergy and Infection Disease/Food Allergy & Anaphylaxis Network criteria for the diagnosis of anaphylaxis in emergency department patients. *J Allergy Clin Immunol.* 2012;129:748–752.

Campbell RL, Li JT, Nicklas RA, et al. Emergency Department diagnosis and treatment of anaphylaxis: a practice parameter. *Ann Allerg Asthma Im*. 2014;113:599–608.

Perina D, Gallo D. Allergic reactions. In: Cone D, ed. *Emergency Medical Services: Clinical Practice and Systems Oversight*. 2nd ed., Vol. 1. West Sussex, United Kingdom. Wiley; 2015: 179–183.

Rowe B, Gaeta TJ. Anaphylaxis, allergies, and angioedema. Tintinalli JE, et al., eds. *Tintinalli's Emergency Medicine: A Comprehensive Study Guide*. 8th ed. New York, NY: McGraw-Hill; 2016: 74–79.

CHAPTER 17

FAILING ASTHMATIC

DAVID POLINER, PHILIP NAWROCKI, AND BENJAMIN J. LAWNER

SETTING

Prehospital

CHIEF COMPLAINT

Respiratory Distress

HISTORY

A 54-year-old male presents to emergency medical services with shortness of breath and chest tightness usually associated with asthma. He reports that he has been using his albuterol inhaler every hour for the past day without relief, and it is now empty. He has frequent asthma exacerbations and was hospitalized a month ago for a similar issue. He has been intubated multiple times in the past.

He has a past medical history of asthma, hypertension, and coronary artery disease.

He has a family history of asthma.

He is a current smoker.

PHYSICAL EXAMINATION

Vital signs: HR 136, BP 108/62, RR 30, SpO$_2$ 86% on room air, temp. 36.8°C.

He appears agitated and is tripoding. He refuses to lay down. Jugular veins are flat, and his trachea is midline. Minimal lung sounds are heard bilaterally, and he is speaking in 1- to 2-word sentences. His cardiac exam is tachycardic but without murmur, rub, or gallop. His abdomen demonstrates paradoxical movements with respirations. He is moving all extremities, and there is no evidence of edema.

DIFFERENTIAL DIAGNOSIS

1. Respiratory failure
2. Severe acute asthma/status asthmaticus
3. Chronic obstructive pulmonary disease exacerbation
4. Acute coronary syndrome
5. Pulmonary embolism
6. Congestive heart failure exacerbation
7. Foreign body aspiration

TESTS

Electrocardiogram: Sinus tachycardia (Figure 17.1)
Waveform capnography: Evidence of bronchospasm (Figure 17.2)

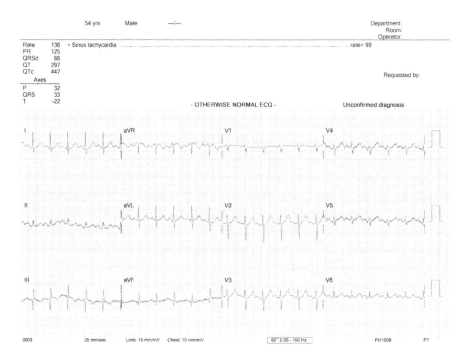

FIGURE 17.1 Electrocardiogram with sinus tachycardia with normal axis and nonspecific ST segment changes.

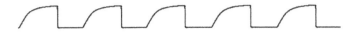

FIGURE 17.2 Obstructive waveform capnography pattern.

CLINICAL COURSE

Oxygen therapy via nasal cannula is initiated with a quick transition to non-rebreather facemask at 15 L/min. Intravenous (IV) access is established, and the patient is placed on the cardiac monitor. He receives albuterol 2.5 mg via nebulizer with minimal improvement in his lung sounds so that faint wheezes are now heard. An immediate second dose of albuterol 2.5 mg with the addition of 0.5 mg ipratropium bromide is given without significant effect. An IV fluid bolus of 20 mL/kg normal saline is started. As a third treatment of nebulized albuterol (2.5 mg) is started, he is given 125 mg methylprednisolone IV. Despite 3 albuterol treatments he continues to speak in 1- to 2-word sentences, displays intercostal retractions, and remains agitated. A trial of noninvasive positive pressure ventilation is begun using continuous positive airway pressure (CPAP) while he sits upright on the stretcher. Initial settings include a positive end-expiratory pressure (PEEP) of 2 cmH$_2$O, with an FiO$_2$ of 100%. He is also started on an infusion of 2 g magnesium sulfate and given a dose of 0.5 mg of 1 mg/mL epinephrine intramuscularly. Albuterol is now continuously administered inline with the CPAP device.

Despite these interventions, he becomes more somnolent, and you note slowing of his respiratory rate and inspiratory effort. Medical control is contacted and requests an additional dose of 0.5 mg of 1 mg/mL intramuscular epinephrine, and PEEP is increased to 5 cmH$_2$O while continuing 100% oxygen for preoxygenation while preparations for rapid sequence intubation are made. While ketamine 2 mg/kg IV and succinylcholine 2mg/kg are drawn up, a nasal cannula is placed on the patient and set to 15 L/min to allow for apneic oxygenation during intubation. Suction is prepared while a folded towel is placed behind the patient's head so that the tragus of the ear is level with the sternal notch to facilitate the best laryngeal view possible. Following medication administration, he is intubated without incident and subsequently loaded into the ambulance for transport to the nearest emergency department. En route, the bag-valve mask is squeezed at a rate to allow for inhalation and then approximately 5 seconds of exhalation to avoid overdistention of the lungs.

On arrival to the emergency department, the patient is connected to a mechanical ventilator and set with a respiratory rate of 10 breaths/min, tidal volume of 6 mL/kg ideal body weight, an inspiratory:expiratory ratio 1:5, FiO$_2$ 100%, and PEEP 5 cmH$_2$O. He is further sedated but not paralyzed and ultimately admitted to the intensive care unit for further management where he is eventually weaned from the ventilator and discharged to home 4 days later.

KEY MANAGEMENT STEPS

1. Recognize symptoms and signs of respiratory distress.
2. Aggressively treat status asthmaticus to avoid intubation by rapidly escalating therapy including continuous positive pressure ventilation, magnesium, epinephrine, and continuous albuterol treatments.
3. Recognize respiratory failure.
4. Optimize intubating conditions and provide for apneic oxygenation.

5. Allow proper expiratory phase in patients with obstructive lung disease who are undergoing positive pressure ventilation.

DEBRIEF

The patient presented to EMS in severe respiratory distress. EMS providers correctly recognized that despite initial therapy the patient displayed signs consistent with worsening respiratory failure including change in mental status, decreased respiratory rate, worsening inspiratory effort, and agitation. Aggressive and escalating treatment is warranted for the asthmatic patient who does not respond to nebulized albuterol, including consideration of intramuscular epinephrine, intravenous magnesium, and noninvasive positive pressure ventilation or intubation (Figure 17.3).

This patient initially displayed several signs of severe respiratory distress including agitation, the "tripoding" position, and decreased lung sounds. Patients who say they have run out of their inhalers, have previously been intubated, or were recently discharged from the hospital are likely poorly controlled asthmatics with the potential to have severe exacerbations. Despite nebulized bronchodilators, the patient continued to show severe respiratory distress. The prehospital providers correctly identified his lack of improvement and escalated therapy by providing a fluid bolus, magnesium bolus, intramuscular epinephrine, and CPAP. His condition rapidly progressed to respiratory failure as evidenced by depression in his mental status and decreased inspiratory rate and effort. This is a critical point to recognize in the care of asthmatic patients as this may lead to respiratory arrest without further intervention.

Noninvasive ventilation has been demonstrated to decrease respiratory rates, hypercapnia, and the need for intubation and overall need for intensive care unit admission especially if administered early. In the case of EMS, this will mean CPAP with initiation of low levels of PEEP at 2 to 3 cmH_2O. This should strongly be considered in patients who display signs of respiratory distress and fail to rapidly improve following initial treatment with bronchodilators. The providers again recognized a deteriorating course despite CPAP and contacted medical control for additional orders and intubation. Intubation is a challenging and dangerous task in a patient with severe respiratory distress and should be avoided if possible as the patient is precipitously close to rapid decompensation and respiratory arrest. Adequate preparation of equipment and suction, proper positioning, preoxygenation, and a defined primary and backup plan are crucial. The intubating assistant should closely observe the patient and monitor for signs of hypoxia or bradycardia as these patients can rapidly progress to cardiac arrest due to hypoxemia and respiratory acidosis. The intubation attempt should be aborted, bag-valve mask ventilation initiated, and placement of supraglottic airway rapidly performed if either bradycardia or hypoxia are noted during the intubation.

Initial postintubation strategies should include adequate sedation and an increased inspiration to expiration ratio to facilitate ventilation and prevention of air trapping. This can be accomplished with bag-valve mask via the slow "squeeze–release–release" mantra. There may be some resistance to initial bag ventilation due to airway resistance but this should not prompt overaggressive squeezing. When placed on a ventilator, the provider should anticipate high pressure alarms due to severe bronchospasm and continue to maintain a low respiratory rate and minimal PEEP to limit the amount of barotrauma.

Aspirated foreign body is an important differential to consider in pediatric patients, especially those who are 1 to 5 years of age. Caregivers may provide a history of foreign body

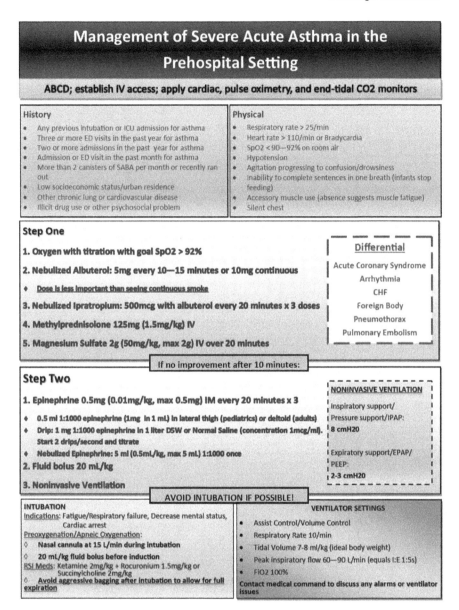

FIGURE 17.3 Acute asthma management summary.

Dalley MT, Ciment A. Severe asthma and COPD. In: Farcy DA, Chiu WC, Marshall JP, Osborn, eds. Critical Care Emergency Medicine. 2nd ed. New York, NY: McGraw-Hill; 2017: 117–128; Suau SJ, DeBlieux PM. Management of acute exacerbation of asthma and chronic obstructive pulmonary disease in the emergency department. Emerg Med Clin North Am. 2016;34(1):15–37; Stanley D, Tunnicliffe W. Management of life-threatening asthma in adults. Contin Educ Anaesth Crit Care Pain. 2008;8:95–99.

ingestion, although often the child presents solely with signs of coughing, choking, or unilateral wheezing and diminished breath sounds. Acute coronary syndrome should be considered with all cases of dyspnea, and any suspicion should prompt acquisition of a 12-lead electrocardiogram. Pulmonary embolism may also be considered, especially in those who are hypoxic, tachycardic, and hypotensive, although this patient's wheezing and a history of reactive airway disease are more consistent with asthma. Congestive heart failure is another important consideration, although more likely to be found with peripheral edema, basilar rales, and a cardiac history. Regardless of etiology, the initial management remains the same with early administration of oxygen therapy, circulatory support with intravenous fluid, consideration of CPAP, and initial bronchodilator therapy if evidence of bronchospasm.

FURTHER READING

Brenner B, Corbridge T, Kazzi A. Intubation and mechanical ventilation of the asthmatic patient in respiratory failure. *Proc Am Thorac Soc.* 2009;6(4):371–379.

Dalley MT, Ciment A. Severe asthma and COPD. In: Farcy DA, Chiu WC, Marshall JP, Osborn, eds. *Critical Care Emergency Medicine.* 2nd ed. New York, NY: McGraw-Hill; 2017: 117–128.

Higgins JC. The crashing asthmatic. *Am Fam Physician.* 2003;67(5):997–1004.

Stanley D, Tunnicliffe W. Management of life-threatening asthma in adults. *Contin Educ Anaesth Crit Care Pain.* 2008;8:95–99.

Suau SJ, DeBlieux PM. Management of acute exacerbation of asthma and chronic obstructive pulmonary disease in the emergency department. *Emerg Med Clin N Am.* 2016;34(1):15–37.

CHAPTER 18

BLUNT CHEST TRAUMA

DANIEL SHOCKET

SETTING

Landing Zone, Empty Parking Lot

CHIEF COMPLAINT

Respiratory Distress

HISTORY

An aeromedical rescue service is called to rendezvous with an ambulance transporting a 27-year-old male involved in a car crash. Ground units indicate the patient is unstable, and the nearest trauma center is approximately 2 hours by ground and 35 minutes by helicopter thus prompting the fire chief to call the aeromedical unit for transport. With the helicopter engine running, the flight crew bring their equipment to the patient who is in the back of an ambulance. Ground emergency medical services (EMS) gives report that the patient was a restrained passenger involved in a side-impact crash on the passenger side. Bystanders stated the vehicle was struck by another car going approximately 40 miles per hour when the driver ran a stop sign. Airbags did not deploy. The patient denies head trauma or loss of consciousness. Per the ground EMS crew, the patient had to be removed from the driver side due to extensive damage to the passenger side. There were no fatalities on scene. The patient was complaining only of pain to his right side until just prior to helicopter arrival when he indicated he could not breathe. He was in an otherwise normal state of health prior to the crash. He endorses severe 10/10, right-sided chest and abdominal pain along with significant shortness of breath. He denies any other complaints. The ground EMS unit has placed the patient in spinal motion restriction, applied oxygen, placed two 16 G intravenous lines to his antecubital fossae, and have 2 L of crystalloid running wide open.

He denies any past medical, surgical, or pertinent family history.

He denies smoking. He endorses alcohol use once per week but denies use today. He denies illicit drug use.

PHYSICAL EXAMINATION

Vital signs: HR 124, BP 90/50, RR 27, SpO_2 92% on non-rebreather mask, temp. 36.5°C.

The patient is found in the back of an ambulance and examination reveals a male who appears of stated age in acute respiratory distress. He is tachypneic with labored and shallow respirations at 27 breaths/min. His airway is intact. O_2 saturation is 92% on non-rebreather mask set to 15 L/min of oxygen. Chest rise appears equal bilaterally, and the nearby helicopter engine and rotors make it too loud to auscultate lung sounds. An ecchymosis is noted to the lateral aspect of the right chest extending from the fifth through eighth ribs. No subcutaneous emphysema is palpable. Radial pulses are thready, and a quick sweep with gloved hands around the torso and extremities find no blood. His abdomen is tender to the right upper quadrant but has no evidence of rebound or guarding. His pelvis is stable. The patient is alert and making eye contact but slow to respond to questions. His Glasgow Coma Scale score is 15, and he spontaneously moves his extremities, which do not have any evidence of deformity or functional limitation.

DIFFERENTIAL DIAGNOSIS

1. Pneumothorax
2. Tension pneumothorax
3. Hemothorax
4. Pericardial effusion
5. Rib fractures
6. Liver laceration

TESTS

No tests were administered.

CLINICAL COURSE

Based on the information obtained by the flight crew and the patient's acute respiratory distress, the team immediately performs a needle decompression thoracostomy to the right side of the chest. A rush of air is heard, and shortly thereafter the patient's respiratory rate improves to 18 breaths/min while SpO_2 increases to 98% and heart rate decreases to 101 with a blood pressure

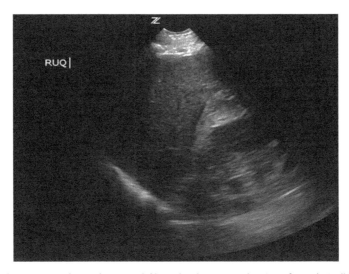

FIGURE 18.1 Right upper quadrant ultrasound. Note the thin vertical stripe of anechoic (black) fluid separating the liver (screen left) and kidney (screen right).

of 110/palp. With the help of ground EMS, the patient is loaded into the helicopter and transport to the trauma center is initiated.

In flight, the patient begins to get diaphoretic and pale. His heart rate increases to 130 and blood pressure falls to 80/palp. His respiratory rate remains 18 breaths/min and SpO_2 98% on oxygen. Reexamination is notable for increasing pain to this right upper quadrant and guarding. An in-flight Focused Assessment with Sonography for Trauma (FAST) exam is performed by the flight crew, which reveals a small amount of free fluid in Morrison's pouch (Figure 18.1) and more significant free fluid in the pelvis (Figure 18.2). The crew begins 2 units of O negative blood and administers tranexamic acid (TXA).

The helicopter arrives at the trauma center and gives report to the emergency department staff. The patient is still alert and talking. Airway and breathing are intact. Blood pressure is 84/46 and heart rate is 120. Free fluid is confirmed by the emergency physician's bedside FAST, and the patient is taken immediately to the operating room for chest tube placement and exploratory laparotomy.

KEY MANAGEMENT STEPS

1. Perform a primary survey prior to a thorough secondary exam.
2. Identify and treat any life-threatening injuries prior to transport.
3. Immediately perform decompression thoracostomy in blunt trauma patients with evidence of tension pneumothorax.
4. Identify and treat presumed hemorrhagic shock.

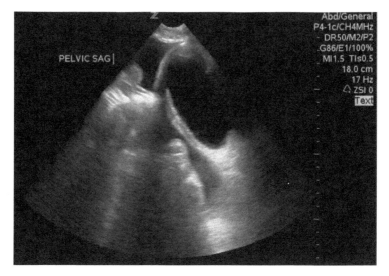

FIGURE 18.2 Pelvic ultrasound. Note the anechoic fluid above and to the left of the fluid-filled bladder and also how that fluid surrounds the rounded loops of bowel to the left side of the image. Normally, bowel would lie adjacent to the bladder and there would be no intervening black fluid.

DEBRIEF

Critical care flight paramedics have an expanded scope of practice compared to most ground transport paramedics. This scope varies depending on the individual flight service, but expanded procedures can include rapid sequence induction for intubation, chest tubes, point-of-care ultrasound, and administration of a wide array of intravenous medications and blood products. On an aeromedical rescue service, one often works in an austere environment and are frequently called to rendezvous with ground units of various experience levels. Given the unique environment of the back of a helicopter, one may not have access to one of the patient's sides and, due to the noise of the engine, often cannot verbally communicate with the patient or use a stethoscope. Thus, it is critical to perform a rapid assessment on the ground prior to transport.

During the primary survey, the patient was noted to be tachycardic, tachypneic, hypoxic, and hypotensive. In the setting of blunt trauma, a tension pneumothorax is high on the differential. With a simple pneumothorax, the patient will likely be tachypneic and hypoxic; however, when air continues to build up in the pleural space and cannot escape, it begins to put pressure on the mediastinal structures. When this occurs, the patient can develop obstructive shock, becoming tachycardic and hypotensive. This is known as a tension pneumothorax and, if not resolved immediately, can result in death. As it is often too loud in the prehospital environment to auscultate the patient's lungs, one must use the mechanism, patient presentation, and clinical picture to initiate a life-saving intervention.

The definitive treatment of a pneumothorax is placement of a chest tube on the affected side. However, if the patient is in extremis, and one is either unable to place a chest tube or cannot place one quickly, a needle decompression thoracostomy is indicated. This procedure involves inserting a large gauge catheter (14 G or greater) into the chest cavity to allow the trapped air to escape. The catheter can be placed either anteriorly in the second intercostal space at the midclavicular line or laterally at the fourth or fifth intercostal space at the anterior axillary line. Some studies have shown that the lateral technique may be successful more frequently than the anterior approach. Regardless of the anterior or lateral approach, the needle should be placed just superior to the rib to avoid lacerating the neurovascular bundle that travels along the inferior aspect of all ribs. Unique to the aeromedical environment is that gases expand with ascent; thus, it is important to be vigilant and aggressively treat a pneumothorax that is resulting in respiratory or hemodynamic compromise.

During flight, the patient was noted to decompensate further. The lack of breathing difficulty, normal respiratory rate, and absence of hypoxia suggested this was not a respiratory issue. Given the mechanism of injury and the patient's grimace to palpation of the abdomen, it was likely the patient was experiencing hypovolemic shock from an intra-abdominal injury. This aeromedical unit had a crew trained in performing point-of-care ultrasound, which allowed for the performance of a FAST exam. This subsequently revealed the presence of free fluid, which, given the patients mechanism and hemodynamic instability, suggested intra-abdominal hemorrhage likely from the liver.

The patient had already received crystalloid fluids by the ground unit and was still hypotensive after 2 L. In the setting of trauma, patient outcomes are better if blood products are given rather than continued crystalloid products. The ideal ratio of packed red blood cells to plasma to platelets are often debated, and the PROMMTT and PROPPR trials have been studying this very thing. Fortunately, blood was available on this helicopter, and 2 units were transfused during flight. Not all aeromedical units carry blood products, and most ground units do not, so the availability of blood products is unique to the ground or air service being used. The flight crew also had available and administered TXA. This medication aids in preventing clot degradation and has been associated with improved outcomes in trauma if given within 3 hours of injury.

Aeromedical transport was appropriately utilized to facilitate this patient's rapid transport to a trauma center. which was indicated based on the mechanism and physical findings. The patient also benefited from an advanced aeromedical service with ultrasound, blood, and TXA administration capabilities. As the patient was still with evidence of hemorrhagic shock on arrival to the emergency department, and the flight crew reported their findings of free fluid in the abdomen, the patient was immediately taken to the operating room rather than needing to obtain further imaging studies. There, the patient could be intubated, receive a chest tube, and begin an exploratory laparotomy nearly simultaneously as the patient is very likely to decompensate further with any delays to rapid intraabdominal hemostasis.

FURTHER READING

Cameron P, Knapp B. Trauma in adults. In: Tintinalli J, ed. *Tintinalli's Emergency Medicine: A Comprehensive Study Guide.* 8th ed. New York: McGraw Hill; 2011:1681–1687.

Holcomb J, Del Junco D, Fox E, et al. The Prospective, Observational, Multicenter, Major Trauma Transfusion (PROMMTT) study: comparative effectiveness of a time-varying treatment with competing risks. *JAMA-Surg.* 2013;148(2):127–136.

Holcomb J, Jenkins D, Rhee P, et al. Damage control resuscitation: directly addressing the early coagulopathy of trauma. *J Trauma.* 2007;62(2): 307–310.

Holcomb J, Tilley B, Baraniuk S, et al. Transfusion of plasma, platelets, and red blood cells in a 1:1:1 vs a 1:1:2 ratio and mortality in patients with severe trauma: the PROPPR Randomized Clinical Trial. *JAMA-Surg.* 2015;313(5):471–482.

Inaba K, Branco B, Eckstein M, et al. Optimal positioning for emergent needle thoracostomy: a cadaver-based study. *J Trauma*. 2011;71(5):1099–1103.

Morrison J, Dubose J, Rasmusson T, et al. Military Application of Tranexamic Acid in Trauma Emergency Resuscitation (MATTERs) study. *Arch Surg*. 2012;147(2):113–119.

Shakur H, Roberts I, Bautista R, et al. Effects of tranexamic acid on death, vascular occlusive events, and blood transfusion in trauma patients with significant hemorrhage (CRASH-2): a randomized, placebo-controlled trial. *Lancet*, 2010;376(9734):23–32.

CHAPTER 19

OUT OF HOSPITAL CARDIAC ARREST

ERIK RUECKMANN

SETTING

Emergency Department Medical Control

CHIEF COMPLAINT

Unresponsive Patient

HISTORY

An ambulance service calls medical control reporting they are on scene of a 62-year-old male patient in cardiac arrest and are requesting an emergency physician for online medical direction. The emergency medical services crew reports that the patient was at a local gym when he was witnessed to collapse. Bystanders immediately started cardiopulmonary resuscitation (CPR), placed an automated external defibrillator, and administered one defibrillation to the patient. Paramedics arrived 3 minutes after receiving the dispatch and found the patient to be in ventricular fibrillation (Figure 19.1) with CPR in progress. They have since placed a basic airway device, continued CPR, administered 1 mg of epinephrine, and defibrillated the patient once. There is no further information available about the patient or their past medical history.

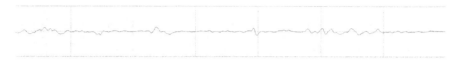

FIGURE 19.1 Initial rhythm strip demonstrating ventricular fibrillation.

PHYSICAL EXAMINATION

Vital signs: HR 0, BP unable to obtain, RR 14 via bag-valve ventilation.

The patient is unresponsive without spontaneous movements. His head is atraumatic, and pupils are 3 mm and reactive bilaterally. There is no jugular venous distension. With bag-valve mask ventilation, there is chest rise and bilateral breath sounds. There is a femoral pulse with CPR. The abdomen is soft but slightly distended, and his skin is cool, not cyanotic, and atraumatic.

DIFFERENTIAL DIAGNOSIS

1. Myocardial infarction
2. Massive pulmonary embolism
3. Electrolyte derangement causing malignant arrhythmia
4. Cardiomyopathy with malignant arrhythmia
5. Aortic dissection with subsequent tamponade
6. Subarachnoid hemorrhage

TESTS

Capnography: 21 mm/Hg (35–45 mm/Hg)

CLINICAL COURSE

The patient remains in ventricular fibrillation, and the paramedics call online medical control to indicate they will be loading and transporting momentarily to the emergency department. The physician instead directs the crew to remain on scene and continue resuscitative efforts with high-quality CPR, intravenous access, crystalloid infusion, intravenous epinephrine and amiodarone, and controlled ventilations. After an additional 10 minutes of efforts and 4 defibrillations, paramedics call back indicating an increase in capnography to 55 mm/Hg with successful return of spontaneous circulation (ROSC). A post-ROSC 12-lead electrocardiogram (ECG) is obtained (Figure 19.2) and reveals an inferior wall ST segment elevation myocardial infarction. The patient is transported to the emergency department and subsequently transferred to the cardiac catheterization suite where the patient undergoes successful percutaneous coronary intervention with stent placement to a culprit lesion located in the proximal right coronary artery. The patient is discharged to home without complication 3 days later.

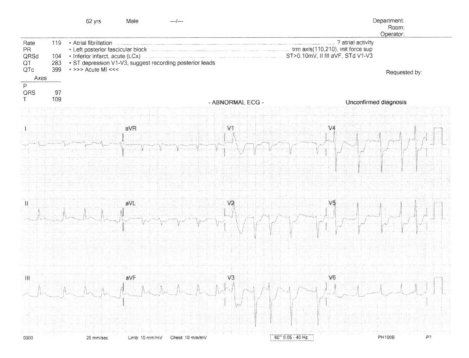

62 yrs   Male   ---/---

Department:
Room:
Operator:

Rate	119	• Atrial fibrillation	? atrial activity
PR		• Left posterior fascicular block	trm axis(110,210), init force sup
QRSd	104	• Inferior infarct, acute (LCx)	ST>0.10mV, II III aVF, STd V1-V3
QT	283	• ST depression V1-V3, suggest recording posterior leads	
QTc	399	• >>> Acute MI <<<	Requested by:

Axes

P	
QRS	97
T	109

- ABNORMAL ECG -   Unconfirmed diagnosis

0000   25 mm/sec   Limb: 10 mm/mV   Chest: 10 mm/mV   60~ 0.05 - 40 Hz   PH100B   P?

FIGURE 19.2 Post-ROSC 12-lead electrocardiogram demonstrating an inferior wall ST segment elevation myocardial infarction.

KEY MANAGEMENT STEPS

1. Out-of-hospital cardiac arrest survival rates are higher with minimal interruptions in CPR and, therefore, should be preferentially resuscitated at the scene.
2. Management of out-of-hospital cardiac arrest should be considered a "care bundle" focusing on high-quality CPR, appropriate ventilation, use of advanced cardiac life ROSC is achieved, one should obtain a 12-lead ECG to assess for evidence of a ST segment elevation myocardial infarction causing the cardiac arrest.
4. Unless unsafe/impractical to do so, the cardiac arrest patient should resuscitated at the scene until ROSC is achieved, at which time the patient may be transported.
5. Should resuscitative efforts be unsuccessful, field termination of resuscitative efforts may be appropriate and preferential to transport.

DEBRIEF

Cardiovascular disease is a leading cause of death in the United States with out-of-hospital cardiac arrest having a 92% mortality rate and accounting for over 350,000 deaths annually. Improving these statistics has been a focus of prehospital resuscitation, which is dependent on a bundle of care interventions to optimize outcome rather than a singular action. These actions must often be followed in the correct order to ensure the best possibility for a positive outcome. Patients who suffer an out-of-hospital cardiac arrest that is witnessed by someone, immediate receive bystander CPR with minimal interruptions, and have arrhythmias amendable to cardiac defibrillation (ventricular tachycardia or ventricular fibrillation) have more favorable outcomes. This bundle of care is centered on maintaining adequate perfusion during the cardiac arrest through high-quality CPR while oxygenation is provided via bag valve ventilation. These actions help maintain adequate cerebral perfusion while interventions to obtain ROSC using defibrillation and medications are implemented.

A central tenant to cardiac arrest management is CPR. For CPR to be successful, it has to be continuous (with minimal interruptions) and of high quality (rate of 100 beats/min and depth of at least 2.5 inches) to maintain adequate cardiac output. Thus, any movement (from floor to stretcher, stretcher to ambulance, etc.) will not allow for effective, continuous, high-quality CPR. This concept is often counterintuitive to both care providers and laypersons as there is a belief that getting off scene quickly is what is appropriate when, in fact, the patient's best chance of survival is remaining in place and providing high-quality uninterrupted CPR along with other interventions to obtain return of spontaneous circulation (ROSC) on scene. Simply put, when possible, the patient should remain where he or she is found while attempting resuscitation until either ROSC is achieved or the efforts are terminated.

While CPR is in progress, targeted interventions are begun with the goal of ROSC. These interventions are detailed in the American Heart Association advanced cardiac life support algorithms and include defibrillation, ventilation, intravenous access, and medication therapy. Of note, airway management and venous access are important in out-of-hospital cardiac arrest; however, high-quality CPR should not be sacrificed for either. Thus, many times basic airway adjuncts and intraosseous venous access devices are used until ROSC is achieved. Cardiac arrest medications often include epinephrine, and in cases of persistent ventricular fibrillation or ventricular tachycardia, amiodarone or lidocaine.

An important tool to gauge resuscitative efforts is waveform capnography. This provides a rough estimate of the state of perfusion and aerobic metabolism of the patient. The normal CO_2 exhaled by a patient is 35 to 45 mmHg, and thus obtaining continuous waveform capnography can assist in gauging the effect of CPR and the presence of spontaneous circulation. A patient in cardiac arrest will have a very low CO_2 as there is no perfusion; high-quality CPR may produce CO_2 levels approaching normal; while a sudden increase in CO_2 is often associated with ROSC. Capnography can also assist the provider in making the difficult decision of terminating efforts because persistently low CO_2 during the resuscitation suggests a poor prognosis.

If ROSC is achieved, a 12-lead ECG should be obtained to evaluate for an acute ischemic cause of the arrest. In this case, the paramedics identified an inferior wall myocardial infarction, which was the likely cause of the ventricular fibrillation and arrest. The patient was promptly taken to the cardiac catheterization laboratory for definitive treatment and did well. In many cases, however, efforts do not result in ROSC and, therefore, termination of resuscitative efforts may be appropriate and is usually based on several factors: Was the cardiac arrest witnessed and was prompt, high-quality bystander CPR provided? Was there a cardiac rhythm that could be defibrillated? Did the patient ever have ROSC? How long has resuscitation gone without ROSC, and does capnography reflect an anaerobic state despite resuscitative efforts? Generally, patients that have received at least 25 minutes of high-quality resuscitation without ROSC, a cardiac rhythm that cannot be defibrillated, and low capnography (<20 mm Hg) have less than a 1% chance of survival and are candidates for termination of efforts.

FURTHER READING

American Heart Association. 2015 American Heart Association guidelines for CPR and ECC. *Circulation*. 2015;132(18 Suppl 2):S313–S314.

Benjamin EJ, Blaha ML, Chiuve SE, et al. Heart disease and stroke statistics—2017 update: a report from the American Heart Association. *Circulation*. 2017;135(10):e146–e603.

Sheak KR, Wiebe DJ, Leary M, et al. Quantitative relationship between end-tidal carbon dioxide and CPR quality during both in-hospital and out-of-hospital cardiac arrest. *Resuscitation*. 2015;89:149–154.

Touma O, Davies M. The prognostic value of end tidal carbon dioxide during cardiac arrest: a systematic review. *Resuscitation*. 2013;84(11):1470–1479.

CHAPTER 20

WEAKNESS

AARON FARNEY

SETTING

Private Rural Residence

CHIEF COMPLAINT

Unresponsive

HISTORY

Emergency medical services (EMS) is dispatched to a private residence for a reported 58-year-old male found down and unresponsive. Upon arrival, the patient's co-workers greet EMS. They inform EMS that the patient did not show up to work today or return phone calls. Concerned, they checked on him at home and found him lying on the kitchen floor, seemingly unresponsive. He was last seen leaving work yesterday at 5:00 pm. He did not seem ill yesterday. It is now 9:00 am the following morning.

His co-workers relate that he took some sick time off last week due to "not feeling well." He had a heart attack 10 years ago and is a smoker. They do not provide any further history. The patient lives alone. There are no signs of forced entry, and nothing in the house appears out of order.

PHYSICAL EXAMINATION

Vital signs: HR 90, BP 200/100, RR 18, SpO$_2$ 86% on room air, temp. 36.5°C.

Examination reveals an overweight adult male laying on the kitchen floor on his right side. He has no external signs of head trauma. Pupils are 5 mm bilaterally and reactive to light; his gaze is deviated to the left. He has sonorous respirations with shallow chest rise. Radial pulse is strong and regular; no murmurs are appreciated. He has no peripheral edema or jugular venous distension. His abdomen is soft, nontender, and nondistended. His extremities are warm and well perfused. He does not respond to verbal stimuli. When a painful stimulus is applied, he withdraws with his left upper and lower extremities, but there is no response from his right side, which is flaccid. At no time does he open his eyes or make any verbal sound.

DIFFERENTIAL DIAGNOSIS

1. Ischemic stroke
2. Hemorrhagic stroke
3. Cervical spine injury
4. Hypoglycemia
5. Drug overdose

TESTS

Blood glucose: 108 mg/dL (70–110 mg/dL)
Electrocardiogram (ECG): Figure 20.1

CLINICAL COURSE

Given the possibility of a fall and abnormal neurological examination, spinal motion restriction is observed and a cervical collar is applied to the patient. A jaw thrust is performed to open the patient's airway, and supplemental oxygen is applied via nasal cannula at 4 L/min. Sonorous respirations continue, and a 30 French nasopharyngeal airway is inserted into the left nare, with resolution of the obstruction and improvement in chest rise. Pulse oximetry improves to 94%. The cardiac monitor is attached to the patient, and an ECG is acquired (Figure 20.1). Intravenous access is established, and the blood glucose is found to be within normal limits.

Based on history and examination, EMS is concerned for a large stroke and determines that rapid transport to a stroke center is indicated. They request helicopter EMS (HEMS) to facilitate bypassing the local primary stroke center and transport to the regional comprehensive stroke center, which is located 2 hours away by ground transport. Shortly thereafter, HEMS arrives and secures the patient's airway by rapid sequence intubation using etomidate and rocuronium, taking care to avoid hypoxia or hypotension. Placement is confirmed with continuous wave-form end-tidal capnography, and air transport is initiated. En route, ventilation is titrated to eucapnea.

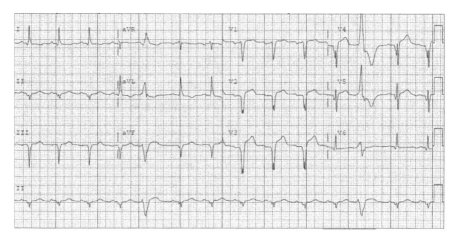

FIGURE 20.1 Sinus rhythm with unifocal premature ventricular contraction. Note the left ventricular hypertrophy with secondary repolarization abnormality.

The patient arrives 20 minutes later at the stroke center, where he undergoes an emergent head computed tomography (Figure 20.2). The patient has evidence of a large subacute ischemic stroke but is deemed not to be a candidate for primary thrombolysis. He is admitted to the neurological intensive care unit and evaluated for possible endovascular interventions. Meanwhile, computed tomography angiogram (Figure 20.3) and magnetic resonance imaging (Figure 20.4) are obtained. Given the abnormal ECG, an echocardiogram is obtained, revealing a severely reduced left ventricular ejection fraction and associated left ventricular thrombus.

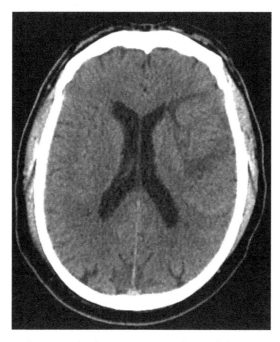

FIGURE 20.2 Head computed tomography demonstrating a subacute left middle cerebral artery territory ischemic stroke without hemorrhage.

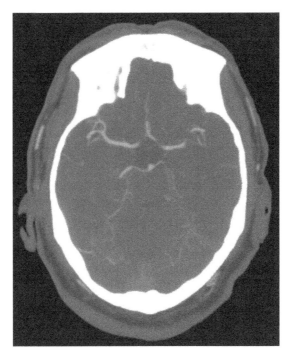

FIGURE 20.3 Head computed tomography angiography demonstrating an abrupt cutoff of the left middle cerebral artery consistent with a large vessel occlusion.

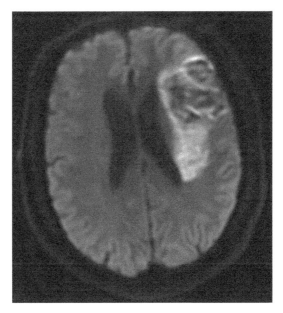

FIGURE 20.4 Head magnetic resonance imaging demonstrating large left middle cerebral artery territory infarct.

KEY MANAGEMENT STEPS

1. Recognize signs of large vessel occlusion (LVO) stroke.
2. Employ spinal motion restriction in unresponsive patients with potential trauma.
3. Utilize basic airway maneuvers to facilitate effective oxygenation and ventilation.
4. Obtain a blood glucose in patients with a suspected stroke.
5. Consider the correct transport destination and appropriate utilization of HEMS.

DEBRIEF

This patient was experiencing a left middle cerebral artery occlusion. This diagnosis is readily apparent by the neurological examination, notable for a dense right-sided hemiplegia and complete aphasia secondary to compromise of the vascular supply to the motor cortex and language areas, respectively. While there are obvious limitations to the history, a careful and thoughtful neurological examination will reveal this diagnosis to the astute provider.

This patient was experiencing a type of stroke known as an LVO. An LVO results from a very proximal clot, resulting in a wide area of ischemic injury that leads to significant functional neurological deficits. With recent advances in invasive stroke interventions, distinguishing an LVO from a non-LVO stroke has become increasingly important. While primary thrombolysis remains the mainstay of acute stroke care, if an LVO is recognized early, it may be amenable to interventional therapies, such as endovascular clot retrieval. Just as with primary thrombolysis, interventions are time-sensitive, and thus the provider's decision to utilize HEMS to facilitate rapid transport given the patient's condition and unknown time of symptom onset.

The prehospital management of an acute stroke involves stabilization of airway, breathing, and circulation; vascular access; measurement of serum glucose and correction of hypoglycemia; cardiac monitoring including ECG acquisition and interpretation; and, most important, rapidly initiating transport to the most appropriate receiving hospital. The cliché "time is brain" is true—transport must not be delayed unnecessarily.

The care of an LVO stroke has additional considerations. Unless local protocols dictate otherwise, EMS should generally transport any patient that is a candidate for primary thrombolysis to the nearest receiving hospital capable of delivering such therapy. If there is no difference in transport time to a comprehensive stroke center or if the patient is not a candidate for primary thrombolysis, the LVO stroke patient should be transported to a comprehensive stroke center for consideration for endovascular intervention. Local protocols and guidance may vary in this area.

Note that an ischemic stroke can be due to either a thrombus, which is a plaque accumulation within the artery, or an embolus, which is a clot thrown into the culprit artery from another location, often the left heart, commonly due to atrial fibrillation. While this distinction may not be relevant in the field, it does carry implications for secondary prevention of a future stroke. In this case, the culprit clot was an embolus thrown from a left ventricle thrombus, which developed in the context of a severely depressed ejection fraction as a result of a previous myocardial infarction, evidenced by available history and by his ECG.

FURTHER READING

Crocco TJ, Tadros A, Davis SM. Stroke. In: Cone DC, Brice JH, Delbridge TR, and Myers JB, eds. *Emergency Medical Services: Clinical Practice and Systems Oversight*. 2nd ed. West Sussex, United Kingdom. Wiley; 2015: 171–178.

Crocco TJ, Tadros, Kothari RU. Stroke. In: Marx J, Hockberger R, and Walls R, eds. *Rosen's Emergency Medicine: Concepts and Clinical Practice*. 7th ed. Maryland Heights, MO. Mosby Elsevier; 2010: 1333–1345.

Powers WJ, Derdeyn CP, Biller J, et al. 2015 American Heart Association/American Stroke Association focused update of the 2013 guidelines for the early management of patients with acute ischemic stroke regarding endovascular treatment: a guideline for healthcare professionals. *Stroke*. 2015; 46: 3020–3035.

SECTION III

EMERGENCY DEPARTMENT

EVIE MARCOLINI

CHAPTER 21

CHEST PAIN

AAMER KHAN

SETTING

Emergency Department

CHIEF COMPLAINT

Chest Pain

HISTORY

A 60-year-old male presents to the emergency department with sudden "tearing" substernal chest pain that radiates to the back and started about an hour and a half prior to his presentation. He denies any recent trauma. He denies shortness of breath but states that he has mild nausea without vomiting. He has had no recent travel or sick contacts. His pain is constant, without aggravating or relieving factors. Emergency medical services reports that the patient had a syncopal episode in the ambulance lasting 5 seconds. He had breakfast about 30 minutes prior to start of symptoms.

He has a past medical history of hypertension and hyperlipidemia.

He is a former smoker with a 40 pack-year history.

His family history is significant for cardiac disease in his father at the age of 70.

PHYSICAL EXAMINATION

Vital signs: HR 120, BP 100/60, SpO$_2$ 99% on room air, temp. 37°C.

Examination reveals a tall, medium-built male who appears to be uncomfortable and constantly repositioning himself due to discomfort. His lungs are clear bilaterally with good air movement. He is tachycardic, and there is an audible diastolic murmur over the right parasternal border over the second intercostal space. He has no chest wall tenderness. His radial pulse is stronger on the left than the right. His abdomen is soft, nontender, nondistended, with normal bowel sounds. There is no lower extremity edema, and skin is warm with good capillary refill in the digits. Neurologic examination reveals grossly normal strength and sensation in all extremities.

DIFFERENTIAL DIAGNOSIS

1. Cardiac ischemia
2. Aortic dissection
3. Pulmonary embolism
4. Pneumothorax
5. Gastroesophageal reflux disease
6. Pneumonia

TESTS

Troponin I: 0.02 ng/mL (0–0.04 ng/mL)

D-dimer: 4,000 ng/mL (<500 ng/mL)

Complete blood count: normal hemoglobin, hematocrit, white blood cell count, and platelets

Chemistry panel: normal sodium, potassium, chloride, bicarbonate, blood urea nitrogen, creatinine, and glucose

Electrocardiogram: sinus tachycardia

Chest X-ray: normal cardiac silhouette, clear lungs; no acute abnormality

Computed tomography angiogram (CTA) of chest, abdomen, and pelvis: dissection flap extending from the aortic root to just proximal to the left subclavian artery

CLINICAL COURSE

Based on history, the patient was placed on oxygen by nasal cannula, a cardiac monitor, and two large-bore intravenous lines were established. After the CTA was reviewed, patient was started on an esmolol infusion, and a specimen sent to blood bank for type and screen. Cardiothoracic surgery consultation was obtained and the patient taken to the operating room. Findings were as noted in the CTA—dissection flap extending from the aortic root to just proximal to the left subclavian artery. The patient had an aortic valve replacement and repair of the aortic arch with graft.

KEY MANAGEMENT STEPS

1. Consideration of aortic dissection in the differential of a patient with chest pain
2. Obtaining serum chemistry (including electrolytes and creatinine), type and screen, troponin, chest X-ray, electrocardiogram, CTA
3. Understanding the urgency of diagnosis in these cases
4. Controlling heart rate and blood pressure
5. Urgent cardiothoracic surgery consultation

DEBRIEF

This patient was experiencing sharp/tearing chest pain from dissection of the aorta. Aortic dissection is characterized by blood entering the medial layer of the vessel wall, after an intimal tear, and creating a false lumen. Risk factors for development of aortic dissection can be divided into conditions that increase aortic wall stress, most commonly hypertension, and aortic media abnormalities, which can be genetic such as Marfan syndrome or inflammatory vasculitis such as Takayasu arteritis.

Typical symptoms will be sudden onset tearing chest pain that will often radiate to the back depending on the location of the dissection, but these symptoms are not always present. Patients can have a variety of presentations including but not limited to a syncopal episode, stroke-like symptoms if extending to the carotid artery, cardiac tamponade if involving the aortic root, pain in the upper extremity depending on the location of the dissection, nausea, and/or diaphoresis.

Abnormal physical examination findings may include:

- Systolic blood pressure difference in extremities
- Focal neurologic deficit
- New murmur

There are two common classification systems for aortic dissection: the Stanford system and the DeBakey system. The Stanford system is more widely used and classifies aortic dissection into two types:

- Type A involves the ascending aorta and can progress throughout the length.
- Type B is distal to the left subclavian artery.

The DeBakey system classifies aortic dissection into three types:

- Type I involves the ascending and descending aorta.
- Type II involves the ascending aorta only.
- Type III involves the descending aorta only.

The key to diagnosing aortic dissection is to consider it, and appropriately following up with a confirmatory study, which would be a CTA.

If suspicion for aortic dissection is low, then D-dimer can be used as a screening tool to exclude aortic dissection. D-dimer is a breakdown product of the coagulation cascade. It can be elevated in a number of conditions including aortic dissection but has a high negative predictive value of 96%. Therefore, if D-dimer is <500 ng/mL, the likelihood of aortic dissection is quite low.

Once aortic dissection is confirmed, heart rate control is important as the tachycardia transmits energy through the vessel causing further shearing forces. There is no specific heart rate goal aside from normocardia. Blood pressure control is also needed and guidelines suggest a goal of 100 to 120 mm Hg. This can be achieved with a beta blocker such as esmolol, which is easily titratable and has a rapid onset and short half-life. Additional control can be achieved with a calcium channel blocker such as nicardipine.

Type A dissections require definitive surgical repair, while type B dissections can be managed surgically or medically depending on the complexity.

FURTHER READING

Acute aortic dissection. Life in the Fast Lane. July 18, 2017. https://lifeinthefastlane.com/ccc/acute-aortic-dissection/

Clinical features and diagnosis of acute aortic dissection. UpToDate. November 7, 2017. https://www.uptodate.com/contents/clinical-features-and-diagnosis-of-acute-aortic-dissection?source=search_result&search=aortic%20dissection&selectedTitle=1~150

Hiratzka LF, Bakris GL, Beckman JA, et al. 2010 ACCF/AHA/AATS/ACR/ASA/SCA/SCAI/SIR/STS/SVM guidelines for the diagnosis and management of patients with thoracic aortic disease. *Circulation.* 2010;121:e266.

Suzuki T, Distante A, Zizza A, et al. Diagnosis of acute aortic dissection by D-dimer: the International Registry of Acute Aortic Dissection Substudy on Biomarkers. *Circulation.* 2009;119(20):2702–2707.

CHAPTER 22

SEVERE HEADACHE

AMAN SHAH

SETTING

Emergency Department

CHIEF COMPLAINT

Headache

HISTORY

A 57-year-old female presents to the emergency department reporting a severe headache that started while she was participating in a high-intensity exercise class approximately 8 hours ago. She was lifting heavy weights that morning when the headache suddenly started. She reports the headache started at 10/10 on the pain scale, associated with diffuse neck pain and stiffness, sensitivity to light, and nausea. She has taken acetaminophen without relief and presents now after the headache has persisted all day. The patient denies history of headaches but notes a brief, less than 1-minute severe headache that occurred 4 days ago and resolved spontaneously. She denies recent trauma, recent illness, or sick contacts.

She has a past medical history of diabetes and hypertension.

She is a former smoker with a 24 pack-year history.

PHYSICAL EXAMINATION

Vital signs: HR 96, BP 194/82, RR 16, SpO$_2$ 97% on room air, temp. 36.3°C.

Patient examination reveals a well-developed, well-nourished female in moderate painful distress. Examination of the head reveals no obvious trauma, pupils are equal and reactive to light and accommodation (the patient reports discomfort when light is shone into her eyes), and bilateral tympanic membranes are normal. There is decreased flexion and extension of neck secondary to patient discomfort. There is no cervical, thoracic, or lumbar spinal tenderness. Heart sounds are normal, the lungs are clear to auscultation, the abdomen is soft and nontender, and the upper and lower extremities have strong distal pulses and normal capillary refill. Neurologic examination demonstrates no focal motor or sensory deficits, intact cranial nerves, normal deep tendon reflexes, and a Glasgow Coma Scale of 15.

DIFFERENTIAL DIAGNOSIS

1. Intracranial hemorrhage
2. Migraine headache
3. Transient ischemic attack
4. Carotid artery dissection
5. Temporal arteritis
6. Meningitis

TESTS

Complete blood count: normal hemoglobin, hematocrit, white blood cell count and platelets
Basic metabolic panel: normal sodium, potassium, chloride, bicarbonate, blood urea nitrogen, creatinine, and glucose
Computed tomography (CT) head: no acute intracranial abnormality

CLINICAL COURSE

The patient was placed on the cardiac monitor and intravenous access was established. She was started on a 1 L intravenous fluid bolus and given 4 mg of morphine sulfate and 4 mg of ondansetron intravenously. Given the severity of the headache, a stat CT head was obtained, which was read by the neuroradiologist as "No acute intracranial abnormality." The patient was then consented for a lumbar puncture (LP), which demonstrated bright red blood in all 4 tubes; laboratory analysis of the cerebrospinal fluid (CSF) was notable for 10,900 red blood cells (RBCs) in tube 1 and 3,425 RBCs in tube 4; the glucose, protein, and white blood cell counts were normal. Neurosurgery consultation was obtained, and the patient was admitted for frequent neurological checks. She was started on a nicardipine drip with a goal of lowering her systolic blood pressure to approximately 140 mm Hg.

KEY MANAGEMENT STEPS

1. Consideration of subarachnoid hemorrhage (SAH) in a patient presenting with an acute onset of a severe headache.
2. Performing a thorough neurologic examination including motor strength, sensory function, cranial nerves, deep tendon reflexes, cerebellar function, and gait.
3. Performing an LP for CSF analysis in patients who have symptoms suggestive of SAH despite a normal CT head.
4. Consultation with neurosurgery about management of suspected SAH with equivocal diagnostics tests, specifically further management and blood pressure control.

DEBRIEF

The patient in this case presented to the emergency department after experiencing an acute-onset, severe headache, neck stiffness or meningismus, and photophobia while physically exerting herself in an exercise class. The acute onset of a maximal severity headache should always place SAH at the top of the differential diagnosis, especially when associated with onset during exertion and symptoms such as nausea, vomiting, brief loss of consciousness, and meningismus. The history of a severe headache within the previous 1 to 3 weeks also raises the possibility of a sentinel bleed. Risk factors for SAH include age greater than 40, hypertension, tobacco use, and a personal or family history of aneurysm and/or SAH. Abnormal connective tissue diseases such as autosomal dominant polycystic kidney disease, neurofibromatosis type 1, and Ehlers-Danlos, among others, are associated with an increased risk of SAH as well.

The etiology of SAH can be traumatic or atraumatic. The leading cause of SAH is trauma, with the location of the bleed to be most likely in the area of impact on the skull. The most common etiology of atraumatic SAH is a ruptured aneurysm. Aneurysms are most commonly located in the circle of Willis (a circulatory anastomosis that supplies blood to the brain), with the anterior communicating and posterior communicating arteries being the most likely involved arteries respectively. Other nontraumatic causes of SAH include arteriovenous malformation and perimesencephalic bleed, the latter describing a SAH typically confined to brainstem with no identified bleeding source despite advanced imaging with angiography.

The standard approach in evaluating patients in whom there is a high suspicion for SAH is a noncontrast head CT (Figure 22.1a). Classically, a head CT with positive findings for SAH will demonstrate hyperattenuation between the sulci and gyri; in lay terms, the CT will show a bright signal (the blood) that outlines the contours of the brain parenchyma (Figure 22.1b).

While the sensitivity of a noncontrast head CT approaches 100% within the first 6 hours after a SAH,[1] the high morbidity and mortality associated with missed diagnoses warrant consideration of an LP in cases with normal CT imaging and a very high clinical suspicion. There are two reasons for performing an LP in patients with suspected SAH: to assess for the presence of RBCs and evaluate opening pressure, with a normal range lying between 10 and 20 cm H_2O.

Regarding the presence of RBCs in the CSF, the classical teaching is that a "steady" number of RBCs in each of the collection tubes signifies a SAH, while an RBC count that decreases from the first to last collection tube represents a traumatic LP and can be used to rule out the diagnosis of SAH. A traumatic tap is caused by the dissection of tissue planes by the LP needle, which can disrupt the venous plexus around the spinal canal. In practice, however, the occurrence of

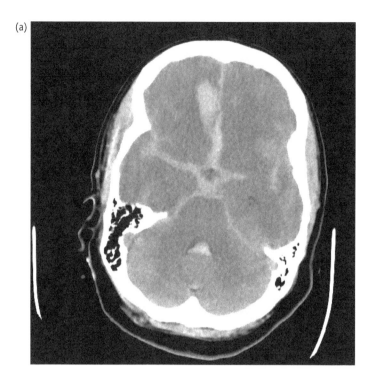

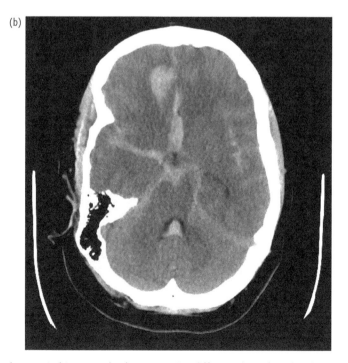

FIGURE 22.1 Head computed tomography demonstrating diffuse subarachnoid and intraventricular hemorrhage with hematoma centered on the anterior interhemispheric fissure and right gyrus rectus.

traumatic tap obscures the diagnosis of SAH and therefore leads to numerous false-positive results. Xanthochromia, which indicates the presence of bilirubin breakdown products from blood in CSF, is a sensitive marker for SAH. It can be used to confirm SAH but may take up to 12 hours to appear. Most clinical labs utilize visual inspection to assess for xanthochromia, which is reported to be 83% sensitive and 96% specific.[2]

The procedure of LP can result in several possible complications, the most common of which is post-LP headache. The pain is thought to be mediated by leakage of the CSF from the dura, causing irritation of fine nerve fibers. Supportive care, including rest and nonsteroidal anti-inflammatory drugs, is the normal treatment; however, persistent headaches can be treated with a blood patch, in which autologous blood is injected into the epidural space to "patch" the hole in the dura from the LP. Other complications include bleeding, infection from nonsterile procedure that can progress to meningitis, and radicular nerve pain from irritation of the spinal fibers by the needle.

All suspected and confirmed cases of SAH should receive neurosurgical consultation. Aneurysmal bleeds can be treated with coil placement and/or surgical clipping. Patients in whom the concern for SAH is high despite negative imaging or negative CSF studies can be admitted to have frequent neurological checks and possible angiography with either CT or magnetic resonance imaging. In the time immediately after a SAH is diagnosed, several factors must be taken into account regardless of neurosurgical availability. Patients on blood-thinning medications should have their coagulopathy reversed as soon as possible; for example, vitamin K and fresh frozen plasma or prothrombin complex concentrate should be administered to patients on Coumadin. The head of the bed should be raised to approximately 30 to 40 degrees to mitigate the risk of increased intracranial pressure, and if there is clinical evidence of elevated intracranial pressure, mannitol should be given. Patients with SAH need strict blood pressure control, with a goal systolic blood pressure of <140 mm Hg. They are also at risk for vascular vasospasm leading to ischemia and will be followed closely for up to 3 weeks in the intensive care unit setting. Patients with SAH should be considered for CSF diversion with ventriculostomy if there is evident hydrocephalus and for seizure prophylaxis if there is significant blood burden or altered mental status. These decisions should be made in concert with neurosurgical consult.

REFERENCES

1. Perry JJ, Stiell IG, Sivilotti MLA, et al. Sensitivity of computed tomography performed within six hours of onset of headache for diagnosis of subarachnoid haemorrhage: prospective cohort study. *Brit Med J.* 2011;343(7817):d4277.
2. Chu K, Hann A, Greenslade J, Williams J, Brown A. Spectrophotometry or visual inspection to most reliably detect xanthochromia in subarachnoid hemorrhage: systematic review. *Ann Emerg Med.* 2014;64(3):256–264.

FURTHER READING

Allely P. Subarachnoid haemorrhage: the ED perspective (blog post). Life in the Fast Lane. December 26, 2017. https://lifeinthefastlane.com/subarachnoid-haemorrhage

Carpenter CR, Hussain AM, Ward MJ, et al. Spontaneous subarachnoid hemorrhage: a systematic review and meta-analysis describing the diagnostic accuracy of history, physical examination, imaging, and lumbar puncture with an exploration of test thresholds. *Acad Emerg Med*. 2016;23(9):963–1003.

Russi CS, Walker L. Headache. In: Marx JA, Rosen P, eds. *Rosen's Emergency Medicine: Concepts and Clinical Practice*. 9th ed. Philadelphia, PA: Elsevier/Saunders, 2018: 153–159.

EYE PAIN

ABBIE SACCARY

SETTING

Emergency Department

CHIEF COMPLAINT

Eye Pain, Vision Difficulty

HISTORY

A 25 kg, 8-year-old boy presents with his parents to the emergency department with severe right eye pain that started the morning prior and has progressively worsened. This evening, the boy began complaining of difficulty seeing the television, prompting his parents to bring him to the emergency department. The patient was evaluated by his pediatrician yesterday and started on Augmentin for presumed preseptal cellulitis. He has taken four doses of the medication without improvement.

Notably, for the past week, the patient has had headaches, rhinorrhea, and cough accompanied by low-grade fevers that his parents attributed to a viral respiratory infection.

The patient has no medical or ocular history and no recent history of trauma to the face or neck.

Medications: Augmentin (amoxicillin with clavulanate potassium) 400 mg/57 mg twice daily and acetaminophen 320 mg every 6 hours for fever and pain

Social history is noncontributory.

Family history is noncontributory.

Review of systems: Positive for fever, headache, double vision, rhinorrhea; no neck stiffness.

PHYSICAL EXAMINATION

Vital signs: HR 95, BP 108/70, RR 18, SpO$_2$ 98% on room air, temp. 37.6°C.

Examination reveals an uncomfortable appearing, well-developed, well-nourished young male. The lower lid of the patients' right eye is notably swollen and erythematous. Ocular exam is as follows: visual acuity 20/20 bilaterally; pain with palpation of the right maxillary sinus; pain with extraocular movement in all directions of the right eye with diplopia reported in all fields by the patient; confrontational fields equal in both eyes; pupils equal and reactive to light and accommodation; external exam significant previously mentioned findings as well as slight injection of right conjunctiva, edema of the upper right eye lid, and slight proptosis of the right eye; funduscopic findings nonconcerning; and intraocular pressures are within normal limits. Transillumination of the right maxillary sinus reveals decreased infraorbital glow. Nasal examination significant for clear rhinorrhea. Throat is clear with mild erythema noted. Neck shows full range of motion with no pain. Breath sounds are clear and equal bilaterally. Heart auscultation reveals regular rate and rhythm with a notable S3. Abdomen is soft and nontender. Peripheral pulses are all +2 with capillary refill <2 seconds.

DIFFERENTIAL DIAGNOSIS

1. Postseptal (orbital) cellulitis
2. Subperiosteal abscess
3. Orbital abscess
4. Preseptal cellulitis
5. Cavernous Sinus Thrombosis

TESTS

Complete blood count: white blood cell count 12.4 k/mm^3; WBC differential: Neutrophils 8120/mm^3

C-reactive protein: 5.3

Computed tomography (CT) sinuses/facial bones (Figure 23.1).

CLINICAL COURSE

The emergency medicine physician immediately started the patient on intravenous (IV) vancomycin and ceftriaxone for treatment of postseptal cellulitis, consulted ophthalmology, and

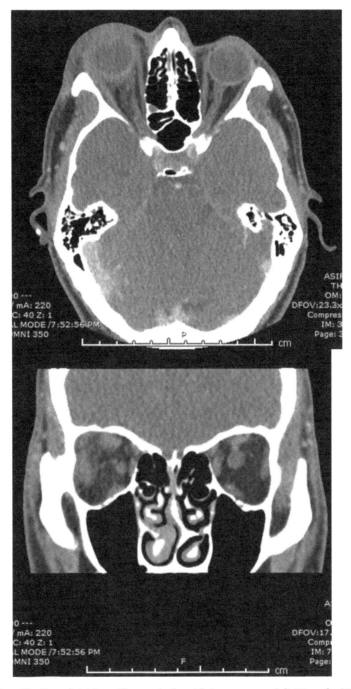

FIGURE 23.1 Opacification of right maxillary and ethmoid sinuses; poor definition of orbital planes in right eye and edema of the right extraocular muscles concerning for postseptal cellulitis; mild proptosis of right globe without gross displacement.

admitted the patient to the pediatric floor. Ophthalmology concurred with the diagnosis of postseptal cellulitis and reevaluated the patient every 12 hours until resolution of eye pain and diplopia. Otolaryngology was also consulted to address the opacified sinuses. Within 24 hours, the patient showed marked improvement, and by admission day 3, the patient's symptoms had completely resolved, and he was discharged home with a 2-week course of clindamycin.

KEY MANAGEMENT STEPS

1. Understanding basic eye anatomy and recognizing the key clinical differences between preseptal and postseptal cellulitis.
2. Obtaining a CT or magnetic resonance imaging of the facial bones and sinuses to definitively diagnose a postseptal cellulitis/abscess.
3. Early administration of IV antibiotics for bacteria that most commonly cause postseptal cellulitis.
4. Admission to the appropriate hospital service and early ophthalmology consultation.

DEBRIEF

Differentiating the relatively benign preseptal cellulitis from the possibly life and vision-threatening orbital cellulitis requires is summarized in Table 23.1.

A basic understanding of eye anatomy is helpful in distinguishing the two. The orbital septum separates the sterile environment of the postseptal anatomy from the preseptal anatomy, which is exposed to the outside environment. The most common cause of preseptal cellulitis is an eyelid problem, usually secondary to trauma or an insect bite, while the most common cause of postseptal cellulitis is a spread of infection from the sinuses, most often the ethmoid sinuses.[1] Polymicrobial infections are most common in postseptal cellulitis with *S. Aureus, S. Pneumoniae,* and anaerobes as the usual culprits. Nontypeable *H. Influenza* should always be considered in children under 5 years old and *Murcomycosis* in diabetics or other immunocompromised patients.[2]

Postseptal cellulitis has an insidious onset, usually heralded by an upper respiratory infection or sinusitis that does not resolve with standard antibiotic care. Fever, facial pain, eye swelling, eyelid edema, and vision loss or diplopia should heighten a clinician's suspicion for postseptal cellulitis.[2] Pain with extraocular movements is the key clinical finding when trying to delineate between preseptal and postseptal infections. A CT scan or magnetic resonance imaging of the sinuses definitively differentiates between the two diseases, and an urgent ophthalmological consult is critical for any suspicion of postseptal disease. Involvement of multiple cranial nerves (especially 3, 4, or 6) is a cavernous sinus thrombosis until proven otherwise and should be worked up as such.

Because postseptal cellulitis can threaten a patient's vision, immediate and aggressive IV antibiotic therapy is always indicated, including broad spectrum coverage for both aerobes and anaerobes. Common choices include a third-generation cephalosporin combined with

Table 23.1 Differentiation between Preseptal Cellulitis and Orbital Cellulitis

	Preseptal cellulitis	Orbital cellulitis
Risk factors	• Local trauma/insect bite • Recent URI or AOM	• Recent URI • Sinus Infection
Pathology	• *S. aureus* • *S. Pneumoniae* • Adenovirus	• Group A strep • *S. Pneumonia* • Gram negative rods • Anaerobes • Nontypeable *H. influenza* • Murcormycosis or aspergillus in immunocompromised patient
Clinical features	• Periorbital swelling • Erythema, warmth, tenderness	• **Ophthalmoplegia** • Diplopia • Headache • Eyelid edema
Physical exam	• Eyelid edema and erythema • Normally reactive pupil • Normal conjunctiva • Painless extraocular movements	• **Pain with extraocular movements** • Decreased visual acuity • Increased IOP • Ptosis
Diagnostic procedures	• CBC • Culture of eyelid wound if evident • CT scan of orbit and sinuses if concern for orbital cellulitis	• CBC • Blood cultures • CT scan if concern for optic nerve involvement or worsening course despite antibiotic therapy
Management	• Mild to moderate: oral antibiotics to cover gram positive and negative bacteria with outpatient follow-up • Severe: admission, IV antibiotics	• Admission • Broad spectrum IV antibiotics • Early ophthalmology and ID consults when available

Note. URI = upper respiratory infection. AOM = acute otitis media. IOP = intraocular pressure. CBC = complete blood count. CT = computed tomography. IV = intravenous. ID = infectious disease.

Vancomycin to cover for methicillin-resistant *Staphylococcus aureus*. Fluoroquinolones may be used for penicillin-allergic patients, and metronidazole or clindamycin may be added for additional anaerobe coverage.[3] A 10- to 14-day course of oral antibiotics should be completed once the patient has improved on IV antibiotic therapy and is stable for discharge home.

With early recognition and aggressive intervention, patients suffering from postorbital cellulitis can have very favorable outcomes. However, depending on the specific infectious organism and the extent of disease at presentation, patients may suffer a number of complications including cavernous sinus thrombosis, meningitis, frontal bone osteomyelitis, or permanent neurological deficits.[1]

REFERENCES

1. Kaiser PK, Friedman NJ. Orbit: infections. In: *The Massachusetts Eye and Ear Infirmary Illustrated Manual of Ophthalmology*. 4th ed. Philadelphia, PA: Saunders/Elsevier; 2014: 10–13.
2. Walker R, Adhikari S. Eye Emergencies. In Tintinalli JE, et al. *Tintinalli's Emergency Medicine: A Comprehensive Study Guide*. 8th ed. New York, NY: McGraw-Hill; 2017: 1558–1559.
3. Vagefi M. Orbit. In: Riordan-Eva P, Augsburger JJ, eds. *Vaughan & Asbury's General Ophthalmology*. 19th ed. New York, NY: McGraw-Hill: 271–283.

CHAPTER 24

SHORTNESS OF BREATH

HARMAN S. GILL

SETTING

Emergency Department

CHIEF COMPLAINT

Shortness of Breath

HISTORY

A 62-year-old male comes in with acute onset shortness of breath associated with chest pain that worsens with deep inspiration. The pain started while at rest approximately 6 hours prior to arrival to the emergency department and is associated with left-sided leg pain and swelling that has been persistent for the last 2 days. The patient has had no fever, cough, recent travels, hemoptysis, sick contacts, hormonal therapy or trauma to the chest.

He has a past medical history of lung cancer and is undergoing chemotherapy. He also had gall bladder surgery 2 weeks prior. He has no prior history of deep vein thrombosis (DVT) or pulmonary embolism (PE).

He is a former smoker with a 10 pack-year history.

He denies family history of cardiac disease.

PHYSICAL EXAMINATION

Vital signs: HR 105, BP 170/80, RR 28, SpO$_2$ 92% on 2 L nasal cannula, temp. 36.8°C.

Examination reveals a well-developed male in moderate respiratory distress. He has no jugular venous distension. His lungs are clear bilaterally with good air movement, his cardiac rate and rhythm are normal; no murmurs, rubs, or gallops are appreciated. His abdomen is soft, nontender and nondistended. His extremities are warm, and well perfused but the left leg appears more swollen than the right. Neurologic examination reveals grossly normal strength and sensation in all extremities, normal gait, and coordination.

DIFFERENTIAL DIAGNOSIS

1. Cardiac ischemia
2. PE
3. Pneumonia
4. Postoperative complication such as perforated viscous
5. Pneumothorax

TESTS

Complete blood count: normal hemoglobin, hematocrit, white blood cell count and platelets

Chemistry panel: normal sodium, potassium, chloride, bicarbonate, blood urea nitrogen, creatinine, and glucose

Troponin I: <0.03 ng/mL (0–0.04 ng/mL), pro-brain natriuretic peptide (proBNP): <450 pg/mL (<50 pg/mL)

Electrocardiogram (ECG): sinus tachycardia with no ST segment changes

Chest X-ray: normal cardiac silhouette, clear lungs; no acute abnormality

Bedside echocardiogram: no pericardial effusion, preserved ejection fraction, no right ventricle (RV) strain, normal aortic flow tract diameter, 2 cm inferior vena cava measurement.

DVT ultrasound: acute occlusive thrombus in left femoral vein.

Computed tomography (CT) PE: large thrombus in right main pulmonary artery consistent with right side lobar PE

CLINICAL COURSE

Based on history and physical exam, the patient was placed on oxygen by nasal cannula, a cardiac monitor, and intravenous access was established. Based on the ECG, PE became more likely than primary cardiac ischemia. This was supported further by the appropriate risk factors in his medical history, physical exam and DVT ultrasound findings consistent with a DVT, unremarkable lab work including a negative troponin/proBNP and chest X-ray/bedside echo that did not show evidence of right heart strain or alternative cardio-pulmonary pathologies. A CT angiogram of his chest confirmed the findings of a PE. The patient was started on weight-based heparin with an initial bolus and admitted to the hospital for further management given his new oxygen requirement.

KEY MANAGEMENT STEPS

1. Consideration of cardiac ischemia in the differential diagnosis of a patient with chest discomfort and shortness of breath.
2. Obtaining serum chemistry (including electrolytes and creatinine), troponin I, proBNP, and chest X-ray in a patient with dyspnea to simultaneously evaluate cardiac and pulmonary etiologies.
3. Recognition of appropriate risk factors and stratification of patients with PE according to the presence of right heart strain/hemodynamic stability as to whether the presentation is more consistent with massive or submassive PE.
4. Decision to admit the patient to the hospital vs outpatient management with lovenox/novel oral anticoagulant (NOAC).

DEBRIEF

This patient was experiencing pleuritic chest pain, dyspnea, and tachypnea with a new oxygen requirement due to a submassive PE. Dyspnea and chest pain are common complaints with a broad differential that emergency physicians encounter on a daily basis. Some etiologies such as PE carry with them a very high morbidity and mortality and require expedited and efficient evaluation and treatment.

In this case and in real life, any person with chest pain and dyspnea should get a prompt ECG and dedicated cardiopulmonary exam. This initial evaluation that is quick is a lot like the primary survey conducted for trauma patients. You can very quickly and efficiently rule out etiologies such as pneumothorax, ST elevation myocardial infarction, bronchospasm, or stridor in a patient with a normal cardiopulmonary exam and a normal ECG. With this basic assessment done you can then proceed sequentially to attain more in terms of risk factors for PE and acute coronary syndrome from your history—much like the secondary survey. This is also the time to search for pertinent positives such as unilateral leg swelling, active oncologic history, and recent surgery from your exam and history. This is then merged with pertinent negatives from your exam and workup such as clear lungs, negative chest X-ray, troponin and proBNP to rule out infectious etiologies and other cardiac etiologies such as non-ST elevation myocardial infarction and heart failure.

For patients who are low risk, clinical decision rules such as the Pulmonary Embolism Rule Out Criteria (PERC)[1] or Wells[2] score can be used to inform the decision on whether to order a D-dimer. The D-dimer is useful in patients with very low risk of having a PE to further decrease the index of suspicion. In the patient in the previously discussed case, for example, the use of a D-dimer would be inappropriate as the clinical gestalt for PE being a likely diagnosis is very high. In fact, it would not be inappropriate to empirically start this patient on heparin even before knowing the result of the CT scan based on the DVT US result alone. You may see some providers do this who are ultrasound-trained and comfortable with the skill of using point-of-care ultrasound to diagnose a DVT and then assume the patient already has a PE (given the chest pain/dyspnea) and empirically treat before getting the results of a CT PE scan.

Tests such as troponin and proBNP, when positive in these patients, are indicators of right heart strain. A point-of-care cardiac ultrasound can assess for RV strain via septal bowing, McConnell sign, sometimes even RV thrombus (Figure 24.1). These findings alongside hemodynamics are modalities that allow the speciation between a massive or submassive PE. This allows the clinician to better appreciate the clinical severity of the patient's presentation and subsequent management.

Standard of care for treatment is weight-based unfractionated heparin, usually started with a bolus followed by a continuous infusion with target partial thromboplastin time range that is 2 to 2.5 times the normal. Some patients do not need to be admitted for PE and can be treated with lovenox[3] or a novel oral anticoagulant.[4] High-risk features include a new oxygen requirement, biochemical, or echo signs of right heart strain, hemodynamic compromise, respiratory insufficiency, and modalities where there are contraindications to heparin therapy (history of heparin induced thrombocytopenia or need for surgical embolectomy). The decision to admit or discharge the patient should always be a shared decision between you, your patient, and your consulting physicians that will be managing this patient beyond the emergency department.

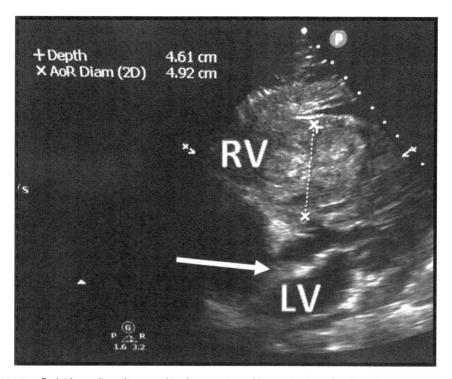

FIGURE 24.1 Bedside cardiac ultrasound in the parasternal long axis view showing a heterogeneous appearing right ventricular mass (thrombus) with intra-ventricular septal flattening (arrow) and impaired left ventricular filling.

REFERENCES

1. Kline JA, Courtney DM, Kabrhel C, et al. Prospective multicenter evaluation of the pulmonary embolism rule-out criteria. *J Thromb Haemost.* 2008;6(5):772–780.
2. Wells PS, Anderson DR, Rodger M, et al. Derivation of a simple clinical model to categorize patient's probability of pulmonary embolism: increasing the models utility with the SimpliRED D-dimer. *Thromb Haemost.* 2000;83(3):416–420.
3. Guyatt GH, Akl EA, Crowther M, Gutterman DD, Schuünemann HJ; American College of Chest Physicians Antithrombotic Therapy and Prevention of Thrombosis Panel executive summary: antithrombotic therapy and prevention of thrombosis, 9th ed.: American College of Chest Physicians evidence-based clinical practice guidelines. *Chest.* 2012;141(Suppl 2):7S–47S.
4. Spyropoulos AC, Turpie AG. Venous thromboembolism management: where do novel anticoagulants fit? *Curr Med Res Opin.* 2013;29(7):783–790.

CHAPTER 25

ABDOMINAL PAIN

ALI KAMRAN

SETTING

Emergency Department

CHIEF COMPLAINT

Abdominal Pain

HISTORY

A 64-year-old male presents to the emergency department with a chief complaint of abdominal pain, nausea, and vomiting for 2 days. The patient reports that he has had intermittent abdominal pain for the past 2 days that is now constant. The pain is associated with nausea and 3 episodes of nonbilious nonbloody vomitus. He describes the pain as 9/10 in severity, crampy, and diffuse in location and worsening over the past 24 hours. He reports having no appetite for the last day and recalls that his last bowel movement was 3 days ago. He denies having had any previous similar episodes of abdominal pain. He also denies any chest pain, shortness of breath, fever/chills, blood per rectum, and urinary changes or trauma. His past medical history includes hypertension, hyperlipidemia, and gastroesophageal reflux disease. His past surgical history includes a rotator cuff surgery at the age of 40 and an open inguinal hernia repair 5 years ago. He smokes 1 pack per day and denies any alcohol or drug use.

PHYSICAL EXAMINATION

Vital signs: HR 110, BP 150/90, RR 16 SpO$_2$ 99% on room air, temp. 37.0°C.

On examination patient is a well-developed, well-nourished thin male in distress laying on the right side with knees bent. Examination of his head and neck reveals bilaterally reactive 5 mm pupils, dry oral mucosa, no jugular venous distention, and midline trachea. His lungs are clear to auscultation bilaterally with good air movement. His cardiac exam reveals a regular rate and rhythm with no murmurs rubs or gallops. His abdominal exam is significant for a round contour with distention, which is slightly more than baseline per patient. Auscultation reveals hypoactive bowel sounds and tympany to percussion, and on palpation the patient's abdomen is rigid with guarding and diffuse pain. The patient has no pain with flank percussion. He has normal appearing genitals without mass or lesions; rectal exam reveals normal tone, normal prostate, and is negative for any gross or fecal occult blood. He is alert, oriented, and cooperative and has no abnormal neurologic findings.

DIFFERENTIAL DIAGNOSIS

1. Bowel obstruction
2. Mesenteric ischemia
3. Cholecystitis
4. Appendicitis
5. Pancreatitis
6. Perforated ulcer
7. Pseudobstruction
8. Malignancy
9. Diverticulitis
10. Abdominal aortic aneurysm
11. Trauma

TESTS

Complete blood count: white blood cell count: 14,000 without elevated neutrophils or bands, normal hemoglobin/hematocrit/platelets

Chemistry panel: sodium 146, potassium 3.1, chloride 114, bicarbonate 22, blood urea nitrogen 15, creatine 0.9, glucose 110, lactate 2.9, lipase normal

Liver function tests: normal alanine aminotransferase/aspartate aminotransferase, normal bilirubin, normal albumin, normal gamma-glutamyl transferase and international normalized ratio

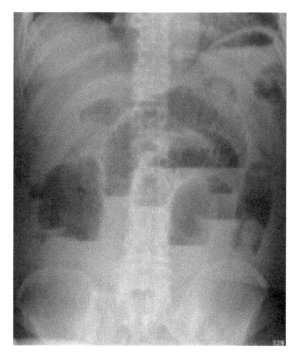

FIGURE 25.1 Upright X-ray of the abdomen consistent with small bowel obstruction, dilated loops of small bowel with air fluid levels are seen in image.

CLINICAL COURSE

Based on the patient's history and physical exam, he was placed on a monitor, intravenous (IV) access was obtained, and he was made nil per os (NPO). Blood work was sent as previously noted, and the patient was provided with analgesia, antiemetic, and crystalloid fluid. A 2-view abdominal X-ray was obtained (upright view shown in Figure 25.1), showing loops of distended small bowel with air-fluid levels without air in the large bowel. General surgery was consulted. At the request of general surgery a computed tomography (CT) of the abdomen and pelvis was obtained with IV contrast, and findings were consistent with a small bowel obstruction (SBO). The patient was taken to the operating room for an exploratory laparotomy.

KEY MANAGEMENT STEPS

1. Obtaining an appropriate history and physical examination to develop a differential consistent with abdominal pathology with a high suspicion for bowel obstruction.
2. Obtaining serum labs to narrow differential
3. Obtaining a 2-view X-ray of abdomen early to narrow the differential and show critical signs
4. Recognizing the high probability of bowel obstruction and providing appropriate analgesia, making patient NPO and obtaining appropriate imaging.
5. Obtaining a stat surgery consult.

DEBRIEF

In a patient presenting with abdominal pain, nausea and vomiting the differential is wide; this patient had a SBO. The key to an accurate diagnosis in this case included a history in which the pertinent positives were previous abdominal surgery, decreased appetite, and no bowel movement in the past 3 days. On physical examination, the pertinent positives consistent with SBO included diffuse pain, distention, hypoactive bowel sounds, and tympany.

When dealing with abdominal pain, one must have a systematic approach given the complexity and the wide differential involving the abdomen. In diffuse abdominal pain such as this patient, the differential includes entities such as: biliary pathology, pancreatitis, appendicitis, ileus, ischemia, diverticulitis, abdominal aortic aneurysm, abscess, perforation, nephrolithiasis, malignancy, traumatic hemorrhage, and pelvic pathology. Thus, it is imperative to obtain an accurate history and physical exam to narrow the differential and plan appropriate testing.

This patient denies any history of alcohol or previous biliary pathology; thus, pancreatitis can be lowered on the differential, although lab work is necessary to exclude this diagnosis given other etiologies of pancreatitis (e.g., gallstones, trauma, steroids, autoimmune, drugs, endoscopic retrograde cholangiopancreatography, scorpion bites, etc.). A normal lipase and a lack of other risk factors make pancreatitis unlikely in this patient. Normal liver function tests on lab studies also lower the likelihood of biliary pathology.

Appendicitis remains high on the differential given diffuse abdominal pain, as appendicitis classically begins in the periumbilical location and then travels to the right lower quadrant and can become diffuse in the setting of perforation, but SBO remains the most likely differential given the rest of the clinical picture in this patient. Other considerations for abdominal pain as previously mentioned remain possibilities but less likely.

When suspecting a SBO time is of the essence and management must occur simultaneously with the workup. As well as obtaining necessary labs as described, the patient should be made NPO, significant electrolyte derangements should be corrected, fluids should be given to correct suspected hypovolemia, and appropriate analgesia should be provided. If signs of abdominal distention are present, the placement of a nasogastric tube for gastric decompression should be considered.

Radiography is necessary to confirm the diagnosis, but surgical consultation should not be delayed if peritoneal signs are present. In a recent study, the sensitivity of plain upright and supine films was 82%.[1] It is reasonable to obtain a 2-view X-ray if SBO is suspected, especially if CT will be delayed, but multidetector CT remains the most accurate test with a sensitivity and specificity of 95%.[2] The use of IV contrast is recommended unless the patient has a contraindication, as it is helpful in assessing for inflammation or ischemia, which are otherwise hard to assess. Oral contrast is also considered in patients obtaining a CT of the abdomen, with the major advantage of ruling out a high-grade obstruction if the contrast passes distally into the decompressed bowel. However, the use of oral contrast is made difficult by a variety of factors including the risk of aspiration in a patient continuing to have nausea/vomiting, patient's inability to tolerate oral contrast, and a longer delay after the patient has taken oral contrast to obtain the CT.

The hallmark finding on CT for a SBO is a dilated (>2.5 cm) proximal small bowel with a decompressed distal small bowel and colon.[2] Other CT signs for SBO include air-fluid levels and a small bowel feces sign (mixture of feculent material mingled with gas bubbles). Recently with improvement in ultrasound technology, an experienced operator can use bedside ultrasound to look for evidence of a bowel obstruction. Ogata et al. found that ultrasound is as sensitive but more specific than plain X-ray in the diagnosis of bowel obstruction.[3] In another recent meta-analysis Taylor et al.[4] reported that ultrasound had better test characteristics than either X-ray or CT.

In summary, abdominal pain in an adult patient carries a wide differential; thus, a focused detailed history and physical examination is of vital importance for an appropriate workup. SBO is an important diagnosis to consider in a patient with a history of previous abdominal surgery, hernias, and/or abdominal neoplasms. Appropriate workup includes obtaining necessary lab work, fluid management, and correction of electrolyte derangements, providing analgesia, bowel rest (NPO), gastric decompression as needed, obtaining appropriate imaging (ultrasound, 2-view X-ray or CT) and initiating a timely surgical consultation.

REFERENCES

1. Thompson W, Kilani R, Smith B, et al. Accuracy of abdominal radiography in acute small-bowel obstruction: does reviewer experience matter? *Am J Roentgenol.* 2007;188(3):W233–W238.
2. Jeffrey RB. Small bowel obstruction. In: Federle MP, Jeffrey RB, Woodward PJ, Borhani AA, eds. *Diagnostic Imaging: Abdomen.* 2nd ed. Salt Lake City, UT: Amirsys; 2010: 44–47.
3. Ogata M., Mateer J. R., Condon R. E. Prospective evaluation of abdominal sonography for the diagnosis of bowel obstruction. *Annals of Surgery.* 1996;223(3):237–241
4. Taylor MR, Lalani N. Adult small bowel obstruction. *Acad Emerg Med.* 2013;20:528–544.

FURTHER READING

Jang TB, Chandler D, Kaji AH. Bedside ultrasonography for the detection of small bowel obstruction in the emergency department. *Emerg Med J.* 2011;28:676–678.

SEIZURE

OLGA KOVALERCHIK

SETTING

Emergency Department

CHIEF COMPLAINT

Seizure

HISTORY

A 23-year-old male is brought in by ambulance after an episode of witnessed seizure-like activity lasting about 7 minutes. A friend provides most of the history due to the patient's condition.

The patient was celebrating the end of final exams when his friends suddenly noticed "he looked out of it." He dropped his drink, became unresponsive, and stiffened up all of his extremities. His friends caught him and lowered him down onto his side; he did not sustain any trauma. Within a few seconds, he developed shaking activity of his entire body, and emergency medical services was called. The patient continued shaking until paramedics arrived about 5 minutes later.

The patient was given 10 mg midazolam intramuscularly and intravenous (IV) access was established by the paramedics. The shaking activity stopped, but the patient was sleepy and confused for the remainder of the way to the hospital.

The patient is a graduate student who completed final exams this morning. He "pulled an all-nighter" with his friend last night. The friend thinks the patient takes some medication, but no additional medical, social, or family history are available.

PHYSICAL EXAMINATION

Vital signs: HR 70, BP 125/85, RR 14, SpO$_2$ 98% on room air, temp. 38.0°C.

Examination reveals a well-developed, well-nourished male in no acute distress. He is resting with his eyes closed. He opens his eyes to voice and follows commands. Examination of his head and neck reveals no signs of trauma. Pupils are equal and reactive to light bilaterally. Mouth examination reveals a 7 mm × 3 mm red lesion on the right lateral aspect of the tongue. His lungs are clear bilaterally with good air movement, and his cardiac rate and rhythm are normal; there are no murmurs, rubs, or gallops. His abdomen is soft, nontender, and nondistended. His underwear is soiled with urine. He has normal peripheral pulses bilaterally, and his capillary refill is <2 seconds. His extremities are warm and well perfused. Neurologic examination is limited by his sleepiness. He has grossly normal and equal strength in all extremities and speaks in a few words at a time. He is disoriented to place, time, and situation.

DIFFERENTIAL DIAGNOSIS

1. Postictal confusion
2. Primary seizure
3. Secondary seizure due to subtherapeutic antiepileptic drug levels, abnormal glucose level, hypothyroidism, drugs/toxins, infection
4. Status epilepticus (SE)
5. Syncope
6. Complex migraine
7. Alcohol withdrawal
8. Psychogenic seizure

TESTS

Fingerstick glucose: 98 mg/dL (normal 70–100 mg/dL)
Complete blood count: white blood cell (WBC) count: 1,7000/μl (normal 3000–12000/μl); normal WBC differential, hemoglobin, hematocrit, and platelet counts
Lactic acid, serum: 6.0 mmol/L (normal 0.0–2.0 mmol/L)
Chemistry panel: normal sodium, potassium, chloride, bicarbonate, blood urea nitrogen, creatinine, glucose, calcium, magnesium, and phosphorus
Liver function tests: normal alanine aminotransferase/aspartate aminotransferase, alkaline phosphate, bilirubin
Toxicology screen: blood alcohol concentration 61 mg/dL (0.061%), remainder negative
Valproic acid level: pending (normal therapeutic range 50–100 μg/mL total valproic acid)
Ammonia level: pending (normal 9.5–49 mcg/dL)
Urine drug screen: pending

CLINICAL COURSE

After ordering labs, additional chart review shows that the patient has a past medical history of seizure disorder, and he is prescribed valproic acid. Additional labs for valproic acid levels and ammonia are added.

Minutes after evaluation, he became unresponsive and developed generalized tonic-clonic activity. He was placed on oxygen by nasal cannula and continuous telemetry monitoring. The seizure activity lasted about 4 minutes before a total of 2 doses of lorazepam were given to stop the seizure. Due to concern for SE, the airway cart was brought to the bedside as an added precaution.

Approximately 10 minutes later he again developed generalized shaking activity. Valproic acid 40 mg/kg IV was administered and the seizure stopped, but he remained altered.

Neurology was called for immediate consultation. He was admitted to the neurology intensive care unit with the diagnosis of SE. He was placed on continuous electroencephalography (EEG) monitoring, which showed epileptiform disturbances but no new occurrences of seizure activity. After several hours, his repeated bloodwork was within normal limits. His mental status gradually returned to baseline, and he was subsequently transferred to the floor.

Once the patient woke up, more history was available. He was diagnosed with epilepsy after a traumatic brain injury several years ago. Despite being compliant most of the time, he skipped "a few doses" of valproic acid during the past week due to stress. He had never "pulled an all-nighter" until this most recent exam. He drinks alcohol rarely, not more than 3 times a year. He admitted to using cocaine for the first time last night as part of celebrating. He was counseled about the risks of these activities in the setting of his seizure disorder.

His initial blood level for valproic acid was subtherapeutic. There was a discussion about starting an additional antiepileptic drug, but ultimately this was not thought to be necessary. The episode was attributed to poor compliance and risky behaviors. His seizures had been well controlled with the same medication for the past year, and he denied having side effects. The patient promised to take his medication regularly and avoid risky behaviors.

The patient was ultimately discharged with close neurology follow-up.

KEY MANAGEMENT STEPS

1. Prioritize the ABCs: airway, breathing, and circulation. During generalized seizure activity, administer supplemental oxygen and prepare suctioning equipment if available.
2. Perform a careful neurologic exam. This will help determine whether additional testing is needed (e.g., computer tomography [CT] scan for new focal deficit) and/or interventions (e.g., monitoring or additional medications for nonconvulsive seizure activity).
3. Obtain a fingerstick glucose early in the workup to identify an easily reversible cause of seizure activity.
4. First-line therapy for seizing patients without IV access is midazolam given intramuscularly. The efficacy is equivalent compared to IV lorazepam and/or diazepam, the two first-line IV therapies of choice for treatment of ongoing seizure (see Table 26.1).

Table 26.1 Seizure and Status Epilepticus Management

Timeline	Therapy	Notes
0–1 min	Airway, breathing, circulation Obtain IV access as quickly as possible Consider supplemental oxygen	Prepare suctioning if available Check blood glucose early
1–5 min	First line medications: o No IV: Midazolam IM 10mg o IV established: - Lorazepam IV, 0.1 mg/kg/dose (max 4 mg/dose) - Diazepam IV, 0.15–0.2 mg/kg/dose (max 10 mg/dose) - Lorazepam and diazepam each may be repeated after a few minutes if not effective right away.	All 3 first-line drugs are considered equally efficacious and are supported by level A evidence
Status epilepticus: if seizure continues after 2 doses of first line medications or >5 min (approx. 5–20 min)	Second-line medications: o Fosphenytoin IV, 20 mg PE/kg (max 1500 mg PE), at 100–150 PE/min o Phenytoin IV, 20 mg/kg loading dose at maximum rate 50 mg/min. o Valproic acid IV, 20–40 mg/kg, at 3–6 mg/kg/min o Levetiracetam IV, 60mg/kg as a single dose (max 4500 mg/dose) o Phenobarbital IV, 15mg/kg as single dose	Second-line agents are to be given once as a single dose There is limited evidence for this stage of treatment; no one agent is preferred Phenytoin administered IV requires careful cardiac monitoring as it has been associated with hypotension and cardiac arrhythmias. It also is associated with more frequent adverse reactions at the infusion site. Thus, fosphenytoin is generally preferred over phenytoin, though both are equally efficacious. Consider intubation if seizure continues after administration of second line medications
Refractory status epilepticus: ongoing seizure after second line therapy or >30 min	Intubation indicated Third-line medications: o Repeat one dose of the second-line drug o Or administer one of the following intravenously: - Midazolam 0.2mg/kg followed by continuous infusion at 0.05–2 mg/kg/hour - Propofol 1–2 mg/kg, start as continuous infusion at 1.2 mg/kg/hour - Pentobarbital 5–15 mg/kg load at <50 mg/min, then 0.5–5 mg/kg/hour - Thiopental 75–250 mg/dose - Phenobarbital 15 mg/kg single dose	Use of third-line therapy warrants emergent EEG monitoring

Note: IM = Intramuscular. IV = intravenously. PE = phenytoin equivalents. Dosages and indications obtained from www.uptodate.com and Glauser T, Shinnar S, Gloss D, et al. Evidence-based guideline: treatment of convulsive status epilepticus in children and adults: report of the Guideline Committee of the American Epilepsy Society. *Epilepsy Curr.* 2016;16(1):48–61.

5. If second-line drug therapy is needed and/or SE is on the differential, prioritize the airway. The patient is likely to require intubation before receiving additional medications.

6. If the patient is intubated for SE and third-line agents are required, the patient will need emergent continuous EEG monitoring to exclude ongoing seizure activity.

7. If a patient with known seizure disorder stops seizing after a short period of time, returns to normal mental status, and has a reasonable explanation for the seizure, he or she can be safely discharged to follow-up with outpatient neurology.

DEBRIEF

A seizure is the clinical manifestation of abnormal electrical activity among neurons. Patients may suffer from recurrent seizures, or epilepsy, typically due to an underlying and fixed condition of the brain. Primary seizures are generally attributed to this condition. Secondary seizures are the consequence of some identifiable and/or reversible condition.[1]

This patient had more than two discrete seizures without complete recovery of consciousness between the episodes, which, by definition, is SE. SE can also be diagnosed when a single seizure lasts more than 5 minutes. Often in SE, after a short period of tonic-clonic activity, seizure activity may be subtle and the diagnosis can sometimes be made only with EEG.[2] It is important to diagnose and treat SE; ongoing electrical activity puts the patient at increased risk of long-term neurologic consequences.[1,2]

Airway, breathing, and circulation take precedence in the management of seizures. Obtaining IV access and providing supplemental oxygen are also critical actions. If available, suctioning should be provided to assist in clearing oral secretions. Nothing should be inserted between the teeth where it might be crushed and lead to additional complications.

There are few universal findings for patients with seizure activity; however, tongue biting, urinary incontinence, and/or a slight increase in blood pressure or body temperature may be commonly detected. Seizure activity may also cause a transient increase in serum glucose, serum lactic acid, and WBC counts without a leftward shift.

Laboratory and imaging studies are individualized to each case. If a patient with well-documented epilepsy presents with a typical seizure episode, a complete workup might consist of finger-stick glucose and serum antiepileptic drug levels. In situations where the history is not clear or in adults with first time seizure activity, more extensive testing is warranted. Generally, this will include glucose, WBC, electrolytes, blood urea nitrogen, creatinine, magnesium, calcium, and a toxicology screen.[1] Prolactin levels are often elevated immediately after a seizure and may be helpful in ruling out pseudoseizure if drawn within 20 minutes of seizure activity.[3] Certain seizure medications affect the liver so liver function tests may be indicated. Valproic acid has been associated with hyperammonemic encephalopathy, so if a patient is on this medication and remains altered without another obvious source, consider checking an ammonia level. A pregnancy test should be included for women of childbearing age. Lumbar puncture may be indicated to workup encephalitis or meningitis in a febrile patient with persistently altered mental status, especially if the patient is immunocompromised. Transient shifts in cerebrospinal fluid cell counts may occur during a seizure and do not necessarily indicate infection. Any infectious workup is further complicated by the fact that there is often concurrent leukocytosis and a slight increase in body temperature.

In adults, noncontrast CT of the head or magnetic resonance imaging of the brain should be considered if any of the following conditions apply: (i) first-time seizure, especially if over age 40 years or (ii) there is a high suspicion for a structural lesion (new focal neurologic deficit, focal seizure onset, change from baseline seizure pattern, or a predisposing history such as recent head injury, sickle cell disease, coagulopathy, cerebral vascular disease, malignancy, HIV infection, AIDS, or travel to an area endemic for cysticercosis). Noncontrast CT reveals large cerebral lesions, but magnetic resonance imaging provides more detailed information and may be appropriate when suspicion is high for intracranial pathology.[4]

While it is not feasible or practical for every patient who presents to the emergency department with seizure, EEG is a useful tool in the diagnostic pathway. EEG can confirm a presumed diagnosis and potentially provide prognostic information for the patient, as certain waveforms are associated with recurrent seizure.[5] Emergency EEG is indicated in a patient who has a persistently altered mental status not otherwise explained by medications or other findings. It is also indicated to detect nonconvulsive SE after administration of general anesthesia medications and/or paralytics.[1]

In a patient with ongoing seizure activity, benzodiazepines are the preferred initial drug of choice. Often patients with known seizure disorder will improve with benzodiazepines. However, if the patient is still seizing after first-line therapy has been given, which includes two doses of either lorazepam or diazepam, second-line therapy includes any of the following administered intravenously: fosphenytoin, phenytoin, valproic acid, levetiracetam, or phenobarbital.[6] See Table 26.1 for the drug names and doses.

Second-line agents are to be given once as a single dose, and no agent is strongly preferred due to a lack of evidence. Each of these medications will decrease the patient's mental status and potentially compromise the airway. A patient requiring these medications will require a higher level of care, and if seizure activity continues, the patient will need to be intubated for airway protection.

Third-line agents for treatment of SE include repeat dose of a second-line drug or administration of an anesthetic agent such as midazolam, propofol, pentobarbital, thiopental, or phenobarbital.[6] If third-line drug therapy is required, consult neurology immediately to arrange emergent EEG monitoring while the patient is in the intensive care unit.

REFERENCES

1. Kornegay JG. Seizures. In: Tintinalli JE, Stapczynski J, Ma O, Yealy DM, Meckler GD, Cline DM. eds. *Tintinalli's Emergency Medicine: A Comprehensive Study Guide.* 8th ed. New York, NY: McGraw-Hill; 2016: 1173–1178.
2. Lowenstein DH, Alldredge BK. Status epilepticus. *New Eng J Med.* 1998;338(14):970–976.
3. Chen DK, So YT, Fisher RS. Use of serum prolactin in diagnosing epileptic seizures: report of the Therapeutics and Technology Assessment Subcommittee of the American Academy of Neurology. *Neurology.* 2005;65(5):668–675.
4. Harden CL, Huff JS, Schwartz TH, et al. Reassessment: neuroimaging in the emergency patient presenting with seizure (an evidence-based review): report of the Therapeutics and Technology Assessment Subcommittee of the American Academy of Neurology. *Neurology.* 2007;69(18):1772–1780.

5. Marks WJ Jr, Garcia PA. Management of seizures and epilepsy. *Am Fam Physician*. 1998;57(7):1589–1600, 1603–1584.
6. Glauser T, Shinnar S, Gloss D, et al. Evidence-based guideline: treatment of convulsive status epilepticus in children and adults: report of the Guideline Committee of the American Epilepsy Society. *Epilepsy Curr*. 2016;16(1):48–61.

EXTREMITY SWELLING

JENNIFER REPANSHEK

SETTING

Emergency Department

CHIEF COMPLAINT

Body Aches

HISTORY

A 23-year-old male presents to the emergency department complaining of severe body aches, which began last night. He states that he starting working out at a "boot camp" gym this week and last exercised yesterday morning. Since last night, he reports diffuse body aches, "I thought I was just sore," but his symptoms have worsened, and he complains of fatigue, generalized weakness, nausea and vomiting twice today, and subjective fever. He also notes that his urine looks dark today but denies dysuria.

He has no significant past medical or surgical history.

He denies smoking, drinks alcohol socially, and denies illicit drug use.

He has no significant family history.

PHYSICAL EXAMINATION

Vital signs: HR 110, BP 110/70, RR 18, SpO_2 98% on room air, temp. 37.8°C.

Examination reveals a well-developed, well-nourished male in who appears uncomfortable. Examination of his head shows no evidence of trauma. He has no scleral icterus or conjunctival pallor. His mucous membranes are dry, and his posterior pharynx is clear. His lungs are clear bilaterally with good air movement, and his cardiac rate and rhythm are normal; no murmurs, rubs, or gallops are appreciated. His abdomen is soft, nontender, and nondistended. His extremities are diffusely tender, lower extremities more so than upper extremities. His soft tissue compartments are soft throughout without pain on passive range of motion, and he has 2+ distal pulses. Neurologic examination reveals grossly normal strength and sensation in all extremities, normal gait and coordination, and normal reflexes.

DIFFERENTIAL DIAGNOSIS

1. Rhabdomyolysis
2. Acute myositis
3. Dermatomysitis
4. Guillain-Barre syndrome

TESTS

Creatine kinase: 3100 IU/L (55–170 IU/L)
Complete blood count: normal hemoglobin, hematocrit, white blood cell count and platelets
Chemistry panel: normal sodium, potassium, chloride, bicarbonate, and glucose
Creatinine 1.70 mg/dL (0.6–1.2 mg/dL), blood urea nitrogen 40 mg/dL (10–20 mg/dL)
Urine dip: large blood, negative leukocytes, nitrites, ketones, and glucose
Urine microscopy: zero red and white blood cells; negative for bacteria
Electrocardiogram: normal
Chest X-ray: normal cardiac silhouette, clear lungs; no acute abnormality

CLINICAL COURSE

Based on history and exam, the patient was placed on a cardiac monitor, electrocardiogram was ordered and intravenous (IV) access was established. Labs including a creatine kinase and urinalysis were ordered, and an IV fluid bolus of 1 L was initiated. The patient's extremity compartments were reevaluated throughout his stay for compartment syndrome. When labs returned, confirming the diagnosis of rhabdomyolysis, the patient received 2 additional liters of normal saline and was admitted for continued rehydration and monitoring of his kidney function.

KEY MANAGEMENT STEPS

1. Consideration of rhabdomyolysis in the differential diagnosis of a patient with myalgia in the setting of intense exercise, drug or alcohol abuse, or crush injuries.
2. Evaluating muscle compartments thoroughly to rule out compartment syndrome.
3. Obtaining laboratory data including urinalysis, chemistry, and creatine kinase to accurately diagnose rhabdomyolysis and appropriately evaluate the extent of renal injury.
4. Prompt initiation of aggressive intravenous fluid resuscitation.

DEBRIEF

The patient was experiencing diffuse myalgia from muscle breakdown secondary to rhabdomyolysis. The classic symptom of rhabdomyolysis is diffuse muscle aches, but the patient can experience localized pain in a specific muscle group, particularly if he or she has compartment syndrome from prolonged pressure to one extremity. Other symptoms of rhabdomyolysis can include dark urine, fever, nausea and vomiting, abdominal pain, tachycardia, and altered mental status in severe cases.

The most frequent causes of rhabdomyolysis are drugs and alcohol, medications, seizure activity, trauma, intense exercise, muscle diseases, and heat illness. It is therefore important to take a complete history in patients with the vague complaint of muscle aches to evaluate for these possible causes of rhabdomyolysis. The evaluation of a patient with suspected rhabdomyolysis should also include a thorough physical examination with attention paid to the patient's muscle compartments. Pain on passive motion is the earliest sign of compartment syndrome, but a muscle compartment with significant swelling, firmness, and extreme pain to palpation should also raise concern for the diagnosis. Distal pulses should be evaluated in all extremities, and an ankle brachial index if there is index of suspicion for compartment syndrome.

Laboratory evaluation should include a creatine kinase, which is diagnostic in patients with rhabdomyolysis. Myoglobin can be assessed but is less accurate for the diagnosis. Because rhabdomyolysis causes the release of myoglobin, a bedside urine dip in the emergency department will be positive for blood, but a lab urinalysis with microscopy will be negative for red blood cells.

The treatment of rhabdomyolysis is primarily focused on early aggressive IV fluid resuscitation. Patients in whom the physician has a high clinical suspicion for rhabdomyolysis should receive a 1 L bolus of normal saline prior to lab results returning if there are no clinical contraindications. A urine output of 200 to 300 mL/hour is an appropriate goal of therapy in the emergency department. Alkalization of the urine or initiation of diuresis with loop diuretics are both controversial practices without good evidence to support them.

Patients who have normal kidney function and urine output, are tolerating oral fluid rehydration after IV fluid resuscitation, and who are otherwise healthy can be considered for discharge home. Most patients with acute rhabdomyolysis require admission to monitor creatine kinase, continue IV fluid resuscitation, and to monitor renal function with creatinine and electrolytes.

FURTHER READING

Counselman FL, Lo BM. Rhabdomyolysis. In: Tintinalli JE, Stapczynski J, Ma O, Yealy DM, Meckler GD, Cline DM, eds. *Tintinalli's Emergency Medicine: A Comprehensive Study Guide*. 8th ed. New York, NY: McGraw-Hill; 2016: 581–583.

Parekh, R. Rhabdomyolysis. In: Walls R, Hockberger R, Gausche-Hill M, eds. Rosen's Emergency Medicine: Concepts and Clinical Practice, 9th Ed. Chapter 119, 1548–1556.e2. Philadelphia, PA: Elsevier Health Sciences; 2018

Nickson C. Rhabdomyolysis (blog post). *Life in the Fast Lane*. October 15, 2017. https://lifeinthefastlane.com/ccc/rhabdomyolysis/

Stone C. Neurologic emergencies; rhabdomyolysis. In: Stone C, Humphries RL, eds. *Current Diagnosis & Treatment Emergency Medicine*. 7th ed. New York, NY: McGraw-Hill; 2011: 620–647.

CHAPTER 28

OVERDOSE

EVIE MARCOLINI AND ANTHONY TOMASSONI

SETTING

Emergency Department

CHIEF COMPLAINT

Lightheadedness, Shortness of Breath, Nausea/Vomiting, Ringing in Ears

HISTORY

A 75-year-old man is brought to the emergency department by his daughter. While she was visiting him, he complained of lightheadedness, nausea, and vomiting. He also had ringing in his ears. He has recently lost his wife of 50 years and hasn't been eating well.

   Prescribed medications: lisinopril 20 mg daily (qd), atorvastatin 40 mg qd, furosemide 40 mg qd, aspirin 81 mg qd
   Social history: lives alone; his wife recently died of a massive intracerebral hemorrhage
   Family history: noncontributory
   Review of systems: he feels hot, short of breath, and has some ringing in his ears. No headache, diarrhea, or abdominal pain.

PHYSICAL EXAMINATION

Vital signs: HR 120, BP 108/70, RR 30, SpO$_2$ 98% on room air, temp. 38.1°C.

The patient appears uncomfortable, diaphoretic, and distressed and has heavy, rapid breathing. He is mildly confused and has some bibasilar crackles in his lungs as well as mild peripheral edema. His neurologic exam is nonfocal, but he is not able to perform a tandem gait because he is lightheaded/unsteady. Pupils are equal and reactive to light and accommodation. He has regular heart sounds without murmur, and his abdomen is soft, nonperitoneal with mild epigastric tenderness. His pulses are equal with slightly delayed capillary refill.

DIFFERENTIAL DIAGNOSIS

1. Diabetic ketoacidosis
2. Acute respiratory distress
3. Hepatic encephalopathy
4. Posterior stroke
5. Toxin (iron, methanol, ethylene glycol, acetaminophen and others)
6. Peptic ulcer disease
7. Ear infection
8. Food poisoning
9. Dehydration
10. Dementia

TESTS

Sodium: 140 mEq/L
Potassium 3.8 mEq/L
Bicarbonate 11 mEq/L
Chloride: 100 mEq/L
Creatinine: 2.0 mg/dL
Glucose: 80 mg/dL

CLINICAL COURSE

On further questioning, the patient revealed that he had been plagued by his arthritis pain over the past 3 weeks and had been taking multiple full-dose aspirin tablets in addition to increasing his dosage of furosemide for persistent ankle edema. Activated charcoal was not indicated since his last ingestion was greater than 4 hours earlier. The medical team suspected salicylate toxicity from a combination of renal insufficiency plus increasing salicylate intake. This was corroborated clinically by hyperpnea, lightheadedness, nausea, vomiting, and tinnitus. Laboratories confirmed the diagnosis:

Salicylate: 52 mg/dL
Arterial blood gas room air: pH 7.39, pCO$_2$ 18 mm Hg, pO$_2$ 125 mm Hg
Urine: pH 5.5 SG 1.035 ketones 2+

The poison center was contacted and following the center's advice the team gave the patient serial 1 mEq/kg bolus doses of sodium bicarbonate followed by an infusion of sodium bicarbonate 150 mEq/L in 5% dextrose in water, which raised the serum pH to 7.53 (goal 7.5–7.6). It was estimated that the patient was at least 4 L volume-depleted, and this was replaced with isotonic crystalloid. Serum potassium was augmented with oral and intravenous potassium infusion and the urine pH rose to 7.5 over the next hours. These steps were taken to ion trap salicylate in the blood (avoiding further distribution to the central nervous system (CNS)) and facilitate urinary excretion of salicylate (a pH-dependent function that improves with urinary alkalinization). The patient was protecting his airway and had no acute respiratory distress. He was transferred to the medical intensive care unit, where his labs were repeated hourly, sodium bicarbonate was bolused to maintain the serum pH ≥7.5 and potassium was administered liberally to keep the urine pH ≥7.5 and the serum potassium <5.0 mEq/L. The patient experienced no further deterioration; serum salicylate levels continued to decline, and the patient's symptoms continued to resolve. His acute kidney injury was noted, and renal function was adequate to keep up with excretion, but the nephrology team was notified at the time of presentation and was asked to stand by for emergent dialysis in case his condition deteriorated.

KEY MANAGEMENT STEPS

1. Recognizing symptoms and history consistent with salicylate toxicity.
2. Consulting the poison center, nephrologist, and intensive care unit early.
3. Fluid resuscitating the patient—patients with moderate to severe poisoning usually require several liters of isotonic fluid to return to baseline hydration and then will have high maintenance fluid requirements. Goal: urine output of approximately 3 cc/kg/hr.
4. Performing gastrointestinal decontamination with activated charcoal if a significant overdose has been ingested within 4 hours (salicylates may be absorbed slowly).
5. Remember that salicylate levels may rise for more 24 hours.
6. Confirming the diagnosis with serum salicylate level—check the units and reference interval ("normal values") since labs may report salicylate levels in different units confounding interpretation.
7. Keeping the blood pH >7.4: Alkalinizing serum and urine, titrating to serum pH 7.45 to 7.55, and remembering that serum pH is more important than urine pH.
8. Following serum salicylate levels to peak and consistent decline. Check blood gases, potassium and urine pH often.
9. Remembering that (i) patients with substantial ingestions who present awake and alert may die within several hours, and (ii) patients with declining salicylate levels may die if allowed to become acidemic.
10. Repleting electrolytes (especially potassium, which will shift intracellularly with bicarbonate administration and drop with volume depletion) and glucose.
11. Avoiding mechanical ventilation when possible; if endotracheal intubation is required, rapid sequence intubation should be preceded by sodium bicarbonate boluses to

assure serum alkalinization and immediately followed by hyperventilation (ex. pCO_2 <20 mmHg)

12. Dialyzing promptly for evidence of neurotoxicity (regardless of level or falling salicylate concentration). Renal failure/insufficiency, cardiovascular instability, and high salicylate levels may also be indications for dialysis. Nearly all patients with salicylate level >100 mg/dL will require dialysis, and elderly patients, those with comorbidities, and those with chronic poisoning may require dialysis at substantially lower levels.

DEBRIEF

Salicylate toxicity can result from acute or chronic poisoning. Salicylates are found in aspirin products and other agents (such as bismuth subsalicylate, methyl salicylate in topical muscle and joint preparations, and other medications). Therapeutic salicylate levels range from 15 to 30 mg/dL. In adults, toxic levels are typically 40 to 50 mg/dL or greater, but chronic toxicity may be present at lower levels. The key to successful treatment of salicylate poisoning is recognizing it and acting early. Understanding the mechanism of toxicity increases awareness of subtle clues to the diagnosis. Salicylates cause platelet dysfunction and gastric mucosal injury and directly affect the chemoreceptor zone of the brain. All of these contribute to nausea, vomiting, and gastric upset. Salicylates also act on the medulla, resulting in hyperpnea and resulting respiratory alkalosis early in the course of poisoning. Finally, salicylates disrupt oxidative phosphorylation, causing metabolic acidosis. The body's response is to attempt respiratory compensation, often resulting in a mixed acid-base disorder. So in the patient with nausea and vomiting a key discriminating observation may be the respiratory pattern—deep and rapid breathing should trigger the question of salicylate overdose and further pursuit of the story. Catching this early is key as salicylate is highly protein bound, metabolized in the liver and excreted by the kidney. As salicylate levels rise, detoxification mechanisms become overwhelmed, and the resulting acidosis promotes accumulation of salicylate in the CNS, the crucial marker for high morbidity and mortality. To emphasize, CNS salicylate concentration is the chief determinant of mortality.

Common early symptoms of salicylate toxicity include hyperpnea, tinnitus, nausea, vomiting, and altered mental status. The most discriminating sign of salicylate toxicity is anion gap acidosis. The most common presentation is a mixed primary respiratory and primary metabolic acidosis. Respiratory acidosis results from the CNS driven hyperpnea, and as ketones and lactate accumulate a primary metabolic acidosis will also become evident. In later presentations, patients can exhibit altered mental status from direct toxicity, lowering of CNS glucose levels and cerebral edema. This can result in seizures if prolonged. Pulmonary edema may develop in severely poisoned patients and generally signifies acute respiratory distress syndrome as opposed to fluid overload. Hypovolemia is common. Ventricular arrhythmia is rare but an ominous sign.

The diagnosis is confirmed by obtaining a serum salicylate level. In the adult, therapeutic levels range 10 to 30 mg/dL, and anything >40 mg/dL is considered toxic. Keep in mind that it may take 5 to 6 hours from ingestion for levels to rise. Lower levels can be associated with toxicity and should be treated aggressively in the setting of signs or symptoms consistent with overdose. Creatinine should be assessed, as a marker for the body's ability to excrete salicylate. Potassium is important to facilitate urinary alkalinization, and lactate is an indicator of anaerobic metabolism. The anion gap will be elevated with toxicity.

The important treatment modalities include activated charcoal if indicated (recent ingestion of tablets), fluid resuscitation, serum (and to a lesser degree urine), alkalinization with bicarbonate, potassium and glucose repletion, and, in severe cases, hemodialysis. Alkalinization is critical, as the resulting increase in pH decreases the rate of diffusion of salicylate into the CNS and also prevents it from returning to circulation in the kidney. Target serum pH should be 7.50 to 7.55 to keep salicylate out of the brain and forestall seizures, coma, respiratory depression (worsening acidosis further), cerebral edema, and brain death. Falling serum pH is treated with sodium bicarbonate boluses of 1 to 2 mEq/kg body weight. Target urine pH should be 7.50 to 8.0, at which point urinary excretion of salicylate is enhanced. Urine pH below target is treated aggressively with potassium administration (even if the potassium is within the normal reference interval) provided the patient is not hyperkalemic. Hemodialysis is indicated in patients with altered mental status, cerebral edema, pulmonary edema, renal failure, liver compromise with coagulopathy, fluid overload, severe academia/electrolyte disturbance, or clinical deterioration despite appropriate management. Mannitol may be administered for evidence of cerebral edema, but neurotoxicity is indicative of the need for immediate dialysis. The decision to dialyze should not be based on salicylate level alone, but a level of ≥90 mg/dL warrants consideration of dialysis in acute overdose while older patients and those with chronic intoxication may require dialysis at lower levels (65 to 70 mg/dL). Additionally, it is prudent to administer vitamin K_1 in moderately to severely salicylate-poisoned patients since the PT/INR often rises as the course progresses. Administration of CNS depressant medications may exacerbate acidemia in these patients by reducing ventilatory drive.

A dreaded symptom in the patient with salicylate toxicity is true respiratory distress. Endotracheal intubation may be dangerous to the salicylate poisoned patient and is only indicated when the patient's respiratory drive cannot keep up with the heightened demand to ventilate CO_2 to maintain acid-base balance. The inherent hyperpnea is the brain's response to metabolic acidosis and is life-preserving. The brief period of apnea during a normal rapid sequence intubation procedure will increase respiratory acidosis can quickly increase diffusion of salicylate anions across the blood brain barrier resulting in heightened toxicity. In cases requiring intubation (determined by respiratory failure or the blood gas showing worsening acidosis), the procedure should be accompanied by ongoing administration of sodium bicarbonate. Intubation should performed as quickly as possible with short-acting sedating or paralytic agents and by the most experienced clinician available. The patient's preintubation minute ventilation is often underestimated and may lead to to rapid decompensation and death if the ventilator is not set to maintain adequate minute ventilation postintubation. Caution must be exercised to avoid barotrauma. Ideally, dialysis (the path to potential salvage of severely ill patients) should be imminent or in progress for most patients ill enough to be intubated. If available, spirometry performed before the point of fatigue and respiratory failure may guide ventilator settings.

Salicylate toxic patients warrant close monitoring in an intensive care unit setting. Endotracheal intubation and mechanical ventilation of the salicylate poisoned patient may result in rapid decline and death unless ventilation is aggressively matched to the patient's disordered physiology and accompanied by prompt dialysis. Astute physical examination, comprehensive history-taking skills, efficient action including alkalinization of the blood, and prompt consultations with toxicology, nephrology, and critical care will afford these patients the best chance of survival.

FURTHER READING

Curry SC. Salicylates. In: Brent J, Wallace KL, Burkhart KK, Phillips SD, Donovan JW. *Critical Care Toxicology: The Diagnosis and Care of the Critically Poisoned Patient*. Philadelphia, PA: Elsevier, Mosby; 2005 pp621-630.

Fertel BS, Nelson LS, Goldfarb DS. The underutilization of hemodialysis in patients with salicylate poisoning. *Kidney Int.* 2009;75:1349–1353.

Hill JB. Salicylate intoxication. *N Engl J Med* 1973; 288:1110–1113.

Lugassy DM. Salicylates. In: Hoffman RS, Howland M, Lewin NA, Nelson LS, Goldfrank LR, eds. *Goldfrank's Toxicologic Emergencies*. 10th ed. New York, NY: McGraw-Hill; 2015:569–591.

O'Malley GF. Emergency department management of the salicylate poisoned patient. *Emerg Med Clin North Am* 2007;25:333–346.

CHAPTER 29

CAT BITE

MARTIN CASEY

SETTING

Emergency Department

CHIEF COMPLAINT

Cat Bite

HISTORY

A 51-year-old right-hand dominant female presents to the emergency department after being bitten by her cat 1 day prior to presentation. She complains of several puncture wounds on her right hand between her thumb and index finger (Figure 29.1). There was initially bleeding from the site, but it resolved with pressure. However, she has developed worsened swelling the past 24 hours and noticed some drainage from one of the punctures. She has limited range of motion in her hand due to pain. She denies any fevers/chills, numbness/tingling, and weakness in her hand. All of her cat's vaccinations are up-to-date.

She has no significant past medical history and does not remember when she had her last tetanus shot.

She drinks alcohol socially on the weekends and does not smoke.

No relevant family history.

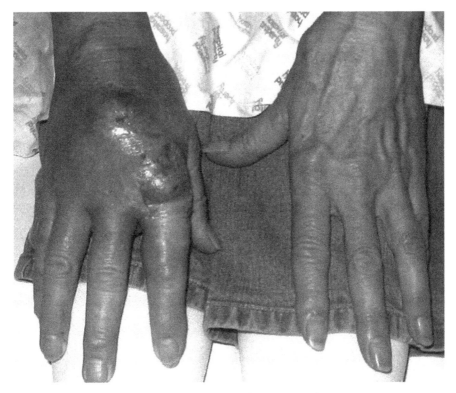

FIGURE 29.1 Pasteurella multicida infection of the hand from an animal bite.

From Morgan, SM. 2010. Oxford Textbook of Medicine. Oxford, England: Oxford University Press.

PHYSICAL EXAMINATION

Vital signs: HR 93, BP 110/70, RR 17, SpO_2 99% on room air, temp. 38.6°C.

Examination reveals a well-developed, well-nourished female in no acute distress. Examination of her hand shows 3 puncture wounds on the dorsal surface of the interdigital space between the first and second fingers. There is significant swelling and erythema around the puncture sites, which are tender to palpation. Fluctuance over the punctate wounds is appreciated. Active and passive range of motion is full throughout. Patient is able to cross her fingers, make the "okay" sign, and abduct against resistance. Sensation is intact in the radial, median and ulnar distributions.

DIFFERENTIAL DIAGNOSIS

1. Puncture wound
2. Infection
3. Retained foreign body
4. Nerve damage
5. Vascular damage

TESTS

Right hand X-ray: positive for soft tissue swelling, no retained foreign bodies

CLINICAL COURSE

The patient's physical exam was concerning for an underlying infection. The wound was copiously irrigated with normal saline, and no foreign bodies were visualized during wound exploration. X-ray corroborated the lack of a retained foreign body and demonstrated no underlying metacarpal fracture. Point-of-care ultrasound showed a large collection fluid under the skin. Given the concern for an underlying infection of the hand, the orthopedic surgery team was consulted. They corroborated the exam and recommended admission for further imaging and wound washout. The patient was given intravenous ampicillin-sulbactam and transferred to the floors for preoperative evaluation. Magnetic resonance imaging showed no extension of the infection into the metacarpals. She was then taken to the operating room for a washout of the abscess. The patient's postoperative course was unremarkable, and she was ultimately discharged to home on a short course of amoxicillin-clavulanate.

KEY MANAGEMENT STEPS

1. Explore the wound to visually determine if there is any exposed bone/tendon involvement or if there is a retained foreign body. Exploration should include assessment through a full range of motion of all digits, since finger position affects tendon position and alignment with the wound.
2. Obtain X-ray to evaluate for foreign body or bony injury.
3. Copiously clean the wound with water, normal saline, or diluted Betadine® (povidone-iodine) solution.
4. Rule out any underlying pathology that may require surgical intervention, such as an open fracture or neurovascular damage.
5. Consider wound closure; many animal bites will be left open given high likelihood of infection.
6. Ask about patient's tetanus status and update if necessary.

DEBRIEF

The patient is experiencing worsened swelling and erythema around her bite wound concerning for infection. While dog wounds have a low risk of infection (about 5%), cat wounds tend to be deeper and have a much higher infection rate (up to 80%). For this reason, patients with a cat bite should be treated with prophylactic antibiotic, regardless of physical exam findings.

Prior to treatment, there are several important steps that must be taken. First, the wound must be explored for foreign bodies that may serve as a nidus of infection. These foreign bodies should be extracted. Especially with deep puncture wounds, visualization of a foreign body may not always be possible. Thus, it is necessary to obtain an X-ray. Any necrotic tissue should be debrided from the wound as well.

After visualization and before X-ray, the wound should undergo copious irrigation to further lower the risk of infection. This can be accomplished with tap water, normal saline, or diluted Betadine® solution. Irrigation under pressure and using copious fluid (>1 L) both decrease the rate of infection. A piston syringe with an 18 or 19 G needle can be used to create adequate pressure. Administering local anesthetic prior to irrigation is recommended as it minimizes discomfort and allows for deeper cleansing.

A patient must be examined for any neurovascular damage that may require further surgical intervention. Motor function of the radial, median, and ulnar nerves is tested by observing the patient's ability to make a thumbs up, "ok" sign, and cross fingers, respectively. Sensation should be tested in all 3 distributions (radial, ulnar, and median nerve) as well. Patients with a swollen hand should also be evaluated for flexor tenosynovitis. Any of the 4 Kanavel's signs increases the index of suspicion for flexor tenosynovitis including (i) finger in slight flexion at rest, (ii) fusiform swelling of the involved finger, (iii) tenderness to palpation along the tendon sheath, and (iv) pain with passive extension (earliest and most important sign).

One must next consider antibiotic therapy for a possible infection. Table 29.1 outlines first-line antibiotic choices by corresponding type of animal bite with amoxicillin-clavulanate being the most commonly used agent. Antibiotic prophylaxis should be given to any bite requiring closure or any high-risk bite. Risk factors for infection include hand bite, delayed presentation of a bite wound (>12 hours), bite near a prosthetic joint, cat bites, punctures wounds, and patients with history of immunosuppression.

Postexposure prophylaxis (PEP) for rabies among cat and dog bites is rarely required, particularly among animals with known immunization history. However, PEP may be considered if a dog's immunization status is unknown or the animal is showing signs of rabies, such as abnormal behavior, ataxia, or seizures. PEP should be strongly considered for bat, raccoon, skunk, and fox bites.

Table 29.1 First-Line Antibiotics for Common Animal Bites

Animal	First-Line Treatment
Cat	Amoxicillin-clavulanate
Dog	Amoxicillin-clavulanate
Human	Amoxicillin-clavulanate
	+/– Acyclovir or valacyclovir (if concerned for herpetic whitlow)
Rat, mouse, squirrel, gerbil	Amoxicillin-clavulanate
Bats, dogs, raccoons, foxes	Rabies immune globulin, rabies vaccine
Monkeys	Acyclovir or valacyclovir (for Herpes B virus)

Source. Table adapted from Quinn J. Puncture wounds and bites. In: Tintinalli JE, Stapczynski J, Ma O, Yealy DM, Meckler GD, Cline DM, eds. *Tintinalli's Emergency Medicine: A Comprehensive Study Guide.* 8th ed. New York, NY: McGraw-Hill; 2016.

FURTHER READING

Ellis R, Ellis C. Dog and cat bites. *Am Fam Physician*. 2014;90(4):239–243.

Moscati RM, Mayrose J, Reardon RF, Janicke DM, Jehle DV. A multicenter comparison of tap water versus sterile saline for wound irrigation. *Acad Emerg Med*. 2007;5:404–409.

Quinn J. Puncture wounds and bites. In: Tintinalli JE, Stapczynski J, Ma O, Yealy DM, Meckler GD, Cline DM, eds. *Tintinalli's Emergency Medicine: A Comprehensive Study Guide*. 8th ed. New York, NY: McGraw-Hill; 2016: 313–319. http://accessemergencymedicine.mhmedical.com.eresources.mssm.edu/content.aspx?bookid=1658&sectionid=109449392. Accessed July 05, 2018.

Sexton, DJ. Infectious tenosynovitis. UpToDate.com. November 2017. https://www.uptodate.com/contents/infectious-tenosynovitis

VERTIGO—POSTERIOR STROKE

USAMA QADRI

SETTING

Emergency Department

CHIEF COMPLAINT

Dizziness

HISTORY

A 55-year-old male presents to the emergency department with a complaint of dizziness that first began 2 days ago and has been worsening. When asked to further describe his symptoms, he states that he feels the room around him spinning to the point that he has to sit down. He does not remember a particular event or trauma that caused his vertigo to begin, and his symptoms are not associated with movement or head position. Throughout this time, he has had nausea and occasional vomiting. The patient also reports that at first he was able to walk but now he feels unsteady and occasionally falls down. He was hoping the symptoms would resolve, but what finally prompted his visit to the emergency department were changes in vision in which he was seeing double, as well as a new headache in the back of his head.

He has a history of diabetes that requires insulin as well as hypertension. He does not always remember to take medications and last visited a doctor 3 years ago. He denies drinking but smokes occasionally and denies any other substance use. He reports that his parents are both alive but in nursing homes, one with a stroke and the other with Alzheimer's disease.

PHYSICAL EXAMINATION

Vital signs: BP 155/80, HR 75, RR 15, SpO_2 94% on room air, temp. 37.1°C.

On physical exam, the patient is an overweight middle-aged man sitting comfortably in the chair. His cardiac exam is normal aside from a systolic murmur in the aortic window. His lungs are clear to auscultation, and his abdomen is soft and nontender. He has good pulses peripherally and no peripheral edema. Given his dizziness, a thorough neurological exam is performed. He is alert and oriented to person, place, and time. Cranial nerve testing reveals no abnormalities. Eye exam shows pupils that are equal and reactive to light with conjugate gaze and intact extraocular movements. However, you do notice a bidirectional nystagmus that does not resolve, vertical skew deviation, and a normal head impulse test. On assessment of his gait, patient is unable to walk without holding the wall for support. He has poor coordination and does not succeed in the finger-to-nose test or in rapid, alternating movements of his hands. He also has a positive Romberg sign though no pronator drift and limited neck mobility. Sensation, motor strength, and reflexes are all preserved.

DIFFERENTIAL DIAGNOSES

1. Posterior stroke or hemorrhage
2. Brainstem mass or tumor
3. Vestibular neuritis
4. Substance use/medication side effects
5. Benign paroxysmal positional vertigo/Meniere's disease

TESTS AND IMAGING

Complete blood count: normal hemoglobin, white blood cell count, platelets
Basic metabolic panel: normal electrolytes, normal blood urea nitrogen, creatinine, and glucose
Computed tomography (CT) head without contrast
Diffusion-weighted magnetic resonance imaging (MRI)

CLINICAL COURSE

Based on the abnormal findings on the neurology physical exam, neurology was consulted, and the patient was sent for a head CT for gross evaluation of any intracranial process. Head CT did not show any hemorrhage, infarction, or mass, but neurology felt there was a high suspicion of stroke. A subsequent MRI was performed that showed evidence of a small infarct in the medial vermis of the left cerebellum. Given the onset of symptoms about 2 days prior, the decision was made to not use tissue plasminogen activator (tPA).

KEY MANAGEMENT STEPS

1. Recognizing the patient is presenting with vestibular syndrome, which includes but is not limited to symptoms of dizziness, vertigo, room spinning, nausea, or vomiting.
2. Obtaining the time course of symptoms, their progressive nature, and conducting a thorough neurological exam including a head impulse–nystagmus–tilt of skew (HINTS) exam when appropriate.
3. Deciding whether dizziness is due to peripheral causes (nonemergent) or central causes (likely emergent).
4. Obtaining appropriate imaging and involving neurology early (head CT versus diffusion-weighted MRI imaging).
5. Deciding whether to administer to tPA for thrombolysis.

DEBRIEF

Dizziness is a very common complaint encountered in clinical practice and is the third most common symptom in patients presenting for evaluation in the emergency department.[1] Classically, the workup for dizziness has emphasized identifying symptoms more precisely as vertigo, lightheadedness, or disequilibrium,[2] but this approach is less effective than one focusing on symptoms' timing and triggers. Moreover, dizziness is now considered as part of a constellation of symptoms that comprise the vestibular syndrome, which also includes vertigo, weakness, nausea, vomiting, near fainting, or disequilibrium, among others. Studies have shown that it is more clinically effective to focus on the timing and triggers of the patient's symptoms, which can be briefly categorized as triggered, episodic, acute, or chronic.[3]

Given that this patient's symptoms presented in the past 2 days, have been continuous, and are not provoked by positional changes, his vestibular syndrome is best described as acute. The differential for acute vestibular syndrome includes less serious, peripheral causes related to inner ear dysfunction (labyrinthitis and vestibular neuritis) as well as more serious central causes such as stroke, aneurysm, or arterial rupture. With patients who present with acute vestibular syndrome, a thorough history and neurological exam are crucial as a number of findings are highly predictive of central causes. These include multiple prodromal episodes of dizziness, headache or neck pain, or any positive neurological signs such as severe gait instability. The HINTS exam is particularly helpful in these patients (Box 30.1)[4] because a single abnormal finding has very high sensitivity and specificity for detecting a central cause such as stroke. The HINTS exam is, in fact, more sensitive than MRI in ruling out stroke in patients with these complaints.[5]

When an emergent central cause is suspected, the next step is to rule out hemorrhage with a noncontrast head CT. Once a hemorrhagic process has been excluded, it is important to activate the stroke code or rapid-response protocol, which will ensure that the neurology team is alerted quickly for the assessment and management of the patient. Timing and early action is also important because the first-line treatment for embolic strokes is the administration of the thrombolytic agent tPA within a narrow window of time—in most cases, 3 hours. Once the stroke code is activated, and tPA is given, the patient is usually transferred to a neurological intensive care unit or similar unit for closer monitoring and supportive management.[6]

BOX 30.1 Bedside Diagnosis of Stroke in the Acutely Dizzy

Patient

HINTS

Head impulse negative
Nystagmus gaze evoked, bilateral, quick phase beats in the direction of gaze
Test for skew positive

INFARCT

Impulse negative
Fast phase alternating (gaze-evoked nystagmus, bilateral)
Refixation on cover test (skew)

OTHER CLUES TO STOKE

- Loss of hearing
- Abnormal pattern of head-shaking induced nystagmus:
    - Early reversal
    - Perverted (vertical nystagmus with horizontal head-shaking)
    - Oppositely directed to spontaneous nystagmus

Source. Leigh RJ, Zee DS. *The Neurology of Eye Movements.* 5th ed. New York, NY: Oxford University Press; 2015: Box 12.4..

REFERENCES

1. Tarnutzer AA, Berkowitz AL, Robinson KA, Hsieh Y-H, Newman-Toker DE. Does my dizzy patient have a stroke? A systematic review of bedside diagnosis in acute vestibular syndrome. *Can Med Assoc J.* 2011;183(9):E571–E592.
2. Stern SD, Cifu AS, Altkorn D. (Eds.) *I Have a Patient with Dizziness How do I Determine the Cause?* In: *Symptom to diagnosis: an evidence-based guide.* New York, NY: McGraw-Hill Education/Medical; 2015: 229–252.
3. Edlow JA. Diagnosing dizziness: we are teaching the wrong paradigm! *Acad Emerg Med.* 2013;20(10):1064–1066.
4. Leigh RJ, Zee DS. *The Neurology of Eye Movements.* 5th ed. New York, NY: Oxford University Press; 2015.
5. Kattah JC, Talkad AV, Wang DZ, Hsieh Y-H, Newman-Toker DE. HINTS to diagnose stroke in the acute vestibular syndrome. *Stroke.* 2009;40(11):3504–3510.
6. Goldman B. Vertigo. In: Tintinalli J, ed. *Tintinalli's Emergency Medicine: A Comprehensive Study Guide.* 8th ed. New York, NY: McGraw-Hill; 2016:1164–1173.

CHAPTER 31

GASTROINTESTINAL BLEED

OLIVER HULLAND

SETTING

Emergency Department

CHIEF COMPLAINT

Hematemesis, Fatigue, Hematochezia

HISTORY

A 72-year-old male presents to the emergency department with a complaint of abdominal pain and hematemesis that began 1 day prior. The pain is crampy in nature, epigastric, and nonradiating. He had 2 episodes of emesis containing bright red blood that morning and had some maroon-colored stools over the past 2 days. He denies fever, constipation, or diarrhea. He has no recent illness or sick contacts. His symptoms have been worsening, and he currently feels lightheaded and fatigued.

He has a past medical history of coronary artery disease, atrial fibrillation, gastroesophageal reflux disease, osteoarthritis, and significant alcohol use.

He drinks 6 to 7 glasses of wine per night. He has had a colonoscopy 2 years prior, which demonstrated polyps but no noted cancer. He is currently anticoagulated with warfarin.

He denies family history of bleeding disorders but has a family history of colon cancer.

PHYSICAL EXAMINATION

Vital signs: HR 102, BP 100/62, RR 18, SpO$_2$ 98% on room air, temp. 36.8°C.

Examination reveals a well-developed thin male in no acute distress. Examination of his head and neck is notable for conjunctival pallor and reveals no jugular venous distension. His lungs are clear bilaterally with good air movement. He is tachycardic with a regular rhythm. His abdomen is soft, tender to palpation in the epigastrium, and nondistended, normal bowel sounds with no noted hepatosplenomegaly. His rectal exam reveals gross bright red blood on the glove as well as maroon-colored stool. His extremities are cool and dry; distal pulses are intact but thready. His skin is pale, with no noted rashes, bruising, or vascular abnormalities. Neurologic examination reveals grossly normal strength and sensation in all extremities, normal gait, and coordination.

DIFFERENTIAL DIAGNOSIS

1. Variceal disease
2. Peptic ulcer disease
3. Gastroduodenal erosions
4. Diverticulosis/diverticulitis
5. Esophagitis
6. Aortoenteric fistula
7. Boerhaave syndrome

TESTS

Hemoglobin, blood urea nitrogen (BUN), prothrombin time/international normalized ratio (PT/INR), complete blood count (CBC), type and cross

CBC: hemoglobin of 6.5 g/dL (normal: 13.5–16.5 g/dL in males), hematocrit of 22% (normal: 39–49%), white blood cell count of 9,500/μL (normal: 4,500–11,500/μL), and platelets 162,000/μL (normal: 150,000–450,000/μL)

Chemistry panel: normal sodium, potassium, chloride, bicarbonate, creatinine, and glucose. BUN 75 mg/dL (normal: 8–20 mg/dL)

PT/INR ratio: 25 seconds (normal: 10–13 seconds), INR of 3.0 normal (<1.1)

Hemoccult/guaiac: positive

Chest X-ray: normal cardiac silhouette, clear lungs; no acute cardiopulmonary abnormality

CLINICAL COURSE

Given the patient's history and altered vital signs, 2 large bore (16 G) intravenous lines were placed, and a bolus (1 L) of crystalloid fluid administered. Based on the physical exam and laboratory evaluations, there was concern for gastrointestinal (GI) bleed. The patient developed worsening hematemesis, prompting transfusion of blood and blood products and reversal agents (packed red blood cells, platelets, vitamin K, prothrombin complex concentrate), endotracheal intubation to secure the airway, and placement of a Sengstaken-Blakemore tube to control bleeding by tamponade while awaiting emergent endoscopy. Octreotide (25–50 µg/hr) was administered, gastroenterology consultation was obtained, and an upper endoscopy demonstrated briskly flowing blood from esophageal varices, which were banded at bedside. Patient was transferred to the medical intensive care unit for further resuscitation, evaluation, and treatment of his variceal disease.

KEY MANAGEMENT STEPS

1. Consideration of location—upper versus lower gastrointestinal bleeding.
2. Early establishment of IV access and transfusion of crystalloid fluid.
3. Obtaining CBC, BUN, PT/INR, type and cross, electrocardiogram.
4. Understanding of transfusion threshold and reversal of anticoagulation.
5. Early consultation with GI for diagnostic and therapeutic endoscopy.
6. Securing the airway at the appropriate time.
7. Placement of Sengstaken-Blakemore tube for unstable massive GI bleeds.

DEBRIEF

This patient's hematemesis, melena, anemia, and fatigue were caused by an esophageal variceal bleed. Typical symptoms of an upper GI bleed include hematemesis, chest pain, abdominal pain, and fatigue, especially in the context of alcoholism and liver disease. Differentiating between upper and lower GI bleed is critical for determining the appropriate algorithm required for treatment and resuscitation. Classically, anything above the ligament of Trietz is considered an upper GI bleed, and anything below the ligament is a lower GI bleed.[1] Hematemesis is more commonly associated with upper GI bleeds. However, it is important to remember that bright red blood in stool, despite having a greater association with lower GI bleeds, can also be secondary to brisk upper GI bleeds and as such may require further workup to determine the location of the bleed.

In all patients with a suspected GI bleed (either upper or lower) it is critical to establish early intravenous access, either two 16 or 18 G IVs with an initial bolus of crystalloid fluids and stat CBC, BUN, and PT/INR. Electrocardiogram is recommended given the reduced oxygen carrying capacity, especially in patients with history of coronary artery disease. Octreotide or somatostatin are splanchnic vasoconstrictors used to reduce portal hypertension and improve endoscopic visualization and hemostasis.[1] Patients with variceal bleeding should be empirically treated with a third-generation cephalosporin or fluoroquinolone to prevent infections such as pneumonia and spontaneous bacterial peritonitis.[2] Chest X-ray can be useful to evaluate for other possible sources of bleeding (e.g., mediastinal widening, hemothorax) and in ruling out pneumomediastinum in patients who have been vomiting or have a history concerning for esophageal damage. Recent research has demonstrated that a restricted transfusion threshold of 7 g/dL of hemoglobin improves outcomes;[3] however, this study excluded patients with massive exsanguination and as such early blood transfusion in a massive GI bleed should still be

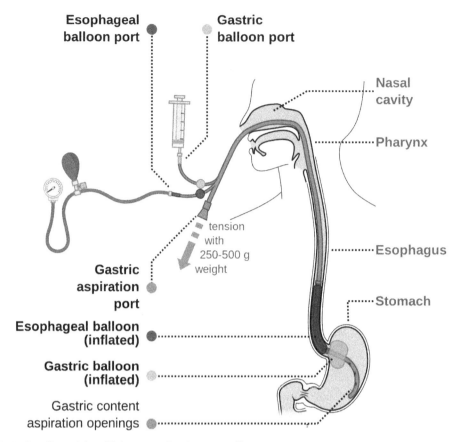

Esophageal balloon port

Gastric balloon port

Nasal cavity

Pharynx

tension with 250–500 g weight

Gastric aspiration port

Esophagus

Stomach

Esophageal balloon (inflated)

Gastric balloon (inflated)

Gastric content aspiration openings

FIGURE 31.1 Sengstaken-Blakemore tube placement diagram.
Creative Commons Attribution-ShareAlike 3.0 Unported, Olek Remesz.

considered. Many upper GI bleeds, especially variceal bleeds, occur in patients with cirrhosis or liver failure, which can exacerbate the bleeding due to a concurrent coagulopathy and should be evaluated with PT/INR. Similarly, it is critical to identify if a patient is anticoagulated—in this case, with warfarin—and administer appropriate reversal agents such as fresh frozen plasma and vitamin K. Endoscopy is both diagnostic and therapeutic, and early endoscopy within 13 hours has demonstrated survival benefits for patients with upper GI bleeds.[4] Unstable patients with difficult to control massive upper GI bleeds should undergo Sengstaken-Blakemore balloon placement for tamponade (Figure 31.1).[5]

REFERENCES

1. Goralnick E, Meguerdichian DA. Gastrointestinal bleeding. In: Marx, John A, Rosen P, eds. *Rosen's Emergency Medicine: Concepts and Clinical Practice*. 9th ed. Philadelphia, PA: Elsevier/ Saunders; 2018: 242–248.
2. Volz K, Sanchez LD. Gastrointestinal emergencies. In: Wolfson AB, ed. *Harwood-Nuss' Clinical Practice of Emergency Medicine*. 6th ed. Philadelphia, PA: Wolters Kluwer; 2015: 537–539.

3. Villanueva C, Colomo A, Bosch A, et al. Transfusion strategies for acute upper gastrointestinal bleeding. *New Engl J Med*. 2013; 368(1):11–21.
4. Lim LG, Ho KY, Chan YH, et al. Urgent endoscopy is associated with lower mortality in high-risk but not low-risk nonvariceal upper gastrointestinal bleeding. *Endoscopy*. 2011;43:300–306.
5. Winters ME. Balloon tamponade of gastroesophageal varices. In: Roberts JR, Custalow CB, Thomsen TW, et al. eds. *Roberts and Hedges' Clinical Procedures in Emergency Medicine*. 7th ed. Philadelphia, PA: Elsevier/Saunders; 2018: 852–858.

FURTHER READING

Morgenstern, Justin. Management of the massive GI bleed (blog post). First10EM. May 23, 2016. https://first10em.com/2016/05/23/management-of-the-massive-gi-bleed/

SECTION IV

INTENSIVE CARE UNIT

JULIE MAYGLOTHLING WINKLE

C H A P T E R   3 2

HYPOTENSION

ANGELA CREDITT

SETTING

Inpatient Unit

CHIEF COMPLAINT

Shortness of Breath

HISTORY

A 68-year-old female with a past history of diabetes, hypertension, and obesity is hospital day 5 after admission for symptomatic cholelithiasis and postoperative day 3 from an open cholecystectomy. Her postoperative course has been complicated by postoperative ileus with persistent nausea and abdominal distension. This evening she developed shortness of breath, productive cough, and an increasing oxygen requirement. She notes persistent abdominal pain that has not worsened or changed. Patient denies chest pain, lower extremity edema, dysuria, hematuria, or any other symptom.

She has a past medical history of diabetes and hypertension and a past surgical history of Cesarean section and cholecystectomy.

She does not smoke or use illicit drugs. She admits to social drinking.

She notes a family history of hypertension and diabetes mellitus.

PHYSICAL EXAMINATION

Vital signs: HR 132, BP 79/52, RR 26, SpO$_2$ 85% on room air, temp. 38.6°C.

Examination reveals an overweight female who appears unwell and is in mild distress. She is lethargic but is able to answer questions and is oriented to person, place, and time. She has normal speech and no focal deficits. Pupils are midsized, equal, round, and reactive to light. Her cardiac exam demonstrates tachycardia with a regular rhythm and no murmur, rubs, or gallops. She is tachypneic with mildly labored breathing without retractions. Upon auscultation of her lungs, she has diminished breath sounds and inspiratory rales in her left base. The patient's abdomen is soft, slightly distended, with appropriate tenderness near her incision site without guarding or rebound tenderness. Her surgical site has no erythema or purulence. There is no costovertebral angle tenderness upon palpation. Her extremities are cool with mottled skin and delayed capillary refill.

DIFFERENTIAL DIAGNOSIS

1. Pneumonia
2. Pulmonary embolism
3. Intra-abdominal or surgical site infection
4. Congestive heart failure
5. Intra-abdominal bleed
6. Urinary tract infection

TESTS

Complete blood count: hemoglobin 11.7 g/dL (12.0–15.0 g/dL), hematocrit 34.2% (35.0–45.0%), white blood cell count 16.7 10^9/L (4.0–11.0 × 10^9/L). Platelets are normal.

Basic metabolic panel: bicarbonate 19 mmol/L (21–33 mmol/L), blood urea nitrogen 26 mg/dL (8–23 mg/dL), creatinine 1.74 mg/dL (0.50–1.00 mg/dL), glucose 246 mg/dL (65–100 mg/dL); normal sodium, potassium, chloride, and calcium

Lactate: 4.6 mmol/L (0.5–2.2 mmol/L)

Urinalysis: normal

Chest X-ray: Figure 32.1

CLINICAL COURSE

Based on the history and physical exam, the patient was placed on supplemental oxygen by nasal cannula. She required 4 L to keep her oxygen saturation above 90%. A second large-bore intravenous (IV) catheter was placed and a bolus of 1 L of normal saline IV fluid was started. Lab work was drawn, including lactate and blood cultures, and an electrocardiogram was obtained, demonstrating sinus tachycardia. The patient was started on broad-spectrum antibiotics to cover

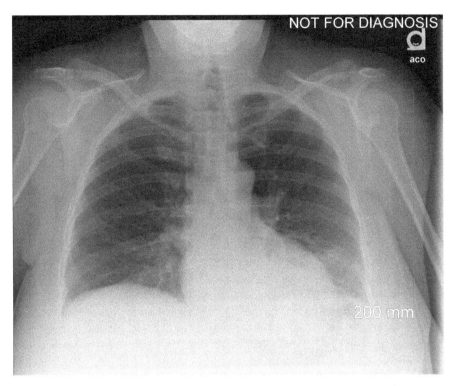

FIGURE 32.1 Chest X-ray. Low lung volumes with patchy air space disease within the left lower lobe.

hospital-acquired infections. A chest X-ray revealed left lower lobe pneumonia. Despite an additional 1 L bolus of crystalloid, her blood pressure remained low. A central line was placed, and she was started on norepinephrine to maintain mean arterial pressure (MAP) >65 mm Hg. A bedside ultrasound was used to assess her volume status and assist in guiding further fluid resuscitation. The patient was then transferred to the intensive care unit for treatment and management of septic shock due to pneumonia.

KEY MANAGEMENT STEPS

1. Identify signs of sepsis, including fever, tachycardia, hypoxia, and altered mental status.
2. Obtain appropriate diagnostic tests, including complete blood count, comprehensive metabolic panel, lactate, blood cultures, chest X-ray, urinalysis, and electrocardiogram.
3. Administer adequate fluid resuscitation based on measured end-points of resuscitation, such as blood pressure and lactate.
4. Draw blood cultures then administer broad spectrum antibiotics within 1 hour of presentation or recognition of sepsis and septic shock.
5. Keep MAP > 65 mm Hg using fluid resuscitation and vasopressors.

DEBRIEF

This patient is hospital day 5, which puts her at risk for hospital-acquired infection. The most common hospital-acquired infections are pneumonia, surgical site infection, gastrointestinal infection, urinary tract infection, and primary blood stream infection. She developed a fever with tachycardia, hypoxia, and tachypnea due to pneumonia. Shortly after symptom onset, she became hypotensive, necessitating the importance of early recognition, intervention, and treatment for septic shock.

Sepsis is a systemic dysregulation in response to infection. Septic shock is defined as sepsis with associated metabolic and circulatory dysfunction causing hypotension resulting in increased mortality.[1]

In 2017, new surviving sepsis campaign guidelines were published. Based on these new guidelines, consider the following recommendations[1]:

- Initial resuscitation should begin immediately with at least 30 mL/kg of IV crystalloid fluid be given within the first 3 hours followed by frequent reassessment of hemodynamic status that includes physical exam, vital signs, urine output, and dynamic variables to predict continued fluid responsiveness. Consider albumin in patients who require a significant amount of fluids.
- It is recommended to maintain MAP >65 mm Hg particularly in patients requiring vasopressors. The first-line vasopressor is norepinephrine. In patients who remain hypotensive despite the use of norepinephrine, vasopressin or epinephrine can be added as second agents. Dopamine should not be used as a vasopressor in patients with septic shock.
- Lactate is a marker of tissue hypoperfusion and increased lactate levels are associated with worse outcomes. Normalization of lactate should be used to guide resuscitation.
- Blood cultures should be drawn prior to starting antibiotics and should include at least 2 sets of cultures. Empiric broad-spectrum IV antibiotics need to be initiated within 1 hour of recognition for both sepsis and septic shock.
- Patients who remain hypotensive despite adequate fluid resuscitation and vasopressors should receive hydrocortisone at a dose of 200 mg IV per day.
- Transfusion with packed red blood cells should occur when hemoglobin is <7.0 g/dL
- Specific anatomic diagnosis of infection should be identified or excluded as quickly as possible. Indwelling catheters, including intravascular devices, should be removed as soon as other vascular access has been obtained.
- In all patients with sepsis or septic shock who require mechanical ventilation, a target tidal volumes of 6 mL/kg should be used, and the head of the bed should be elevated to 30° to 45°. In patients with sepsis-induced adult respiratory distress syndrome, plateau pressures should be limited to 30 cm H_2O, patients should be in a prone position if possible, and high versus low positive end-expiratory pressure should be used.
- Keep glucose <180 mg/dL. Begin administering insulin when glucose levels are >180 mg/dL.

REFERENCE

1. Rhodes A, Evans LE, Alhazzani W, et al. Surviving sepsis campaign: international guidelines for management of sepsis and septic shock 2016. *Crit Care Med*. 2017;45(3):486–552.

FURTHER READING

Jui J. Chapter 89: Septic shock. In: Tintinalli JE, Cline DM, Ma JO, Cydulka RK, Meckler GD, Thomas SH, Handel DA. *Tintinalli's Emergency Medicine: A Comprehensive Study Guide*. 7th ed. China: McGraw-Hill; 2011:431–435.

Nickson, Chris. Early goal directed therapy in septic shock (blog post). Life in the Fast Lane. February 14, 2014. https://lifeinthefastlane.com/ccc/early-goal-directed-therapy-in-sepsis/.

Weingart, Scott. Practical evidence podcast 015—Surviving Sepsis Campaign (SSC) guidelines 2016 (in 2017). EMCrit Blog. January 22, 2017. https://emcrit.org/practicalevidence/ssc-guidelines-2016/

HYPOXIA

DREW CLARE

SETTING

Intensive Care Unit

CHIEF COMPLAINT

New-Onset Hypoxia in an Intubated Patient

HISTORY

A 26-year-old female with no known past medical history is admitted to the trauma intensive care unit after being involved in a major motor vehicle collision. On arrival to the emergency department, she was unresponsive with Glasgow Coma Scale of 3. She was intubated immediately for airway protection. Her vital signs were within normal limits, and her initial physical exam was remarkable for a large scalp laceration. Chest X-ray, focused assessment with sonography for trauma (FAST) exam, and labs were normal, and her head computed tomography (CT) revealed a small subdural hematoma. Her C-spine and abdominal CT were negative for traumatic injury. Shortly after arrival to the intensive care unit, her oxygen saturation decreased to 80%. She had no previous episodes of hypoxia either before or after the intubation. Subsequently, her heart rate increased from the 90s to the 120s, and her blood pressure decreased from 130/84 to 95/43. Further history is limited as the patient is intubated and sedated.

PHYSICAL EXAMINATION

Physical examination reveals a young female who is intubated and sedated. Head and neck exam reveals the prior mentioned scalp laceration and an appropriately placed cervical collar with no underlying hematoma. The endotracheal tube is secured at 23 cm at the teeth, which was the original position. Her chest wall is stable to palpation, and she has asymmetric chest rise on inhalation. She has absent breath sounds on the right and normal breath sounds on the left. Her cardiovascular exam is significant for tachycardia. Her abdomen is soft and nondistended. Her pelvis is stable. She has no gross musculoskeletal deformity, instability, or edema. Neurological exam reveals a Glasgow Coma Scale of 3T, and pupils are 4 mm and sluggish bilaterally.

DIFFERENTIAL DIAGNOSIS

1. Airway obstruction
2. Pneumothorax
3. Mucus plug/atelectasis
4. Aspiration or infection
5. Pulmonary embolus

TESTS

A limited bedside thoracic ultrasound is performed revealing lung sliding on the left, absence of lung sliding on the right. Switching to M-mode on the right chest revealed a "barcode sign."

CLINICAL COURSE

After first confirming that the endotracheal tube was in place and patent and that oxygen was appropriately hooked up, the patient was removed from the ventilator and was manually ventilated with a bag-valve mask. There was increased resistance to bagging. An attempt was made to suction the airway through the endotracheal tube with no mucus or foreign body found. A bedside ultrasound was performed revealing the following image (Figure 33.1).

This was interpreted as a lack of lung sliding on the right, which is concerning for pneumothorax. In the setting of worsening hemodynamics, the clinicians suspected tension pneumothorax. An emergent chest tube was placed, and the patient's oxygen saturation and hemodynamics improved immediately. A subsequent chest X-ray was obtained confirming proper placement of the chest tube and expansion of bilateral lungs.

KEY MANAGEMENT STEPS

1. Recognize the acute clinical decline including hypoxia, tachycardia, and hypotension.
2. Start assessment with airway, breathing, circulation (ABCs).

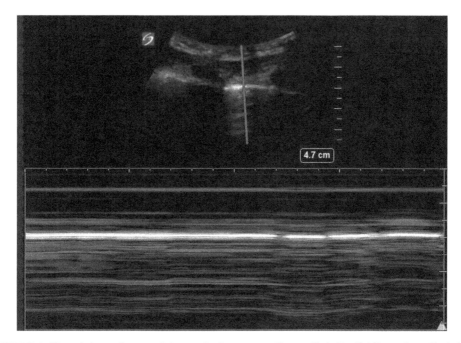

FIGURE 33.1. M-mode lung ultrasound demonstrating pneumothorax. Note the flat lines above the bright white pleural line (representing normal subcutaneous tissue and chest wall), and the flat lines below the pleural line, representing lack of lung sliding. In the setting of normal pleural sliding, the area below the pleural line would appear grainy, not smooth and flat.

3. Perform lung ultrasound to evaluate for possible pneumothorax.
4. Chest tube insertion.
5. Obtaining a chest X-ray to confirm proper chest tube position, resolution of pneumothorax.

DEBRIEF

This case involves a young, previously healthy trauma patient who clinically deteriorates shortly after intubation. The reason for this is expansion of her previously occult pneumothorax (initial chest X-ray was negative, and CT scan of chest was not obtained). It is important to understand that the transition to positive pressure ventilation associated with intubation and mechanical ventilation can drastically worsen a pneumothorax. Anteroposterior (AP) chest radiographs have reported sensitivities as low as 50% for identifying a pneumothorax. Due to this poor sensitivity, patients with a previously normal AP chest X-ray are at risk for developing a delayed pneumothorax or hemothorax. This supports the importance of performing an extended FAST exam (eFAST) in trauma, to include scanning the anterior lung to assess for pneumothorax. Although there are several possible causes of hypoxia in an intubated patient, the diagnosis was made more likely by the absence of breath sounds on one side and associated tachycardia and hypotension. It was quickly confirmed with a limited bedside ultrasound demonstrating absence of lung sliding, which is indicative of a pneumothorax.

Ultrasound has a sensitivity of 93.8% and a negative predictive value of 99.9% in the evaluation of a pneumothorax. This is much greater than that of an AP chest X-ray. To perform a limited bedside thoracic ultrasound, the high-frequency linear probe should be used. Place the probe on the anterior chest wall with the indicator toward the patient's head. Identify the ribs by their posterior shadowing and then find the bright white pleural line running horizontally just deep to the ribs. In a normal lung, this pleural line will be seen sliding with ventilation. If the sliding is subtle, it may be difficult to visualize. In this case, switch to M-mode through the pleural line. On the screen, there will be many sharp, linear lines superficial to the pleural line. Deep to the pleural line should appear grainy, as this is the lung moving with each breath. This is called the "seashore sign." In a pneumothorax, the lines below the pleural line are equally as sharp as those above. This is called a "barcode sign," or "stratosphere sign" (Figure 33.1).

It is also important to consider other possible causes of postintubation hypoxia. Equipment should always be evaluated, making sure the oxygen is hooked up correctly, and mechanical ventilation settings are appropriate. Mucous plugging can lead to decreased ventilation of certain portions of the lung. This is addressed with deep suctioning and chest percussion. Worsening lung disease such as chronic obstructive pulmonary disease or pneumonia can cause hypoxia as well and pulmonary contusions in the setting of chest trauma may also be present. The patient should be treated accordingly. Another possible cause of hypoxia, especially in this particular patient with associated tachycardia and hypotension, is a pulmonary embolism. This can be evaluated with bedside ultrasound (to asses for acute right ventricular strain), as well as a CT scan if feasible. A helpful mnemonic for some of the possible causes of post intubation hypoxia is DOPE.

Displacement of the endotracheal tube
Obstruction of the airways (mucus plug, lung disease)
Pneumothorax, pulmonary embolism
Equipment malfunction

FURTHER READING

Bersten AD, Soni N. *Oh's Intensive Care Manual*. 7th ed. Butterworth-Heinmann; 2014.

Blaivas M, Lyon M, Duggal S. A prospective comparison of supine chest radiography and bedside ultrasound for the diagnosis of traumatic pneumothorax. *Acad Emerg Med*. 2005;2:844–849.

ALTERED MENTAL STATUS

CYNTHIA OLIVA

SETTING HISTORY

Medical-Surgical Floor

CHIEF COMPLAINT

Altered Mental Status

HISTORY

A 72-year-old male with multiple comorbidities is hospital day 3 after being admitted for right lower extremity cellulitis. He initially presented to the emergency department with complaints of fever, chills, pain, and redness of his right thigh and was admitted for intravenous (IV) antibiotics and pain control. It is 1 am when nursing staff alerts you that patient is agitated and combative. They report he is disoriented to time, place, and situation. He is yelling the name "Mary." The patient has removed all of his monitoring and is attempting to get up out of bed.

He has a past medical history of hypertension, coronary artery disease, chronic obstructive pulmonary disease, obstructive sleep apnea, and diabetes.

He has a past surgical history of cholecystectomy and 1 cardiac stent.

He is a former smoker with a 25 pack-year history. He is a widow with no children.

He has a family history of hypertension.

Current medications include vancomycin, aspirin, atorvastatin, metoprolol, neutral protamine hagedorn insulin, Lantus, morphine as needed, and Benadryl at bedtime for sleep aide.

PHYSICAL EXAMINATION

Vital signs: HR 101, BP 170/84, RR 24, SpO$_2$ 88% on room air, temp. 36.8°C. Examination reveals a thin, agitated, elderly male in moderate distress. His head and neck are atraumatic, but his face appears flushed with nasal flaring. There is no nasal cannula in place. No jugular venous distension noted. He is slightly tachycardic but no murmurs, rubs, or gallops. Capillary refill is less than 2 seconds. He is tachypneic with intercostal retractions, paradoxical breathing, and diminished air movement bilaterally with faint expiratory wheezing. No rales are appreciated. His abdomen is soft, nontender, and nondistended. He has a 5 cm × 4 cm area of erythema consistent with cellulitis over right anterior thigh. No purulence, fluctuance, or crepitus is palpated over this region. There is no lower extremity edema or calf tenderness. His extremities are warm. Neurologic examination is limited by his agitation, but he is moving all extremities equally with no obvious focal deficits. No facial droop is noted. Speech is understandable although he does not appropriately answer questions and is noted to be cussing to himself.

DIFFERENTIAL DIAGNOSIS

1. Hypoglycemia
2. Sepsis
3. Opiate overdose
4. Delirium
5. Hypoxia
6. Hypercarbia
7. Cerebrovascular accident
8. Metabolic derangement (electrolyte abnormalities, renal dysfunction, hypothyroidism)

TESTS

Blood glucose 132.

Complete blood count: normal hemoglobin, hematocrit, and platelets. White blood cell count 13, which is down from 18 at admission.

Chemistry panel: sodium 140, potassium 3.9, chlorine 102, HCO$_3$ 26, blood urea nitrogen 30, creatine 1.3, glucose 130, anion gap 9, albumin 3.5

Arterial blood gas: pH 7.21 (7.35–7.45), PaCO$_2$ 68 mm HG (35–45 mm Hg), PaO$_2$ 70 mmHg (80–100 mm Hg).

Electrocardiogram (ECG): sinus tachycardia with normal intervals. No ST segment elevation; left ventricular hypertrophy noted. Consistent with previous ECG on admission, troponin I: 0.02 ng/mL (0–0.04 ng/mL).

Portable chest X-ray: hyperinflated lungs with cardiomegaly. No pleural effusions or pulmonary edema noted. No focal consolidations.

CLINICAL COURSE

Supplemental oxygen was administered by face mask with improvement of his oxygen saturation to 95% but no change in his agitation. Arterial blood gas revealed an acute respiratory acidosis secondary to hypercarbia. Chart review revealed the patient received a total of 8 mg morphine in the past 12 hours. He was given 0.4 mg naloxone IV with no change in mental status. A trial of bilevel positive airway pressure was attempted, but he was too agitated to tolerate the mask, which he kept trying to remove. He was successfully intubated using rapid sequence induction and transferred to the intensive care unit.

KEY MANAGEMENT STEPS

1. Consideration of broad differential diagnosis in a patient with altered mental status (AMS).
2. Obtaining appropriate labs and imaging for potential diagnoses contributing to patient's decompensation.
3. Recognition of hypercarbia on arterial blood gas.
4. Appropriate airway management.
5. Transfer patient to intensive care unit.

DEBRIEF

This patient was experiencing AMS from hypercarbia. Hypercarbia should be suspected in patients who are at risk for hypoventilation and have limited pulmonary reserve who present with worsening mental status. This patient has many risk factors for developing hypercarbia, including history of chronic obstructive pulmonary disease and obstructive sleep apnea. When the patient was evaluated, it was noted that oxygen was not in place. In addition, he received narcotic pain medication, which may have a sedative effect, making him more somnolent and decreasing his respiratory drive. Attempting noninvasive positive pressure ventilation is a reasonable first step. In some cases, judicious use of an anxiolytic or dissociative agent may facilitate patient compliance with noninvasive ventilation. For example, administration of ketamine has been described for this purpose. However, if a patient is unable to tolerate bilevel positive airway pressure despite best efforts, definitive airway management with endotracheal intubation is warranted.

The differential diagnoses for an elderly, hospitalized patient presenting with AMS is very broad. One commonly overlooked and easily identified cause of AMS is hypoglycemia. A point-of-care fingerstick glucose should be obtained in all patients presenting with AMS. In this case, the patient was euglycemic.

Other possible diagnoses causing AMS include acute coronary syndrome, stroke, sepsis, electrolyte abnormalities, and delirium. To evaluate for acute coronary syndrome, an ECG and troponin should be ordered. A detailed neurologic exam is warranted to evaluate for signs of stroke. To evaluate for sepsis, vital signs should be closely monitored for tachycardia, tachypnea, fever, or hypothermia in addition to obtaining appropriate tests (a complete blood count to evaluate for leukocytosis or leukopenia, urinalysis for infection, and chest X-ray to evaluate for pneumonia). Delirium is a serious disturbance in mental abilities that results in confused thinking and reduced cognition. Delirium can be difficult to diagnose and should be considered only after organic causes have been ruled out.

FURTHER READING

Cydulka R. Chronic obstructive pulmonary disease. In: Tintinalli J, ed. *Tintinalli's Emergency Medicine Manual*. 7th ed. New York, NY: McGraw-Hill; 2012: 475–480.

Davidson AC, Banham S, Elliot M, et al. BTS/ICS guideline for the ventilator management of acute hypercapnic respiratory failure in adults. *Thorax*. 2016;71:ii1–ii35.

Han JH, Wilber ST. Altered mental status in older emergency department patients. *Clin Geriatr Med*. 2013;29(1):101–136.

Jeffrey AA, Warren PM, Flenley DC. Acute hypercapnic respiratory failure in patients with chronic obstructive lung disease: risk factors and use of guidelines for management. *Thorax*. 1992;47(1):34–40.

FEVER

SARAH MORGAN

SETTING

Intensive Care Unit

CHIEF COMPLAINT

Fever

HISTORY

A 64-year-old female has been hospitalized for 1 week following a diverticular gastrointestinal bleed. On hospital day 1, she required placement of a right internal jugular central venous catheter for volume resuscitation and blood transfusion, as well as an indwelling urinary catheter for strict monitoring of urine output. Her gastrointestinal bleeding has resolved. She is now hospital day 5 with a documented fever of 38.8°C (101.8°F). She has associated chills, lethargy, and fatigue. No cough or shortness of breath and no abdominal pain or pelvic pain are reported. Her symptoms have been worsening throughout the day, and she is now developing confusion.

    She has a past medical history of diverticulosis.

    She does not smoke, drink alcohol, or use illicit drugs.

    Family history is positive for diabetes in her mother and high cholesterol in her older brother.

PHYSICAL EXAMINATION

Vital signs: HR 124, BP 88/52, RR 22, SpO$_2$ 97% on room air, temp. 38.9°C.

Examination reveals an ill-appearing woman in mild distress. Examination of her head is normal. Neck examination shows a right-sided central line covered with a clean, dry dressing, surrounding skin is erythematous but not tender, and there is no induration or discharge. Lungs are clear bilaterally with good air movement; she is tachypneic but is not using accessory muscles of respiration. She is tachycardic with a regular rhythm. No murmurs, rubs, or gallops are appreciated. Her abdomen is soft and nontender. Bowel sounds are present and active. She has no lower extremity edema or rash. She has an indwelling urinary catheter, and the urine is dark. Neurologic exam reveals a drowsy woman oriented but slow to respond to questions without nuchal rigidity or focal deficits in strength or sensation.

DIFFERENTIAL DIAGNOSIS

1. Central line associated blood stream infection (CLABSI)
2. Catheter-associated urinary tract infection (CAUTI)
3. Hospital-acquired pneumonia (HAP)
4. Diverticulitis

TESTS

Complete blood count: white blood cells 21 (3.7–11.6), hemoglobin and platelets normal.

Chemistry panel: blood urea nitrogen 30 (8–23) and creatinine 2.2 (0.5–1.0); remainder of chemistry panel normal.

Lactate: 6.4 (0.5–2.2).

Blood cultures: drawn from central line and peripheral stick (pending).

Urinalysis: hazy and dark, negative for leukocyte esterase, nitrites, white blood cells 4 (0–5); no bacteria seen.

Rectal occult blood: negative.

Chest X-ray: mild bibasilar atelectasis, no focal consolidation.

CLINICAL COURSE

Based on the history, blood and urine cultures were obtained, and the patient was immediately started on broad-spectrum antibiotics to cover hospital-associated pathogens including *Pseudomonas* and methicillin-resistant *Staphylococcus aureus* (MRSA). She was given 3 L of intravenous fluid resuscitation based on her hemodynamics and elevated lactate level. Her central line was removed, and new central access was placed at a different site given progression to shock refractory to fluids and need for vasopressor support. Over the next 24 hours, the patient's hemodynamics stabilized, and she was able to wean off of vasopressors. Her initial blood cultures grew MRSA; however, subsequent blood cultures showed clearance of infection.

Central access and the urinary catheter were removed after the patient was off of vasopressors for 24 hours. A peripherally inserted central catheter line was placed after finalized blood culture clearance was confirmed. She completed 14 days of intravenous vancomycin from the date of the first negative blood culture.

KEY MANAGEMENT STEPS

1. Consideration of most likely sources of infection in the patient who develops fever while in the intensive care unit (ICU).
2. Obtaining a complete blood count, lactate, and blood cultures prior to empiric antibiotics.
3. Rapid source control with removal (and, if needed, replacement) of indwelling lines.
4. Appropriate empiric antibiotics for hospital associated pathogens started within 6 hours of first noting infection.

DEBRIEF

This patient developed septic shock secondary to a CLABSI. CLABSI is defined by the Infectious Disease Society of America and critical care guidelines as a blood stream infection, which develops in a patient with a central venous catheter in place for >48 hours, with no other obvious source of infection. Source control is key in managing patients with concern for CLABSI. Most guidelines will allow the central line to stay in place if the patient is hemodynamically stable while confirmatory blood cultures are pending; however, if the patient is hemodynamically unstable, the central catheter should be removed immediately, and, if needed, a new catheter should be placed at a different site with a fresh stick. CLABSI is associated with an increased morbidity and mortality as well as increased hospital length of stay. The incidence of CLABSI is directly proportional to the number of days a central line is in place (see Figure 35.1). Thus, important prevention techniques include removal of all invasive lines and catheters as soon as possible.

Another important diagnosis for consideration is CAUTI. Most patients in the ICU setting have a urinary catheter in place either due to hemodynamic instability or for close monitoring of urinary output. CAUTI has an approximate incidence of 10/1,000 catheter days, with 1% to 5% of these cases developing secondary bacteremia. As with central lines, urinary catheters should be removed at the earliest possible juncture to avoid CAUTI development.

HAP is the other most commonly encountered cause for infectious fever in the ICU and occurs after a patient has been hospitalized greater than 48 to 72 hours. The most common symptoms are fever, cough, and increased secretions. Most frequently associated microorganisms are MRSA, methicillin-resistant *Staphylococcus aureus*, pseudomonas, *Streptococcus pneumoniae*, and *Haemophilus influenza*. In the patient in this case, a clear chest X-ray with no associated symptoms of pneumonia made HAP a less likely diagnosis.

Investigation of fever in the ICU necessitates quick evaluation and management. Although fever may be due to a noninfectious source, >50% of fevers in the ICU setting are related to infection and critically ill patients already in the ICU are at risk for rapid decompensation to septic shock, end-organ damage, and mortality. Blood cultures, respiratory culture, and urinalysis

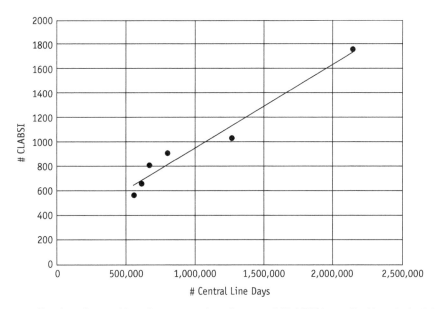

FIGURE 35.1. Number of central line days vs. number of reported CLABSI in medical/surgical adult ICU patients.

Data from the 2013 National Healthcare Safety Network (NHSN) report, data available via the CDC website. https://www. cdc.gov/nhsn/datastat/index.html

with urine culture, complete blood count, lactate, and chest X-ray are good initial diagnostic evaluations. Antibiotics should be chosen based on the antibiogram of the region; however, initial broad-spectrum coverage to include MRSA and *Pseudomonas* is appropriate, with de-escalation as cultures and sensitivities come back. Antibiotics and source control should be initiated as soon as possible to prevent further morbidity and mortality.

FURTHER READING

Burton D, Edwards J, Horan T, Jernigan J, Fridkin S. Methicillin-resistant *Staphylococcus aureus* central line-associated blood stream infections in US intensive care units, 1997–2007. *J Am Med Assoc.* 2009;301(7):727–736.

Marik P. Fever in the ICU. *Chest.* 2000;117(3):855–869.

Rehbman T, deBoisblanc, B. Persistent fever in the ICU. *Chest.* 2014;145(1):158–165.

National Healthcare Safety Network Centers for Disease Control and Prevention. Annual reports. July 2017. https://www.cdc.gov/nhsn/datastat/index.html

AGITATION

MEGAN RASHID

SETTING

Intensive Care Unit

CHIEF COMPLAINT

Altered Mental Status

HISTORY

A 90-year-old woman presents to the intensive care unit (ICU) after a ground-level fall. She lives alone and performs all of her activities of daily living independently at baseline. She walks 2 miles a day and has no significant past medical history other than high blood pressure, for which she takes lisinopril. Her computed tomography scans are negative except for fractures of ribs 5 to 7 on the left. She is admitted to the ICU for closer monitoring of her respiratory status. She is placed on oxycodone for analgesia for her rib fractures.

Overnight, she becomes agitated and loud, yelling that the bedside nurse has tried to harm her. She pulls out her intravenous line and tries to get out of bed, obligating the team to place her in restraints.

PHYSICAL EXAMINATION

Vital signs: HR 105, BP 172/94, RR 26, SpO_2 96% on 2 L nasal cannula oxygen, temp. 36.8°C.

Physical exam shows an elderly woman in some acute distress with multiple bruises on her left chest and abdomen. Her neurological exam is nonfocal. She has no facial droop; she is moving all extremities equally. She is agitated, confused, and not following commands, but her speech is clear. She is in sinus tachycardia, but no extra heart sounds are appreciated. She is tachypneic, with lungs clear to auscultation bilaterally. Her abdomen is soft and nontender, and her extremities are warm and well-perfused.

DIFFERENTIAL DIAGNOSIS

1. Delirium
2. Dementia
3. Myocardial ischemia
4. Cerebrovascular accident/transient ischemic attack
5. Inadequate ventilation (hypoxia/hypercarbia)
6. Infection
7. Medication administration

CLINICAL COURSE

This patient had an electrocardiogram and troponins that were negative for cardiac ischemia. A head computed tomography and neurological exam were negative for stroke. An arterial blood gas demonstrated no hypoxia or hypercarbia. An evaluation for infection including chest X-ray, urinalysis, and complete blood count was also unremarkable. Basic metabolic panel, thyroid stimulating hormone, and liver function tests showed no evidence of electrolyte abnormalities, renal dysfunction, or other metabolic derangement. She was treated with a low dose of intramuscular haloperidol, which alleviated her symptoms. She was placed on scheduled acetaminophen orally, and lidocaine patches were applied to her chest wall with improvement in her pain control. Additional narcotic pain medication was not needed. She had no further episodes of agitation throughout her hospitalization.

KEY MANAGEMENT STEPS

1. Life-threatening causes of symptoms must be ruled out.
2. Treatment should proceed while appropriate workup is being initiated.
3. Identifying patients at high risk for ICU delirium, and subsequently attempting to prevent it, can decrease the incidence of delirium.

DEBRIEF

Delirium is an acute change in global cognitive function characterized by attention deficits and disordered thinking combined with fluctuating changes in behavior (Table 36.1).[1] This patient had a very typical presentation for the hyperactive form of ICU delirium. However, hypoactive delirium is actually the most common form of hospital-acquired delirium and is responsible for 57% of the cases, though it often goes undiagnosed.

Recognition and prompt treatment are important, as the presence of delirium is an independent risk factor for increased length of stay, post-ICU cognitive dysfunction, and mortality. The most reliable tool for diagnosis is the Confusion Assessment Method for the ICU (CAM-ICU), and it is used widely in ICUs for screening at-risk patients. Risk factors include advanced age, baseline cognitive impairment, psychiatric/medical comorbidities, malnutrition, sensory impairment, and sleep deprivation, making geriatric patients the most susceptible population. Treatment is aimed at prevention, and, to that end, the Society of Critical Care Medicine endorses the ABCDEF bundle, which includes interventions that help reduce delirium, improve pain management, and reduce long-term consequences for adult ICU patients[2]:

A: Assess, prevent, and manage pain. Assess pain frequently, treat pain within 30 minutes of detection, and reassess response to intervention. Nonopioid medications such as acetaminophen or ibuprofen can help decrease the amount of opioids administered.

B: Both spontaneous awakening trials and spontaneous breathing trials. Daily sedation interruption decreases duration of mechanical ventilation.

C: Choice of analgesia and sedation. Treat pain first, then consider nonbenzodiazepine sedation, such as haloperidol, dexmedetomidine, or propofol.

D: Delirium—assess, prevent, and manage. The CAM-ICU is a validated screening tool for delirium. Interventions include sleep enhancement, reducing deliriogenic medications, structured reorientation, and adequate oxygenation.

Table 36.1 Risk Factors for Development of Intensive Care Unit Delirium

Risk Factors—Intensive Care Unit Delirium		
Patient Characteristics	Environment	Comorbidities
Age	Sensory impairment/lack of assistive devices (eyeglasses, hearing aids)	Cognitive impairment/ psychiatric disease
Alcohol/nicotine abuse	Psychoactive/sedative medications	Pre-existing cardiopulmonary disease
High illness severity score	Lack of visible sunlight/reorientation	
Malnutrition	Physical restraints	
	Tubes and catheters	
	Isolation	

E: Early mobility and exercise. Early physical and occupational therapy results in better functional outcomes at hospital discharge, shorter duration of delirium, and more ventilator-free days.

F: Family management and empowerment. The Society of Critical Care Medicine advocates for an open ICU model to keep patients and their families actively involved in decision-making, which can reduce length of stay, and increase patient satisfaction, quality, and safety.

Implementation of the ABCDEF bundle has the potential to improve clinical outcomes, including ventilator- and delirium-free days.[2]

REFERENCES

1. Marino P. Disorders of consciousness—delirium. In: *The ICU Book*. 4th ed. Wolters Kluwer: Philadelphia, PA; 2014:801–804.
2. Barr J, Fraser GL, Puntillo K, et al. Clinical practice guidelines for the management of pain, agitation, and delirium in adult patients in the intensive care unit. *Crit Care Med*. 2013;41(1):263–306.

DYSPNEA

MICHAEL JOYCE

SETTING

Surgical Ward

CHIEF COMPLAINT

Difficulty Breathing

HISTORY

A 65-year-old female who underwent lysis of adhesions for small bowel obstruction under general anesthesia is admitted to the floor for postoperative care. On postoperative day 2, she is started on a clear liquid diet, which she has tolerated without issue. Before afternoon rounds, the patient begins to complain of sudden onset of difficulty breathing with chest discomfort. The difficulty breathing is associated with painful inspiration. The nurse placed a nasal cannula with no improvement. The chest discomfort is described as heavy and tight. There is no associated diaphoresis, vomiting, or abdominal pain.

She has a past medical history of hypertension and hyperlipidemia.

She is an everyday smoker of 1 pack per day.

She denies family history of lung disease.

Current medications: heparin 5000 units subcutaneous every 8 hours, oxycodone 5 mg orally as needed severe pain every 6 six hours, esomeprazole 40 mg daily

PHYSICAL EXAMINATION

Vital signs: HR 116, BP 118/72, RR 28, SpO$_2$ 94% on room air, temp. 38.3°C.

Examination reveals an alert female in mild respiratory distress. Examination of her head and neck is normal and reveals no jugular venous distension. Her respiratory effort appears labored, lungs are clear, and equal bilaterally with no rales or rhonchi. She is tachycardic with no murmurs, rubs, or gallops. Her abdomen is soft with no rebound or guarding; there is a well-healing abdominal incision and the dressing is clean, dry, and intact. She has 1+ edema on the right lower extremity and no edema to her left lower extremity. Neurologic exam reveals normal strength and sensation to all extremities.

DIFFERENTIAL DIAGNOSIS

1. Pulmonary embolism
2. Pneumonia
3. Pneumothorax
4. Myocardial infarction
5. Aspiration

TESTS

Troponin I: 0.18 ng/mL (0–0.04 ng/mL).

Brain natriuretic peptide (BNP): 280 pg/ml (0–50 pg/mL).

Complete blood count: normal hemoglobin, hematocrit, white blood cell count, and platelets.

Chemistry panel: normal sodium, potassium, chloride, bicarbonate, blood urea nitrogen, creatinine, and glucose.

Electrocardiogram (ECG): sinus tachycardia with no ST elevation (Figure 37.1).

Chest X-ray: normal cardiac silhouette, clear lungs. No acute abnormality.

Bedside cardiac ultrasound: Figure 37.2.

Computed tomography (CT) angiography chest: Figure 37.3.

CLINICAL COURSE

Based on the history and sudden clinical decline, the patient was immediately placed on nasal cannula oxygen, a cardiac monitor, and secondary intravenous (IV) access was established. ECG revealed sinus tachycardia. A diagnosis of pulmonary embolism was considered. An immediate bedside ultrasound showed a large dilated right ventricle. Given these findings, systemic anticoagulation was immediately administered with heparin bolus and maintenance infusion. The patient's blood pressure remained stable and a CT scan revealed a large right-sided pulmonary embolism. CT surgery was consulted to evaluate for possible thrombectomy, but given her stable vital signs, the decision was made to continue anticoagulation.

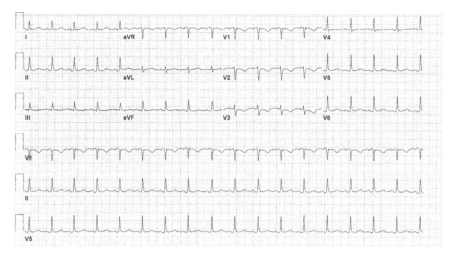

FIGURE 37.1. Electrocardiogram: sinus tachycardia. Note T wave inversions in lead V_1–V_4.

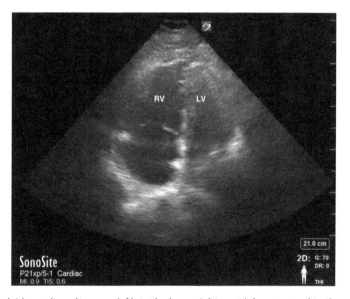

FIGURE 37.2. Bedside cardiac ultrasound: Note the large right ventricle compared to the normal-sized left ventricle.

KEY MANAGEMENT STEPS

1. Consideration of pulmonary embolism in a postoperative patient with sudden onset of shortness of breath.
2. Initiation of anticoagulation when clinical suspicion is high and confirmatory tests are pending.
3. Obtain troponin, BNP, serum chemistry (including electrolytes and creatinine), and level 1 chest X-ray in a patient with acute decompensation.

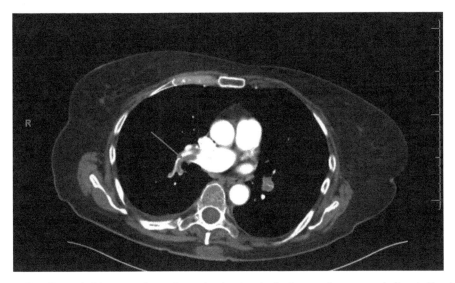

FIGURE 37.3. Computed tomography angiography chest: note the large pulmonary embolism in the right main pulmonary artery (arrow).

4. Appropriate early consultation with cardiothoracic surgery for potential thrombectomy considering risk of IV tissue plasminogen activator (tPA) in postoperative patient.

DEBRIEF

This patient developed sudden onset shortness of breath caused by a pulmonary embolism. These emboli usually form in the deep venous system as a response to predisposing factors such as endothelial injury, stasis, turbulent blood flow, and hypercoagulability. This patient was at risk due to her recent surgery and subsequent immobilization in the hospital. This patient was on prophylaxis for deep vein thrombosis/pulmonary embolism, and thus her risk was very low at 0.1%,[1] but, given the severity of the complications if missed, the diagnosis cannot be overlooked and must be considered in any patient with sudden onset shortness of breath and risk factors.

When a pulmonary embolism is suspected, it is important to remember that the first step should be anticoagulation to prevent any worsening of the clot. This can be initiated in a patient for whom suspicion is high and before confirmatory tests have been completed. Use of a continuous heparin infusion (80 units/kg bolus with 18 units/kg/hr infusion) allows for easy termination of anticoagulation should the final diagnoses be different or for any bleeding complications. Another option would be therapeutic dosage of low molecular weight heparin (Lovenox) at 1 mg/kg every 12 hours. However, in the patient who is at risk for bleeding, shorter acting and potentially reversible unfractionated heparin is a more prudent choice. Anticoagulation does not prevent the patient from receiving more advanced therapies such as thrombolytics or thrombectomy surgery, and thus there should be no delay in administration.

IV tPA has shown benefit in patients with large hemodynamically compromising pulmonary emboli. However, a relative contraindication to tPA is recent major surgery due to the potential to bleed at the surgical bed.[2] In this case, the patient improved with systemic anticoagulation and the decision was made to avoid the potential risks associated IV tPA. Had the patient become further hemodynamically compromised, IV tPA could have had life-saving effects and must be considered.

Bedside ultrasound has the ability to help assist in the diagnosis of pulmonary embolism in a rapid fashion. A limited echocardiogram showed a dilated right ventricle, indicating elevated pulmonary artery pressure further suggesting an obstruction in outflow (Figure 37.2).

Laboratory analysis can also aid in the diagnosis. With acute obstruction of the pulmonary system, the heart will be under increased stress. The right ventricle will dilate, and release BNP. With the increased workload and strain, troponin may be mildly to moderately elevated.

Chest X-ray is rarely revealing of any specific findings in pulmonary embolism; however, the absence of alternative diagnosis such as pneumothorax or consolidation is helpful.

ECG in pulmonary embolism usually reveals sinus tachycardia but is not specific for the disease. A right ventricular strain pattern of T wave inversions in leads V_1 to V_4 is the most specific finding but only found in 30% to 35% of patients.[3] This patient had both sinus tachycardia and a right ventricular strain pattern.

The gold standard for diagnosing a pulmonary embolism is CT pulmonary angiography. Contrast material is injected into a large IV and images obtained when the contrast is in the pulmonary vasculature, allowing the physician to determine if there are any filling defects. It is important to consider that the patient must first be hemodynamically stable before attempting to obtain this study.

Thrombectomy performed by cardiothoracic surgery is an option for large pulmonary embolism and should be considered for all patients with pulmonary embolism that has hemodynamic changes.

REFERENCES

1. Kerkez MD, Ćulafić ĐM, Mijač DD, Ranković VI, Lekić NS, Stefanović DŽ. A study of pulmonary embolism after abdominal surgery in patients undergoing prophylaxis. *World J Gastroenterol.* 2009;15(3):344–348.
2. Fugate JE, Rabinstein AA. Absolute and relative contraindications to IV rt-PA for acute ischemic stroke. *Neurohospitalist.* 2015;5(3):110–121.
3. Burns, E. The ECG in pulmonary embolism (blog post). Life in the Fast Lane. October 2017. https://lifeinthefastlane.com/ecg-library/pulmonary-embolism/ 9

FURTHER READING

Noble V, Nelson P. *Manual of Emergency and Critical Care Ultrasound.* 2nd ed. Cambridge, England: Cambridge University Press; 2011.

CHAPTER 38

ANEMIA

KATHLEEN LI

SETTING

Intensive Care Unit

CHIEF COMPLAINT

Dizziness

HISTORY

A 54-year-old male is hospital day 5 after being admitted for unstable angina. He underwent cardiac catheterization with drug-eluting stent placement 3 days prior. He describes progressively worsening dyspnea and dizziness over the past 2 days. Today, he felt dizzy walking to the bathroom and almost passed out and also reports mild chest pain. He denies abdominal pain, nausea, vomiting, or diarrhea but, on further inquiry, admits that his stool this morning was unusually dark.

He has a past medical history of hypertension, hyperlipidemia, coronary artery disease, and a stomach ulcer 20 years ago. He has no past surgical history.

He is a former smoker with a 30 pack-year history.

He reports family history of cardiac disease.

He is taking aspirin 81 mg, ticagrelor, metoprolol, and simvastatin daily.

PHYSICAL EXAMINATION

Vital signs: HR 110, BP 106/64, RR 24, SpO$_2$ 100% on room air, temp. 35.9°C.

Examination reveals a well-developed, well-nourished male who is mildly diaphoretic but in no acute distress. Examination of his head and neck reveals conjunctival pallor. His lungs are clear bilaterally with good air movement; he is mildly tachycardic with a regular rhythm; no murmurs, rubs, or gallops are appreciated. His abdomen is soft, nontender, and nondistended. Rectal tone is normal, with dark brown stool that is guaiac positive. He has no lower extremity edema bilaterally with good peripheral pulses. His extremities are warm and well-perfused. Neurologic examination reveals grossly normal strength and sensation in all extremities, normal gait, and coordination.

DIFFERENTIAL DIAGNOSIS

1. Symptomatic anemia
2. Myocardial infarction
3. Sepsis
4. Arrhythmia
5. Pulmonary embolism

TESTS

Complete blood count: hemoglobin 5.5 g/dL (13.9–16.3 g/dL), hematocrit 14.4% (32%–52%). White blood cell count and platelets are normal.

Chemistry panel: blood urea nitrogen 33 mg/dL (6–23 mg/dL); normal sodium, potassium, chloride, bicarbonate, creatinine, and glucose.

Prothrombin time, international normalized ratio, and activated partial thromboplastin time: normal.

Troponin I: <0.01 ng/mL (0–0.04 ng/mL).

Type and cross: blood type A; rhesus factor positive; antibody negative.

Electrocardiogram: sinus tachycardia, no ischemic ST changes or T wave inversions.

Chest X-ray: normal cardiac silhouette, clear lungs. No acute abnormality.

CLINICAL COURSE

Based on this change in the patient's clinical status, he was upgraded to the intensive care unit. He was started on a proton pump inhibitor infusion and then transfused a total of 3 units of crossed red blood cells with improvement in his chest pain and blood pressure and an increase in his hemoglobin from 5.5 to 8.0. Gastroenterology was consulted, and the patient underwent esophagogastroduodenoscopy, which revealed an 8 mm duodenal ulcer (Figure 38.1). Stool *Helicobacter pylori* antigen was found to be positive, and the patient was started on triple therapy

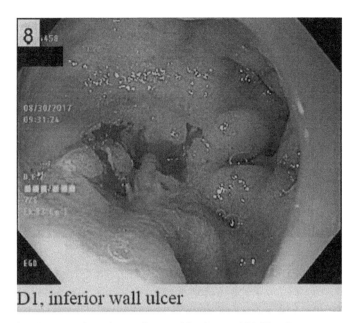

D1, inferior wall ulcer

FIGURE 38.1 Duodenal ulcer with evidence of recent bleeding and friable edges.

(clarithromycin, amoxicillin, and pantoprazole). In conjunction with cardiology, decision was made to discontinue aspirin while continuing ticagrelor therapy.

KEY MANAGEMENT STEPS

1. Recognize risk factors for blood loss anemia.
2. Obtain serum complete blood count, coagulation factors, type and cross, and troponin I in a patient with suspected acute blood loss anemia.
3. Determination of transfusion threshold and amount.
4. Appropriate early consultation with gastroenterology based on patient's symptomatic severe anemia and guaiac positive stools.

DEBRIEF

This patient was experiencing dizziness and shortness of breath from symptomatic anemia from a bleeding duodenal ulcer. His bleeding risk was elevated due to recent initiation of dual antiplatelet therapy.

Anemia can present with a wide spectrum of (often nonspecific) symptoms, including fatigue, chest pain, shortness of breath, dizziness, and syncope. The most common cause of anemia is blood loss. Therefore, it is important to inquire about potential bleeding sources such as hematochezia, melena, vaginal bleeding, recent surgery, or trauma, as well as about risk factors that are associated with bleeding—aspirin, nonsteroidal anti-inflammatory drugs, anticoagulants, bleeding disorders, or cirrhosis.

Patients with suspected or confirmed acute blood loss anemia should have two large-bore intravenous lines placed and be placed on a cardiac monitor to observe for hemodynamic instability. A decision must be made whether to acutely treat the anemia with transfusion of blood products and, if the bleeding is ongoing or the anemia is severe, address the source of bleeding urgently. In addition, for patients who are therapeutically anticoagulated, the risks and benefits of reversal of anticoagulation also needs to be resolved.

Patients who are hemodynamically unstable with active bleeding or have other signs of hemorrhagic shock should be transfused regardless of hemoglobin level. Massive transfusion protocol, which is a rapid infusion of a balance of red blood cells, plasma, and platelets, should be considered. For hemodynamically stable patients, the risks and benefits of transfusion need to be considered. A number of randomized trials have demonstrated a lower hemoglobin transfusion threshold of 7 g/dL to be safer than a more liberal threshold of 10 g/dL.[1] Most clinical guidelines for transfusion now recommend consideration of a patient's clinical status (volume status, symptoms, duration or extent of anemia, signs of shock) in addition to the hemoglobin level.[2]

Despite the benefits of transfusion, it is associated with multiple risks. There is risk of human error resulting in a transfusion reaction, most commonly an acute hemolytic reaction, from receiving incorrectly matched blood. Febrile nonhemolytic reactions and allergic reactions are also possible. Additionally, transmission of communicable diseases such as HIV and hepatitis are possible, although this risk, with modern blood banking techniques, is now exceeding remote. Finally, metabolic derangements can occur with transfusion, such as hypocalcemia and hyperkalemia.

More commonly, especially in the critically ill population, transfusion of packed red blood cells is associated with increased risk of infection, including wound infections, sepsis, and pneumonia; increased incidence of multiple organ failure; and increased risk of acute lung injury. In addition, transfusions are associated with longer intensive care unit and hospital length of stay, more complications, and increased mortality. These effects are dose-dependent, meaning the more units of blood that are transfused, the higher the risk of complications.

REFERENCES

1. Corwin HL, Gettinger A, Pearl RG, et al. The CRIT study: anemia and blood transfusion in the critically ill—current clinical practice in the United States. *Crit Care Med*. 2004;32(1):39–52.
2. Napolitano LM, Kurek S, Luchette FA, et al. Clinical practice guidelines: red blood cell transfusion in adult trauma and critical care. *Crit Care Med*. 2009;37(12):3124–3157.

FURTHER READING

Villanueva C, Colomo A, Bosch A, Concepcion M, Hernandez-Gea V, Aracil C. Transfusion strategies for acute upper gastrointestinal bleeding. *New Engl J Med*. 2013;368(1):11–21.

ABDOMINAL DISTENTION

MEGHA RAJPAL

SETTING

Burn Intensive Care Unit

CHIEF COMPLAINT

Burn

HISTORY

A 28-year-old male is admitted to the burn intensive care unit after being involved in a house fire. He suffered partial and full thickness burns to his anterior chest, abdomen, face, and bilateral upper extremities that total 31% of his total body surface area (TBSA). He was intubated on initial presentation for concern of inhalation injury. It has been 16 hours since the fire, and he has been receiving aggressive intravenous fluid resuscitation per the Parkland formula (4 mL/kg × %TBSA).

The nurse calls to inform you that the patient is having low urine output for the past 2 hours. He had previously urinated 75 to 100 mL/hr, but for the past 2 hours he has made only 30 mL total. In addition, she states that the ventilator alarm has been indicating increased peak pressures, but the ventilator settings have not changed since admission.

He has no significant past medical or surgical history. He is a social drinker and smoker.

PHYSICAL EXAMINATION

Vital signs: HR 110, BP 90/60, RR 18, SpO_2 95% on synchronized intermittent mechanical ventilation, rate 12, tidal volume 600, positive end-expiratory pressure 5, pressure support ventilation 10, FiO_2 80%, temp. 38.3°C, weight 70 kg.

Examination reveals a well-developed male who is intubated and sedated on continuous infusions of propofol and fentanyl. He has partial and full thickness burns covering his anterior chest and abdomen, parts of right and left arms, and most of the face, with some intraoral burns and visible soot in his nares. He is tachycardic with palpable peripheral pulses. His lung exam demonstrates diffuse rhonchi with mild rales at the bases. His abdomen is minimally distended and firm to palpation. His Glasgow Coma Scale score is 8T when sedation is turned off (opens eyes and localizes to painful stimulus). He has a Foley catheter in place that is draining minimal clear urine.

DIFFERENTIAL DIAGNOSIS

1. Acute lung injury
2. Abdominal compartment syndrome (ACS)
3. Intra-abdominal hypertension (IAH)
4. Hypovolemia
5. Acute kidney injury
6. Sepsis

TESTS

Complete blood count: normal hemoglobin, hematocrit, white blood cell count, and platelets.
Chemistry panel: sodium: 135, potassium: 5.0, chloride: 100, bicarbonate: 25, blood urea nitrogen: 22, creatinine: 1.9, glucose: 96.
Arterial blood gas: pH: 7.2, pCO_2 50, pO_2 60, HCO_3, 25 Lactate 5.0.

CLINICAL COURSE

The Foley catheter was flushed and a bladder scan demonstrated a decompressed bladder. The bladder pressure was checked and found to be elevated at 26 mm Hg. Peak pressures on the ventilator were also found to be elevated at 36 mm H_2O. Acute ACS was suspected, and surgery consulted for abdominal decompression. The patient was placed in a supine position without elevation of the head of the bed to reduce the abdominal pressure. Fluid resuscitation was slowed, and an nasogastric tube was inserted. The tidal volume and inspiratory flow rate on the ventilator were decreased.

KEY MANAGEMENT STEPS

1. Appreciate that patients receiving aggressive fluid resuscitation are at risk for development of IAH and ACS.
2. Recognize the clinical signs of ACS including low urine output, increased peak pressures, decreased tidal volumes, and hypotension.
3. Knowledge of the risk factors, presenting signs, and a high degree of suspicion are necessary to effectively diagnose and treat ACS.

DEBRIEF

A severe burn is any burn encompassing over 20% TBSA, excluding superficial burns. At the extremes of age, <20% may be considered severe as they are at greater risk of morbidity and mortality. The TBSA is calculated using the rule of nines (Figure 39.1). The patient presented in this case had partial and full thickness burns covering about 31% TBSA and thus had severe burns. After ABCs and secondary survey, fluid resuscitation becomes a priority, and the Parkland formula is used to guide resuscitation:

- Adults: Lactated Ringer's solution 4 mL × weight (kg) × %TBSA burned.
- Children: Lactated Ringer's solution 3 mL × weight (kg) × %TBSA burned.
- Half of the volume is administered over the first 8 hours, and the other half over the next 16 hours.

While the Parkland formula is a good guide at initial resuscitation efforts, one must consider the patient's cardiorespiratory status and urine output (0.5–1 mL/kg/hr) to appropriately direct resuscitation. Despite the appropriate use of the Parkland formula, it may overestimate fluid resuscitation in some patients and predispose them to the development of ACS.

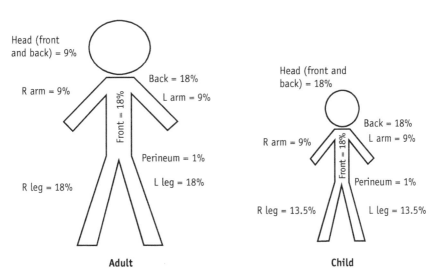

FIGURE 39.1 The rule of nines assesses the percentage of burn and helps guide treatment decisions.

Intra-abdominal pressure (IAP) is the steady state pressure within the abdominal cavity. Normal abdominal pressure is about 5 to 7 mm Hg. IAH is sustained IAP >12 mm Hg and ACS is sustained IAP >20 mm Hg with new organ failure. Measurement of bladder pressure is the gold standard to screen for IAH and ACS. Intra-abdominal perfusion pressure is defined as mean arterial pressure minus IAP; when IAP increases, the perfusion pressure decreases and this leads to reduced blood flow to the abdominal viscera.

Primary ACS results from injury or disease within the abdominal cavity. Our patient had secondary ACS caused by fluid resuscitation in a burn victim. Although burn patients most frequently suffer from ACS, any patient requiring aggressive fluid resuscitation is at risk. The patient developed clinical signs of ACS including a tense abdomen, hypotension, high peak pressures on vent, low urine output, and elevated creatinine. As IAP rises, multiple organ systems are affected including renal, gastrointestinal, hepatic, and cardiopulmonary.

Renal impairment occurs secondary to direct compression of renal parenchyma and renal vein impairing venous drainage. The gastrointestinal tract is extremely sensitive to increased IAP, which causes decreased mesenteric blood flow and mucosal perfusion and compression of mesenteric veins. The liver's ability to clear lactic acid is also reduced with IAH.

Mechanically ventilated patients with elevated IAP have increased peak pressures, hypoxemia, and hypercarbia due to reduced chest wall compliance and elevation of diaphragm causing extrinsic compression of the lung. IAH also decreases cardiac output and causes hypotension by impairing cardiac function and reducing venous return by compression of the inferior vena cava.

The definitive treatment for acute ACS is decompressive laparotomy with temporary abdominal wall closure. In the interim, supportive care should be provided by nasogastric and rectal drainage to reduce IAP. The patient should be placed in supine position and adequate pain control, sedation, and ventilatory support should be provided to relax the abdominal wall and improve ventilation and oxygenation. Fluid administration should be decreased or held.

FURTHER READING

Ivatury RR, Diebel L, Porter JM, Simon RJ. Intra-abdominal hypertension and the abdominal compartment syndrome. *Surg Clin N Am*. 1997;77(4):783–800.

Malbrain ML, Cheatham ML, Kirkpatrick A, et al. Results from the International Conference of Experts on Intra-abdominal Hypertension and Abdominal Compartment Syndrome. I. definitions. *Intens Care Med*. 2006;32(11):1722–1732.

Richards WO, Scovill W, Shin B, Reed W. Acute renal failure associated with increased intra-abdominal pressure. *Ann Surg*. 1983;197(2):183–187.

Tintinalli JE, Stapczynski JS, Ma OJ, Cline DM, Meckler GD, Yealy DM, eds. *Tintinalli's Emergency Medicine*. 8th ed. New York, NY: McGraw-Hill, 2016.

TACHYCARDIA

STEPHEN MILLER

SETTING

Medicine Inpatient Unit

CHIEF COMPLAINT

Heart Palpitations and Dizziness

HISTORY

A 58-year-old male with a history of chronic systolic heart failure with reduced ejection fraction, hypertension, and high cholesterol is admitted to the inpatient medicine floor with a chronic heart failure exacerbation. He states he has been short of breath with minimal exertion, unable to lay flat at night, and has noted increased edema to his lower extremities for the past 4 days. The patient also states he had an episode of heart palpitations and syncope the day prior to being admitted to hospital. Since admission earlier in the day, he has been treated with 1 inch of nitroglycerin paste to his chest and intravenous Lasix for diuresis treatment. While on the floor, the patient develops sudden onset of heart palpations associated with chest pain, worsening shortness of breath, and dizziness.

He has past medical history of hypertension, heart failure with reduced ejection fraction (25%), diabetes, high cholesterol, and myocardial infarction 8 months ago He is a smoker with a 39 pack-year history His father died from a myocardial infarction at age 63.

PHYSICAL EXAMINATION

Vital signs: HR 168, BP 92/54, RR 23, SpO$_2$ 91% on room air, temp. 36.8°C.

Examination reveals a well-developed, well-nourished male in acute distress. His skin is diaphoretic. Examination of his head is normal; his neck exam demonstrates jugular venous distention. His cardiac exam has a tachycardic rate, regular rhythm, and no murmurs are appreciated. He is visibly tachypneic and lung exam reveals bilateral crackles in the bases. His abdomen is obese without distention or tenderness. He has 2+ pitting bilateral lower extremity edema. His extremities are warm and well perfused. Neurologic examination reveals grossly normal sensation and strength in all extremities. He is alert and oriented.

DIFFERENTIAL DIAGNOSIS

1. Ventricular tachycardia (VT)
2. Supraventricular tachycardia (SVT) with aberrant conduction
3. Cardiac ischemia
4. Electrolyte abnormality
5. Congestive heart failure exacerbation

TESTS

Electrocardiogram (ECG): Figure 40.1.
Troponin I 0.88 ng/mL (0–0.04 ng/mL).
Brain natriuretic peptide 875 pg/mL (<100 pg/mL).
Complete blood count: normal hemoglobin, hematocrit, white blood cell count and platelets.

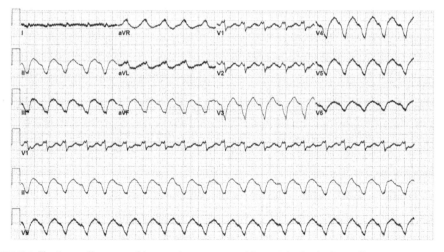

FIGURE 40.1 Electrocardiogram: wide complex monomorphic ventricular tachycardia.

Chemistry panel: potassium 3.2 mEq/L (3.5–4.8 mEq/L), glucose 189 (65–100 mg/dL), magnesium 1.4 mg/dL (1.8–2.8 mg/dL), normal sodium, chloride, bicarbonate, blood urea nitrogen, creatinine, and phosphorous.

Chest X-ray: enlarged cardiac silhouette, mild pulmonary edema bilaterally, no infiltrates.

CLINICAL COURSE

Given the patient's significant history of cardiac disease and the wide complex tachycardia seen on ECG, the patient was placed on a cardiac monitor, nasal cannula oxygen was titrated to oxygen saturation >94%, and defibrillator pads were placed on his chest in an anterior–posterior fashion and connected to the defibrillator. Despite having a palpable pulse, he was determined to be unstable due to his chest pain, shortness of breath, and low blood pressure. He was given 2 mg of intravenous versed for sedation and underwent synchronized cardioversion at 100 Js. With one shock, he was successfully converted into sinus rhythm. He was given 150 mg of amiodarone over 10 minutes and started on an amiodarone infusion. Potassium chloride and magnesium sulfate were administered to achieve normal serum potassium and magnesium levels. The cardiology service was consulted and the patient was transferred to the cardiac intensive care unit for further evaluation and treatment. The next day, he had an automatic implantable cardioverter-defibrillator placed.

KEY MANAGEMENT STEPS

1. Recognize a change in cardiac rhythm with wide complex tachycardia.
2. Place the patient on a cardiac monitor and appropriately place defibrillator pads.
3. Identify a sustained VT resulting in an unstable patient in need of electrical cardioversion.
4. Administration of antiarrhythmic medication and evaluate the etiology of VT.
5. Cardiology consult and transfer the patient to intensive care unit.

DEBRIEF

VT is a wide QRS complex (>120 ms), regular rhythm, with a rate greater than 100 beats/min (most commonly 150–200 beats/min). It can be monomorphic (uniform) or polymorphic (multiple QRS morphologies). VT can be nonsustained (≥3 ventricular complexes that last <30 seconds) or sustained (lasting >30 seconds or associated with hemodynamic compromise). Most commonly, VT occurs in the presence of structural heart disease and can be life-threatening by impairing cardiac output and leading to acute cardiac failure.

There are several key management decisions that must be made when responding to a patient with suspected VT.

- VT versus SVT: While a rule of thumb is that any new-onset symptomatic wide complex tachycardia is VT until proven otherwise, monomorphic VT needs to be distinguished from an SVT with aberrant conduction. Specific ECG findings, such as atrioventricular dissociation, presence of capture or fusion complexes, are suggestive of VT. A history of structural heart disease also makes VT more likely.

- Patient stability: Any evidence of hemodynamic compromise in the setting of a wide complex tachycardia requires electrical synchronized cardioversion. Initial shock should be at 100 J going up to 200 J (biphasic) or 360 J (monophasic). If feasible, consideration of sedation and/or pain control should be initiated prior to cardioversion. Antiarrhythmic medications should be considered, even in patients requiring electrical cardioversion.
- Medical therapy: If the patient is stable without hemodynamic compromise, acute chest pain, or altered mental status, and the diagnosis of VT is presumed, an antiarrhythmic can be started without cardioversion. Amiodarone is the drug of choice initially with dosing of 150 mg bolus and infusion at 1 mg/min × 6 hours followed by 0.5 mg/min. Other pharmacologic agents to consider are procainamide or lidocaine.
- Evaluation for underlying etiology of VT: Common etiologies of VT can be ventricular scarring from previous myocardial infraction and ongoing structural heart disease. New cardiac ischemia, hypoxia, and electrolyte abnormalities should also be considered. Medications that can prolong the QT interval and substance abuse are also potential inciting factors. Assessment should include appropriate lab testing, including troponin and a comprehensive metabolic panel. Correction of electrolyte abnormalities, in particular potassium, magnesium, and calcium should be a priority. It is also important to address any hypoxia with oxygen therapy, noninvasive, or invasive airway management.
- Polymorphic VT: Torsades de pointes or "twisting of the points" is a wide complex polymorphic tachycardia with a changing amplitude and an axis that twists around the baseline. While similar etiologies as monomorphic VT should be considered, this can occur in the setting of prolonged QT interval. Special consideration should be given to medications or conditions that affect the QT interval. Overdrive pacing and intravenous magnesium sulfate are additional treatments to consider.

FURTHER READING

Al-Khatib SM, Stevenson WG, Ackerman MJ, et al. 2017 AHA/ACC/HRS guideline for management of patients with ventricular arrhythmias and the prevention of sudden cardiac death. *J Am Coll Cardiol*. 2017. doi: 10.1016/j.jacc.2017.10.054.

Burns, E. Ventricular tachycardia—monomorphic (blog post). Life in the Fast Lane. November 22, 2017. https://lifeinthefastlane.com/ecg-library/ventricular-tachycardia/

Yealy DM, Kosowsky JM. Dysrhythmias. In: Walls RM., Rosen P, eds. *Rosen's Emergency Medicine: Concepts and Clinical Practice*. 9th ed. Philadelphia, PA: Elsevier/Saunders; 2017: 929–958.

FOCAL WEAKNESS

JORDAN TOZER

SETTING

Surgical/Orthopedic Ward

CHIEF COMPLAINT

Slurred Speech, Focal Weakness

HISTORY

A 64-year-old female is postoperative day 2 from a total knee replacement. Since returning from the operating room, she has experienced nausea and vomiting and has been unable to take any of her scheduled medications. At 2:00 pm, she experienced sudden onset of slurred speech and right-sided weakness. She has almost total loss of motor function on the right side and a sharply increasing headache. She denies any associated vision changes, left-sided weakness or paresthesias, chest pain, or shortness of breath. On chart review, you see that she is scheduled for lisinopril 40 mg daily, clonidine 0.2 mg 3 times daily, and metformin 1000 mg twice daily, all of which have been held due to her nausea and vomiting.

She has a past medical history of hypertension and diabetes.

She is a current smoker with a 40 pack-year history.

She has a family history of myocardial infarction and cerebrovascular accident.

PHYSICAL EXAMINATION

Vital signs: HR 95, BP 215/110, RR 18, SpO$_2$ 98% on room air, temp. 36.8°C.

Examination reveals a well-developed well-nourished female in mild distress. Examination of her head and neck is normal. Her lungs are clear bilaterally with good air movement, and her cardiac rate and rhythm are normal; no murmurs, rubs, or gallops are appreciated. Her abdomen is soft, nontender, and nondistended. She has no lower extremity edema and strong peripheral pulses are noted throughout. Her extremities are warm and well-perfused. Neurologic examination reveals a symmetric face and midline tongue. The rest of her cranial nerves are intact. Her speech is extremely slurred and nearly unintelligible. Her peripheral strength is noted to be 1/5 in the right upper and lower extremity and 5/5 in the left upper and lower extremity. Her sensation is dulled to light touch on the right side and preserved on the left side.

DIFFERENTIAL DIAGNOSIS

1. Acute hemorrhagic stroke
2. Acute ischemic stroke
3. Hypoglycemia
4. Hypertensive encephalopathy
5. Seizure

TESTS

Point-of-care blood glucose: 181 mg/dL.

Electrocardiogram (ECG): normal sinus rhythm with voltage criteria for left ventricular hypertrophy, no ischemic changes from prior ECG.

Complete blood count: normal hemoglobin, hematocrit, white blood cell count, and platelets.

Chemistry panel: normal sodium, potassium, chloride, bicarbonate, blood urea nitrogen, creatinine, glucose.

Prothrombin time 13.8 seconds, international normalized ratio 1.2, partial thromboplastin time 36 seconds.

Chest X-ray: no acute cardiopulmonary process.

Noncontrast head computed tomography: Figure 41.1.

CLINICAL COURSE

The patient was placed on a continuous cardiac monitor, and intravenous access was confirmed. After hypoglycemia was excluded as a culprit for the patient's acute neurologic deficits, an emergent head computed tomography (CT) was done to further evaluate the cause. The CT demonstrated a large left intraparenchymal hemorrhage. Rapid blood pressure management was achieved with an intravenous infusion of nicardipine with a goal systolic blood pressure

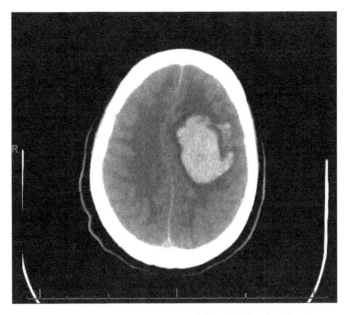

FIGURE 41.1 Head computed tomography. Note the large left-sided, bright-white intraparenchymal density indicative of hemorrhage.

of <140. Neurosurgery was consulted, and the patient was taken to the neurosurgical intensive care unit for ongoing blood pressure management and frequent serial neurologic examinations.

KEY MANAGEMENT STEPS

1. Consideration of hypoglycemia in the differential diagnosis of the patient with new neurologic changes.
2. Obtaining an emergent noncontrast head CT in a patient with stroke-like symptoms.
3. Recognition of an intracranial hemorrhage on the head CT, which is highly suggestive of hypertensive spontaneous hemorrhagic stroke.
4. Early and rapid blood pressure management with a parenteral, titratable agent.
5. Appropriate early consultation with neurosurgery.

DEBRIEF

This patient experienced new neurologic deficits caused by an expanding intraparenchymal hemorrhage, likely secondary to severe hypertension. Typical signs and symptoms of intracranial hemorrhage include headache, nausea, vomiting, elevated blood pressure, and neurologic deficits. The severity of deficit and rapidity of symptom progression are attributable to size and rate of brain volume affected by hemorrhage, respectively. Therefore, these patients can quickly progress through obtundation to complete unresponsiveness early in their clinical course, requiring escalation of care to include airway protection, sedation, and ventilator management.

When a patient presents with stroke-like symptoms, it is important to obtain a blood glucose to rule out hypoglycemia as an easily reversible cause. Routine labs should be sent following the establishment of intravenous access. Complete blood count, electrolytes, cardiac biomarkers, coagulation studies, serum drug screen, and ECG should be ordered. Following that, rapidly obtaining a noncontrast head CT will delineate hemorrhagic from ischemic stroke, as acute intracranial blood will appear bright white (Figure 41.1).

Most commonly, hemorrhagic strokes are caused by severe hypertension that causes small, aging blood vessels to rupture. Other causes of intracranial hemorrhagic include ruptured intracerebral aneurysms, bleeding arteriovenous malformations, bleeding secondary to malignancy, and trauma. In conjunction with neurology and neurosurgery consultants, CT angiography can be considered to further evaluate intracranial bleeding.

There are several critical management decisions that must be considered in the case of hypertensive hemorrhagic stroke:

1. Acute blood pressure management. Blood pressure reduction may reduce further hemorrhage expansion and therefore severity of neurologic deficit, leading to improved outcomes. However, reduction in blood pressure can also reduce cerebral perfusion pressure and therefore potentially worsen deficits, especially in the case of already elevated intracranial pressure (ICP): cerebral perfusion pressure = mean arterial pressure – ICP. There is no compelling evidence for strictly defined blood pressure goals; however, the most recent American Heart Association/American Stroke Association guidelines state systolic blood pressure <140 is safe and preferred.[1] Parenteral, easily titratable agents such as labetalol, nicardipine, or clevidipine are recommended.

2. Reversal of anticoagulation. Coagulation studies should be obtained in every case of intracranial hemorrhage, regardless of cause. If the specific anticoagulant is known and/or coagulation derangements are noted, targeted reversal agents should be administered as soon as intracranial hemorrhage is confirmed. Platelets should also be repleted in the case of thrombocytopenia. Generally accepted goals are international normalized ratio <1.3, partial thromboplastin time <35 seconds, and platelets >100,000.

3. ICP management. Increased ICP, expanding hemorrhage, and impending herniation should be considered in patients with mental status change or rapidly declining neurologic function. Several simple management steps to reduce ICP should be done in all patients, including head of bed elevation to 30°, adequate analgesia/sedation in intubated patients, and avoidance of hypotonic fluids. More severe cases, those with intraventricular hemorrhage, hydrocephalus, or Glasgow Coma Scale score <8 should be considered for aggressive treatment including osmotic diuresis with mannitol or hypertonic saline, neuromuscular blockade, and/or ventriculostomy placement.

4. Neurosurgery consultation. Neurosurgical consultation or transfer to an appropriate facility should be done urgently. Surgical intervention for ICP monitoring, external ventricular drain placement in the setting of intraventricular hemorrhage or ventricular obstruction, and hemorrhage evacuation can be considered on a case-by-case basis and may affect functional outcomes.

REFERENCE

1. Hemphill JC 3rd, Greenberg SM, Anderson CS. Guidelines for the management of spontaneous intracerebral hemorrhage: a guideline for healthcare professionals from the American Heart Association/American Stroke Association. *Stroke*. 2015;46(7):2032–2060.

FURTHER READING

Crocco TJ, Meurer WJ. Stroke. In: Walls RM, Rosen P, eds. *Rosen's Emergency Medicine: Concepts and Clinical Practice*. 9th ed. Philadelphia, PA: Elsevier/Saunders; 2017: 1241–1255.

Dastur CK, Yu W. Current management of spontaneous intracerebral hemorrhage. *Stroke Vasc Neurol*. 2017;2(1):21–29.

Kim JY, Bae HJ. Spontaneous intracerebral hemorrhage: management. *J Stroke*. 2017;19(1):28–39.

SECTION V

MEDICINE FLOOR

ALLEN TRAN

PALPITATIONS

COLIN TURNER

SETTING

Inpatient Medicine Ward

CHIEF COMPLAINT

Palpitations

HISTORY

A 62-year-old woman was admitted 1 day ago with congestive heart failure. She has improved with intravenous diuretics.

On postadmission day 1, she develops palpitations, which she describes as a feeling of her "heart racing." The palpitations have persisted for 45 minutes and are accompanied by light headedness and a feeling of anxiety. They began abruptly while changing position in bed. She has had similar palpitations on rare occasions over the last several years, but those episodes lasted less than a minute before self-terminating.

Her past history includes heart failure with preserved ejection fraction, hypertension, and a tubal ligation. Her current medications are furosemide 40 mg intravenous daily and ramipril 10 mg daily.

She is a nonsmoker and drinks 1 to 2 glasses of wine weekly.

Her father had a myocardial infarction at age 67; there is otherwise no family history of cardiac disease.

PHYSICAL EXAMINATION

Vital signs: HR 180, BP 104/64, RR 18, SpO$_2$ 98% on room air, temp. 36.7°C.

General inspection reveals a well-appearing but anxious lady. Examination of the head and neck shows rapid, regular pulsation of the internal jugular vein. Equal breath sounds are heard bilaterally, with no crackles or other adventitious sounds. The apical impulse is not palpable in the left lateral decubitus position. On cardiac auscultation, heart sounds are regular and rapid, with no extra heart sounds or murmurs. The abdomen is soft and nontender, with no masses or organomegaly. Peripheral pulses are palpable throughout, there is no leg edema, and the extremities are warm and well-perfused.

DIFFERENTIAL DIAGNOSIS

1. Atrioventricular nodal re-entrant tachycardia (AVNRT)
2. Sinus tachycardia
3. Atrioventricular re-entrant tachycardia (AVRT)
4. Atrial tachycardia
5. Atrial flutter with fixed conduction
6. Inappropriate sinus tachycardia
7. Sinus node re-entrant tachycardia

TESTS

Complete blood count: normal hemoglobin, white blood cell count, and platelets.
Chemistry panel: normal creatinine, sodium, potassium, chloride, total CO$_2$, and glucose.
Electrocardiogram (ECG): Figure 42.1.

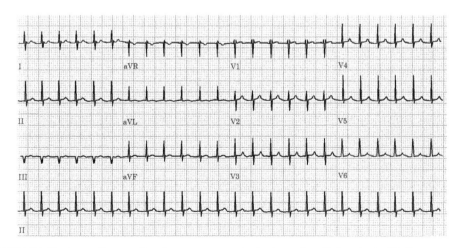

FIGURE 42.1 Electrocardiogram. Regular narrow-complex tachycardia with heart rate 180. P waves are not clearly discernible. A pseudo-R' wave can be seen in some leads, representing atrial activation.

CLINICAL COURSE

The patient was placed on a cardiac monitor. A standard Valsalva maneuver was performed, but her tachycardia persisted. Next, a modified Valsalva maneuver with supine repositioning was performed. This did not terminate her tachyarrhythmia. Adenosine 6 mg was administered intravenously, followed rapidly by a normal saline flush. Cardiac monitoring showed reversion to sinus rhythm; 12-lead ECG was performed, which confirmed normal sinus rhythm with heart rate 80. Her symptoms resolved.

KEY MANAGEMENT STEPS

1. Recognition of the differential diagnosis for regular, narrow-complex tachycardia.
2. Attempting nonpharmacologic maneuvers to terminate AVNRT.
3. Administering adenosine as a first-line pharmacologic step in the presence of a regular, narrow-complex tachycardia.

DEBRIEF

This patient was experiencing a hemodynamically stable, regular, narrow-complex tachycardia. The most common paroxysmal supraventricular tachycardia is AVNRT, which represents about 60% of paroxysmal supraventricular tachycardias[1] and occurs more commonly among younger populations (with incidence peaking in the second to fourth decades); it is more common in women than in men. Symptoms begin and terminate abruptly and most commonly include palpitations, light headedness, and shortness of breath.[2] Although not typically associated with underlying structural heart disease,[3] those with coincident heart disease may additionally experience symptoms of ischemia or congestive heart failure.

The differential diagnosis is that of a regular, narrow-complex (QRS <120 msec) tachycardia. Sinus tachycardia is the most common of these, but the history of abrupt onset and lack of an underlying triggering condition argue against sinus tachycardia. AVRT due to conduction through an accessory pathway, such as in Wolff-Parkinson-White syndrome, can present similarly to AVNRT. Evidence of pre-excitation on a baseline sinus rhythm ECG (a shortened PR interval and/or the presence of delta waves) suggests AVRT rather than AVNRT. However, signs of pre-excitation may not be seen if the accessory pathway is concealed (the pathway only allows for retrograde conduction).

AVNRT may begin suddenly after a premature atrial contraction, and the heart rate is typically 120 to 220 beats/min. Due to near simultaneous atrial and ventricular activation, the P wave is often buried within the QRS complex. If P waves can be discerned, the P wave axis is usually negative, which reflects retrograde atrial activation.

The patient presenting with suspected AVNRT should be placed on cardiac monitor, and a 12-lead ECG obtained. Although rarely necessary for AVNRT, urgent electrical cardioversion should be performed in the event of symptoms or signs of clinical instability such as hypotension, ischemia, or heart failure. In the absence of these features, nonpharmacologic maneuvers should be attempted. A standard vagal maneuver can be performed by having the supine or semi-recumbent patient exhale forcefully against a closed glottis for 10 to 15 seconds; the effect can also be accomplished by asking the patient to blow into a 10 mL syringe with sufficient force to move the plunger.[4] The REVERT trial found that use of a modified Valsalva maneuver, wherein the patient performs a Valsalva maneuver in the semi-recumbent position and is then placed supine with the legs elevated to 45° for 15 seconds was more effective than the standard Valsalva maneuver in terminating supraventricular tachycardia (with success rates of 43% versus 17%).[5]

Pharmacotherapy is the next step if nonpharmacologic measures fail or cannot be performed. Adenosine, as an intravenous push over one to two seconds followed rapidly by a normal saline flush, is effective approximately 80% of the time. The initial dose is 6 mg, and a 12 mg dose can be given subsequently if the first was unsuccessful. Adenosine administration requires cardiac and blood pressure monitoring. Side effects include transient anxiety, chest discomfort, shortness of breath, and facial flushing. Asthma is considered a contraindication due to potential bronchoconstriction, and adenosine should also be avoided if acute myocardial ischemia is suspected.

If vagal maneuvers and adenosine have been ineffective, other atrioventricular nodal blocking agents can be used. In the acute setting, intravenous beta blockers (such as metoprolol or the rapidly titratable esmolol) or calcium channel blockers (diltiazem or verapamil) can be used.

REFERENCES

1. Michaud GF, Stevenson WG. Supraventricular tachyarrhythmias. In: Kasper D, Fauci A, Hauser A, Longo D, Jameson J, Loscalzo J. eds. *Harrison's Principles of Internal Medicine*. 19th ed. New York, NY: McGraw-Hill; 2014:1476–1489.
2. Knight BP, Link MS, Downey BC, eds. Atrioventricular nodal reentrant tachycardia. In: Post T, ed. UpToDate. September 26, 2017. https://www.uptodate.com/contents/atrioventricular-nodal-reentrant-tachycardia
3. Olgin JE, Zipes DP. Specific arrhythmias: diagnosis and treatment. In: Mann DL, Zipes DP, Libby P, Bonow RO, eds. *Braunwald's Heart Disease: A Textbook of Cardiovascular Medicine*. 10th ed. Philadelphia, PA: Elsevier; 2015:748–797.
4. Smith G, Boyle MJ. The 10 mL syringe is useful in generating the recommended standard of 40 mmHg intrathoracic pressure for the Valsalva manoeuvre. *Emerg Med Australas*. 2009;21(6):449–454.
5. Appelboam A, Reuben A, Mann C, et al. Postural modification to the standard Valsalva manoeuvre for emergency treatment of supraventricular tachycardias (REVERT): a randomised controlled trial. *Lancet*. 2015;386(10005):1747–1753.

NO URINE OUTPUT

ALISON RODGER

SETTING

Inpatient Medicine Ward

CHIEF COMPLAINT

No Urine Output

HISTORY

An 87-year-old man was admitted to the geriatric inpatient unit after a fall for further workup of the fall and physiotherapy. A Foley catheter was placed in the emergency department and subsequently removed on post admission day 2.

Two days after Foley removal, he now has lower abdominal pain and no urinary output for the past 18 hours. He denies back pain, fever, or chills, but he admits to having had dysuria the day before.

He has a past medical history of benign prostatic hypertrophy (BPH) with baseline symptoms of nocturia and a weak urinary stream.

His medications include acetaminophen as needed and vitamin D 1,000 units daily.

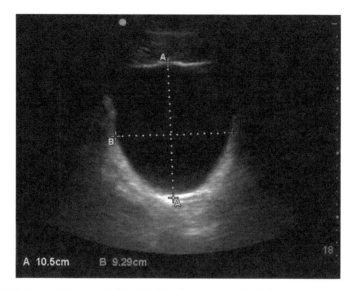

FIGURE 43.1 Point-of-care ultrasound of the bladder (transverse view), demonstrating urinary retention. Most ultrasound machines can calculate bladder volume automatically based on 3D measurements, but one simple formula for bladder volume estimation is length × width × height × 0.75.

PHYSICAL EXAMINATION

Vital signs: HR 80, BP 130/70, RR 16, SpO_2 98% on room air, temp. 37.7°C.

Examination reveals an 87-year-old man who is in mild distress. He is grimacing, indicating that he is in pain. Examination of his head and neck is normal. His lungs are clear bilaterally with good air movement. His cardiac rate and rhythm are normal and no murmurs, rubs, or gallops are appreciated. Jugular venous pressure is 3 cm above the sternal angle, and there is no peripheral edema. He has lower abdominal distention, and his lower abdomen is dull to percussion and tender to palpation. Bowel sounds are present. Rectal exam shows normal rectal tone and an enlarged, smooth prostate. Neurologic examination reveals normal strength and sensation in all extremities, symmetric 2+ reflexes in the upper and lower extremities, negative Babinski (toes down-going), normal gait, and normal coordination.

Figure 43.1: Bedside bladder ultrasound (transverse view).

DIFFERENTIAL DIAGNOSIS

1.   Acute urinary retention (may be of neurologic, obstructive, infectious, inflammatory, traumatic etiology, or medication induced)
2.   Anuria from acute renal failure (may be of prerenal, renal or postrenal etiology)
3.   Appendicitis and intra-abdominal sepsis
4.   Abdominal aortic aneurysm

TESTS

Complete blood count: white blood cell count 15×10^9/L (3.5–12×10^9/L), normal hemoglobin, and platelets.

Chemistry panel: serum creatinine 155 μmol/L (50–110 μmol/L) from a baseline of 80 μmol/L. Normal sodium, potassium, chloride, bicarbonate, blood urea nitrogen, and glucose.

CLINICAL COURSE

Based on the history, physical exam, and bedside point of care ultrasound results, urgent bedside catheter decompression with a 16 F dual lumen Foley was completed. Urine was sent for urinalysis and culture. His symptoms of pain improved, and his vitals were stable over the following hour. Urinalysis revealed the presence of pyuria, nitrites, and bacteria. A diagnosis of acute urinary retention secondary to cystitis with underlying risk factor of BPH was made. As a consequence of the urinary retention, he had mild acute kidney injury. While waiting for urine culture results, empiric antibiotics were initiated. Outpatient urology consult was ordered, and tamsulosin 0.4 mg orally once daily was started. After several days, his urinary catheter was removed, and a trial of void was successful. He was discharged without a catheter.

KEY MANAGEMENT STEPS

1. Consider acute urinary retention in the differential diagnosis for a patient with reduced urine output, particularly in the presence of lower abdominal (suprapubic) pain.
2. Neurologic emergencies must be considered as a cause for acute urinary retention, and a neurologic exam including an assessment of rectal tone should be considered. Other causes include obstructive etiology, infectious and inflammatory causes, medication induced, or traumatic.
3. Urethral catheterization is the first-line treatment for acute urinary retention (never force a catheter if difficulty encountered). This is followed by treatment of the underlying cause(s).
4. Obtain serum chemistry, urinalysis, urine culture, urine electrolytes, urine creatinine, and urine osmolality in a patient with urinary retention to assess for prerenal causes of decreased urine output or consequences of infection or retention.
5. Consider urologic consultation based on urinary retention in a patient with a known history of BPH.

DEBRIEF

This patient with a known history of BPH developed anuria from acute urinary retention due to cystitis. Typical symptoms of acute urinary retention include sudden onset lower abdominal pain and no urine output. It is possible, but less likely, that acute urinary retention will present as an acute kidney injury as the only presenting feature.

Anuria can be approached similarly to acute kidney injury. A standardized approach that considers prerenal, renal, and postrenal causes should be employed. Prerenal causes for anuria include decreased effective circulating volume (e.g., hypovolemia, congestive heart failure, sepsis), renal vasoconstriction (e.g., nonsteroidal anti-inflammatory drugs, angiotensin-converting enzyme inhibitors, hepato-renal syndrome), and large vessel disease (e.g., thrombosis, vasculitis, dissection). Renal etiologies include acute tubular necrosis, acute interstitial nephritis, small vessel disease and glomerulonephritis. A postrenal etiology, such as acute urinary retention, must be ruled out in acute onset anuria. Risk factors for developing acute urinary retention include older age (especially men), BPH, prostate cancer, urethral stricture, diabetes, bed rest, surgery, and certain medications. In contrast to acute urinary retention, chronic urinary retention develops over a long period, is painless, and may be associated with overflow incontinence.

When approaching a patient with anuria and a suspected postrenal etiology, a neurologic emergency must always be considered, and a complete neurologic assessment is warranted with subsequent imaging if suspecting a spinal cord lesion. A digital rectal exam to assess rectal tone is indicated in these cases. Signs and symptoms of prostatitis should be sought in males. In females, a pelvic exam to assess for prolapse is necessary. A complete blood count, blood chemistry, urinalysis, urine culture, and bladder ultrasound are required as part of the initial workup. Prostate-specific antigen is not generally measured in the acute setting of urinary retention as levels are often falsely elevated.

Prerenal (i.e., poor blood delivery to the glomeruli) causes of anuria should also be considered. After a volume assessment that suggests hypovolemia, a fluid challenge monitoring for improvement of urine output and creatinine can be performed to aid in the diagnosis. A low urine sodium and a fractional excretion of sodium greater than 2% supports a prerenal etiology. Hypercalcemia needs to be ruled out as it can result in hypovolemia and vasoconstriction. A complete medication review should be performed with temporary or permanent discontinuation of any medications that can lead to poor renal flow. Renal artery imaging can be considered when suspecting the less common cases of renal artery disease. Treatment of prerenal acute kidney injury involves treatment of the underlying cause that led to hypovolemia and restoration of euvolemia.

Once urinary retention is identified, urinary catheterization should be completed immediately to decompress the bladder. Identification and treatment of the underlying cause and removal of provocation factors should follow. In this case, treatment of the cystitis with appropriate antibiotics is crucial, in combination with treatment of the underlying BPH, which acted as a risk factor for acute urinary retention.

FURTHER READING

Hernandez DH, Tesouro RB, Castro-Diaz D. Urinary retention. *Urologia*. 2013;80(4):257–264.

Khastgir J, Klan A, Speakman M. Acute urinary retention: medical management and the identification of risk factors for prevention. *Nat Clin Pract Urol*. 2007;4(8):422–432.

Marshall JR, Haber J, Josephson EB. An evidence-based approach to emergency department management of acute urinary retention. *Emerg Med Pract*. 2014;16(1):1–24.

Selius BA, Subedi R. Urinary retention in adults: diagnosis and initial management. *Am Fam Physician*. 2008;77(5):643–650.

Verhamme KMC, Sturkenboom MCJM, Stricker BH, Bosch R. Drug-induced urinary retention: incidence, management and prevention. *Drug Safety*. 2008;31(5):373–388.

CHAPTER 44

FEVER

GLENN PATRIQUIN

SETTING

Acute Care Inpatient Ward

CHIEF COMPLAINT

Fever

HISTORY

An 81-year-old woman was admitted 6 days ago through the emergency department after a fall while bowling, having sustained a broken hip. Her management consists of open reduction and internal fixation on day 1, followed by titrating analgesics and physiotherapy prior to discharge. Overnight, she develops a fever of 38.1°C. She complains of a 1-day history of pelvic discomfort but denies shortness of breath, chest pain, abdominal or flank pain, and back pain. She has no hip pain or leg swelling. She has had an indwelling urethral catheter since admission.

She has hypertension, treated with enalapril, and diet-controlled diabetes. There is no contributory family history.

She is a retired teacher, who lives independently in her own house. She does not smoke, and rarely drinks alcohol.

PHYSICAL EXAMINATION

Vital signs: HR 110, BP 120/62, RR 20, SpO$_2$ 94% on room air, temp. 38.3°C.

Examination reveals a fit-looking older woman in no overt distress. There is no meningismus. She has normal heart sounds with no extra sounds or murmurs, and has no stigmata of infective endocarditis. Her lung sounds are clear except for fine bibasilar crackles. Her abdomen is soft, with suprapubic tenderness on deep palpation. A urethral catheter is connected to a closed system. She has no tenderness on percussion of her spine or costovertebral angles. Her surgical wound is closed without erythema or drainage. Her extremities are warm, with palpable pulses, and her lower limbs are nottender or swollen. She has one peripheral intravenous catheter on the dorsal hand which is noninflamed. Her neurological exam reveals normal power, tone, and coordination, and she is oriented to time and place.

DIFFERENTIAL DIAGNOSIS

1. Cather-associated urinary tract infection
2. Blood stream infection
3. Hospital-associated pneumonia
4. Surgical site infection
5. Venous thromboembolism

TESTS

Complete blood count: normal hemoglobin, hematocrit, and platelets. Elevated white blood cell count at 15.4×10^9/L.

Chemistry panel: normal sodium, potassium, chloride, bicarbonate, blood urea nitrogen, creatinine, and glucose.

Chest X-ray: plate-like atelectasis at bases bilaterally, but no consolidation or abnormalities of the cardiac silhouette.

Urinalysis: 150 white blood cells/hpf, trace blood; leukocyte esterase- and nitrite-positive.

CLINICAL COURSE

Based on the patient's history of new onset fever and pelvic discomfort in the setting of an indwelling urinary catheter, an infection from a urinary source was suspected. Prior to starting antibiotics, the urinary catheter was removed, and a mid-stream urine was sent for culture and sensitivities. The catheter was not replaced as it was deemed unnecessary. Two sets of blood cultures were obtained, and the patient was treated with intravenous antibiotics. Her empiric regimen was narrowed to specifically cover the isolate from her urine, 10^5 colony forming units (CFUs)/mL of *Escherichia coli*. Her fever and pelvic discomfort resolved over the following 24 hours. Her blood cultures were negative, and she completed a 7-day course of antibiotics.

KEY MANAGEMENT STEPS

1. Consideration of CAUTI in a patient with an indwelling catheter and signs or symptoms suggestive of infection.
2. Avoiding premature diagnostic closure by considering alternative diagnoses for fever in a hospitalized patient with urinary catheter and pyuria.
3. Obtaining midstream urine after removing the urinary catheter to guide antimicrobial management.
4. Recognizing that urinary catheters are risk factors for infections, should only be used with a clear indication, and for the shortest time necessary.

DEBRIEF

This patient had fever and pelvic discomfort due to CAUTI. Infections of the urinary tract are among the most common HAIs. Essentially all hospital-acquired UTIs are associated with urinary catheter use, an intervention that was used for over 20% of inpatients in a recent point-prevalence study in the United States.[1]

It is important to note that findings of bacteriuria and pyuria alone in this catheterized patient are not sufficient to make a diagnosis of CAUTI, and this may lead to premature diagnostic closure. Asymptomatic bacteriuria, present in more than 20% of women over 80 years old, does not require treatment, except for during pregnancy and prior to urologic instrumentation.

According to the Infectious Diseases Society of America,[2] a diagnosis of CAUTI is made based on:

- Indwelling urethral or suprapubic catheter, intermittent catheterization, or removal of a catheter within the previous 48 hours.
- Symptoms or signs compatible with urinary tract infection with no other identified source of infection.
- $\geq 10^3$ CFU/mL of ≥ 1 bacterial species in a single urine specimen.

Catheters should be used only for specific indications and should not be used for convenience in a patient who could otherwise void voluntarily as they are a risk factor for HAIs. The incidence of CAUTI increases with increasing number of days of urinary catheter use.[3] Clinicians should limit the use and duration of catheters, with daily reassessments, removing them as soon as they are no longer indicated.

The typical bacteria associated with CAUTI are members of the Enterobacteriaceae, such as *E. coli* and *Klebsiella*, as well as *Pseudomonas* and *Enterococcus spp*. Empiric treatment should be based on local susceptibility patterns and guidelines, and definitive treatment is based on antimicrobial susceptibility testing by the microbiology laboratory. The recommended treatment duration for CAUTI depends on the patient's initial response to therapy. For patients with prompt resolution of symptoms, seven days is the preferred duration; this can be extended to between 10 and 14 days in those with a delayed response, even after discontinuation of the catheter.

REFERENCES

1. Magill SS, Edwards JR, Bamberg W, et al. Multistate point-prevalence survey of health care–associated infections. *N Engl J Med.* 2014;370:1198–1208.
2. Hooton TM, Bradley SF, Cardenas DD, et al. Diagnosis, prevention, and treatment of catheter-associated urinary tract infections in adults: 2009 international clinical practice guidelines from the Infectious Diseases Society of America. *Clin Infect Dis.* 2010;50:625–663.
3. Pratt R, Polk BF, Murdock B, Rosner B. Risk factors for nosocomial urinary tract infection. *Am J Epidemiol.* 1986;124:977–985.

FURTHER READING

Hooton, TM. Nosocomial urinary tract infections. In: Mandell GL, Bennett JE, Dolin R, eds. *Mandell, Douglas, and Bennett's Principles and Practice of Infectious Diseases.* 7th ed. Philadelphia, PA: Churchill/Livingstone/Elsevier; 2010: 3725–3737.

Nicolle LE, Bradley S, Colgan R, Rice JC, Schaeffer A, Hooton TM. Infectious Diseases Society of America guidelines for the diagnosis and treatment of asymptomatic bacteriuria in adults. *Clin Infect Dis.* 2005;40:643–654.

CHAPTER 45

CHEST PAIN

ANDREW CADDELL

SETTING

Inpatient Medicine Ward

CHIEF COMPLAINT

Chest Pain

HISTORY

A 76-year-old male patient is postadmission day 4 for pneumonia. He had been improving and ambulating with physiotherapy. He has developed 30 minutes of retrosternal chest pain, associated with diaphoresis, nausea, and presyncope. It does not radiate, change with position, or worsen with inspiration. His fever on initial presentation has subsided. He denies shortness of breath, orthopnea, paroxysmal nocturnal dyspnea, and palpitations. His nurse notes his systolic pressure fell from 160 to 110 after being given a single nitroglycerin spray.

His history is significant for dyslipidemia and a "cardiac murmur," which was investigated years ago.

He is a lifelong nonsmoker. He has no significant alcohol consumption.

He denies family history of cardiac disease.

PHYSICAL EXAMINATION

Vital signs: HR 110, BP 110/90 (bilaterally), RR 18, SpO$_2$ 98% on room air, temp. 36.8°C.

Examination reveals an elderly gentleman in no acute distress. His head and neck examination is normal. His peripheral pulse is normal, although he has a brachioradial delay. His central pulse is delayed and weak. His jugular venous pressure is 2 cm above the sternal angle with normal waveform. His precordium has a sustained apical impulse but is otherwise normal. He has a normal S1 and soft S2. There is a loud III/VI systolic ejection murmur that radiates to the carotids. It is not accentuated in the left lateral decubitus position. It increases with a Valsalva maneuver. There are no extra heart sounds. His lungs have inspiratory crackles to the left base. His abdomen is benign. He has trace lower extremity edema bilaterally with good peripheral pulses. His extremities are warm and well-perfused.

DIFFERENTIAL DIAGNOSIS

1. Aortic stenosis
2. Hypertrophic cardiomyopathy
3. Cardiac ischemia
4. Congestive heart failure
5. Resolving pneumonia
6. Gastroesophageal reflux disease
7. Pulmonary embolism
8. Aortic dissection

TESTS

High sensitivity troponin T: 30 ng/L (baseline 30 ng/L; N <14 ng/L).

Complete blood count: normal hemoglobin, hematocrit, white blood cell count and platelets.

Chemistry panel: normal sodium, potassium, chloride, bicarbonate, blood urea nitrogen, creatinine, and glucose.

Electrocardiogram: Figure 45.1.

Chest X-ray: Resolving left lower lobe pneumonia.

CLINICAL COURSE

Based on the history and examination the patient was placed on a cardiac monitor, intravenous access was obtained, and transitioned to a unit with higher monitoring. Due to the presumed severe aortic stenosis, very cautious use of low-dose intravenous nitrates was given, in combination with low-dose fentanyl, until he was pain free. Serial electrocardiogram failed to demonstrate ischemic changes. Serial troponins remained 30.

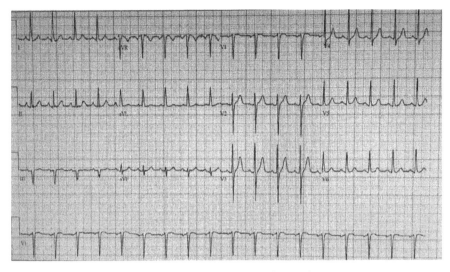

FIGURE 45.1 Electrocardiogram. Sinus tachycardia with no ischemic changes.

An urgent echocardiogram was completed the next morning. It demonstrated severe aortic stenosis with a peak velocity of 4.5 msec, mean gradient of 50 mm Hg, and valve area 0.86 cm^2. He had preserved left ventricular systolic function and moderate concentric left ventricular hypertrophy.

With a new diagnosis of symptomatic severe aortic stenosis, cardiology was consulted, and he underwent inpatient cardiac catheterization. It demonstrated no significant fixed coronary artery disease. An uncomplicated aortic valve replacement was done by cardiovascular surgery the following week.

KEY MANAGEMENT STEPS

1. Generate a differential diagnosis for an adult patient with chest pain.
2. Recognize physical exam findings of aortic stenosis and assess severity.
3. Be cautious with the use of vasodilators in patients with severe aortic stenosis.
4. Appropriate consultation with cardiology/cardiovascular surgery for valve replacement.

DEBRIEF

This patient was experiencing discomfort related to his severe aortic stenosis (AS). Typical symptoms of severe AS include chest pain, heart failure symptoms (dyspnea, orthopnea, paroxysmal nocturnal dyspnea), and presyncope/syncope.[1] Chest pain can be from underlying ischemic heart disease. In the absence of significant coronary artery disease, another cause of chest pain includes increased oxygen demand secondary to compression of the coronary arteries from increased left ventricular muscle mass and increasing oxygen demand. Also, shortened diastole from tachycardia can reduce coronary perfusion and result in chest pain.

Aortic stenosis causes narrowing of the aortic valve. It is commonly caused by congenital valve abnormities (i.e., bicuspid aortic valve), progressive degenerative calcification of the valve, or rheumatic fever. As the stenosis of the valve worsens, the pressure gradient between the left ventricle and aorta is increased to maintain forward flow. The increased pressure generated in the left ventricle leads to compensatory concentric hypertrophy.

Patients develop symptoms at varying degrees of stenosis. In general, symptoms don't begin until the stenosis is severe (defined as an aortic valve area <1 cm^2, maximum aortic transvalvular velocity ≥4 msec, or mean pressure gradient ≥40 mm Hg). Physical exam findings of AS may be present regardless of severity of AS. A 1997 review of physical exam findings found the following to have the highest positive likelihood factors[2]:

1. Slow rate of rise of the carotid pulse
2. Mid- to late peak intensity of the murmur
3. Decreased intensity of the second heart sound

Medical management of symptomatic AS is challenging. In the presence of the fixed outlet obstruction of AS, vasodilators (such as nitroglycerin) must be used with caution. Because the cardiac output is limited by the obstruction, vasodilation can lead to a precipitous drop in systolic blood pressure, as seen in the previously described case.[3] The vasodilation can be exaggerated in patients who use nitroglycerin after exercise, as exercise also causes vasodilation. Similarly, beta blockers (reducing contractility) and diuretics (reducing preload) should also be used with caution as they can cause hypotension. All changes should be small and incremental to avoid acute worsening.

The definitive management of AS is surgical. In general, surgery is indicated if the patient has any of the following[4]:

1. Symptomatic severe AS
2. Asymptomatic, very severe AS
3. Asymptomatic, severe AS undergoing another cardiovascular surgery (e.g., valve surgery, coronary artery bypass graft)
4. Severe AS with a reduced left ventricle ejection fraction (<50%)

Among frail patients, transcatheter aortic valve implantation (TAVI) is a reasonable alternative to open surgery where a bioprosthetic valve is placed via catheter over the native valve. TAVI has shown similar results to surgical interventions, and better results than medical therapy alone, in patients who are at high[5] and intermediate[6] surgical risk. The decision between TAVI or surgical aortic valve replacement is a complex one, typically involving interventional cardiology, cardiovascular surgery, radiology, and, in some cases, geriatrics.

REFERENCES

1. Aortic stenosis: MSD manual professional version. September 2016. http://www.msdmanuals.com/professional/cardiovascular-disorders/valvular-disorders/aortic-stenosis.
2. Etchells E, Bell C, Robb K. Does this patient have an abnormal systolic murmur? *J Am Med Assoc.* 1997;277(7):564–571.

3. Medical management of symptomatic aortic stenosis. UpToDate. August 12, 2015. https://www.uptodate.com/contents/medical-management-of-symptomatic-aortic-stenosis?source=search_result&search=aortic%20stenosis&selectedTitle=3~150.

4. Jamieson WR, Cartier PC, Allard M, et al. Surgical management of valvular heart disease 2004. *Can J Cardiol.* 2004;20(Suppl E):7E–120E.

5. Smith CR, Leon MB, Mack MJ, et al. Transcatheter versus surgical aortic-valve replacement in high-risk patients. *N Engl J Med.* 2011;364(23):2187–2198.

6. Leon MB, Smith CR, Mack MJ, et al. Transcatheter or surgical aortic-valve replacement in intermediate-risk patients. *N Engl J Med.* 2016; 374(17):1609–1620.

FURTHER READING

O'Gara PT, Loscalzo J. Aortic valve disease. In: Kasper D, Fauci A, Hauser S, Longo D, Jameson J, Loscalzo J, eds. *Harrison's Principles of Internal Medicine.* 19th ed. New York, NY: McGraw-Hill; 2014.

ABDOMINAL PAIN

RACHELLE BLACKMAN

SETTING

Inpatient Medicine Ward

CHIEF COMPLAINT

Abdominal Pain

HISTORY

A 34-year-old male with known Crohn's disease is admitted to the medical teaching inpatient floor with a 3-day history of epigastric abdominal cramping with 5 to 8 bloody bowel movements per day. He is started on intravenous (IV) hydration and steroids for an inflammatory bowel disease (IBD) flare. Today on post admission day 2, he complains of acute central abdominal pain with new nausea and vomiting. He denies fever. Bowel movements are less frequent, but they are still bloody.

He was a previous smoker with a 5 pack-year history but quit 2 years ago.

His mother has ulcerative colitis.

PHYSICAL EXAMINATION

Vital signs: HR 105, BP 115/80, RR 18, SpO$_2$ 98% on room air, temp. 37°C.

Examination reveals a thin male in distress. Head and neck exam is normal with a jugular venous pressure of 2 cm. His lungs are clear bilaterally with good air movement. Cardiovascular examination reveals a sinus rate and rhythm without murmur, rubs, or gallop. His abdomen is mildly distended with generalized tenderness to light and deep palpation in all four abdominal quadrants. There is mild guarding and rebound tenderness. There are no palpable masses. There is no hepatomegaly, splenomegaly, or signs of chronic liver disease. His extremities are warm with palpable pulses. Neurological examination is grossly normal.

DIFFERENTIAL DIAGNOSIS

1. Small or large bowel obstruction/perforation
2. Crohn's flare
3. Acute splanchnic venous or arterial thrombosis
4. Ileus
5. Diverticulitis

TESTS

Complete blood count: hemoglobin 100 g/L (120–160 g/L), white blood cell count 12×10^9/L ($4–12 \times 10^9$/L), platelets 500×10^9/L ($150–350 \times 10^9$/L) with a low hematocrit.

Chemistry: lactate 2.5 mmol/L (0.0–2.0 mmol/L), pH acidotic with bicarbonate of 18 mmol/L (22–30 mmol/L), normal alkaline phosphatase, alanine aminotransferase, aspartate aminotransferase, amylase, bilirubin, electrolytes, blood urea nitrogen, creatinine, and glucose.

Abdominal X-ray: new onset ileus.

Computed tomography (CT) abdomen: Figure 46.1.

CLINICAL COURSE

Based on worsening abdominal tenderness and new vomiting despite treatment, a CT scan was ordered, demonstrating acute symptomatic inferior mesenteric vein thrombosis with ileus. Due to ongoing gastrointestinal bleeding, IV unfractionated heparin (UFH) was initiated and general surgery were consulted. Considering symptoms of ileus, patient was placed on restricted nil per os diet with IV hydration and pain control. His abdominal symptoms improved over the next few days with anticoagulation alone.

KEY MANAGEMENT STEPS

1. Consideration of splanchnic vein thrombosis (SVT) in the differential diagnosis of a patient with IBD and acute onset abdominal pain.

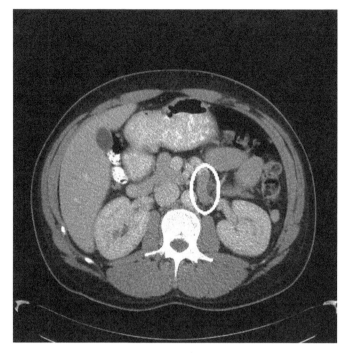

FIGURE 46.1 Computed tomography abdomen. Note inferior mesenteric vein (IMV) thrombosis (circled), as evident by hypodense material within the vein and distension of the IMV.

2. Obtaining a serum lactate and an abdominal X-ray as part of the initial workup in patients who may have bowel ischemia.

3. Consideration of advanced imaging modalities if suspicious for mesenteric thrombosis. CT scan allows for diagnosis of SVT and investigates for other causes.

4. Initiation of anticoagulation in the setting of acute symptomatic SVT, with short acting UFH as treatment if there is potential for abdominal surgery or if the patient is at high risk for bleeding.

5. Early consultation to general surgery if there are concerns for bowel ischemia based on CT findings and blood work.

DEBRIEF

This patient developed acute worsening abdominal pain in the setting of an active IBD flare, due to acute SVT of the inferior mesenteric vein. Symptoms of SVT can be variable, from asymptomatic to acute abdominal pain, nausea, vomiting, and/or gastrointestinal bleeding, depending on the timing and extent of thrombus.

SVT is a rare presentation, affecting up to 2% of thrombosis diagnoses annually. It includes thrombosis of the mesenteric veins, splenic vein, portal veins, and hepatic venous thrombosis (Budd–Chiari syndrome). Most are diagnosed incidentally on imaging; however, complications can be severe including splenic or bowel ischemia.[1]

Many cases are idiopathic. Risk factors for SVT have been identified as the following[2-4]:

- Solid tumor (22%–27%) or hematologic malignancy (i.e., myeloproliferative neoplasm)
- Liver cirrhosis
- Intra-abdominal sepsis
- IBD
- Diverticulitis
- Local abdominal surgery or trauma
- Thrombophilic conditions

When SVT is considered, it is important to obtain complete blood count, electrolytes, liver panel, and blood gas for lactate and pH. Abdominal imaging can begin with X-ray; however, further imaging such as CT scan with contrast should be considered if there is any concern for bowel ischemia.

The CHEST guidelines recommend at least 3 months anticoagulation therapy for all acute and symptomatic SVT, so long as thrombocytopenia and/or active gastrointestinal bleeding is under control.[5] Prolonged treatment may be considered if there are ongoing thrombotic risk factors, such as malignancy. For asymptomatic SVT diagnoses, avoid anticoagulation unless:

- Extensive and acute thrombosis
- Progression of thrombosis on follow up imaging
- Ongoing malignancy or chemotherapy

Anticoagulant choice as per CHEST guidelines:

- UFH: consider if unstable, high bleeding risk, or requiring procedures that need immediate breaks in therapy
- Low molecular weight heparin: consider if malignancy related thrombosis, liver disease, or thrombocytopenia
- Vitamin K antagonist
- Direct oral anticoagulants: no strong clinical evidence to support. Therefore, any use would be off-label.

REFERENCES

1. Cohen, D. Splanchnic venous thrombosis: ACP Expert Analysis. *ACP Hospitalist*. October 2016. https://acphospitalist.org/archives/2016/10/splanchnic-venous-thrombosis.htm
2. Ageno W, Beyer-Westendor J, Garcia D, et al. Guidance for the management of venous thromboembolism in unusual sites. *J Thromb Thrombolysis*. 2016;41:129–143.
3. Riva N, Donadini M, Dentali F, et al. Clinical approach to splanchnic vein thrombosis: risk factors and treatment. *Thromb Res*. 2012;130(Suppl 1):S1–S3.
4. Acosta S and Björck M. Mesenteric vascular disease: venous thrombosis. In: Coronenwett J, Johnston K, Rutherford R, eds. *Rutherford's Vascular Surgery*. 8th ed. Philadelphia, PA: Saunders/Elsevier; 2014: 2414–2420.
5. Kearon C, Akl E, Comerota A, et al. Antithrombotic therapy for VTE disease: antithrombotic therapy and prevention of thrombosis, 9th ed: American College of Chest Physicians evidence-based clinical practice guidelines. *CHEST*. 2012;141(Suppl 2):e419S–e494S.

CHAPTER 47

ALTERED MENTAL STATUS

JACLYN LEBLANC

SETTING

Inpatient Medicine Ward

CHIEF COMPLAINT

Altered Mental Status

HISTORY

A 76-year-old female was admitted to hospital a week ago for pneumonia requiring oxygen and intravenous antibiotics. She initially improved but developed vomiting and diarrhea 2 days after admission. Clostridium difficile was ruled out; dimenhydrinate was added for symptom relief. On day 4, she developed new intermittent confusion, which was felt to be secondary to dimenhydrinate, and it was stopped the following day. The vomiting and diarrhea persisted, as did her confusion, and the patient has had little oral intake in the last week. She completed her 7-day course of antibiotics last evening.

Today, on day 8, she was found to be quite somnolent. Approximately 1 hour later, she seized for 2 minutes. She has no fever or chills. Current medications include amlodipine and enoxaparin 40 mg subcutaneously every 24 hours.

She has a past medical history of hypertension.

She is a lifelong nonsmoker. She consumes 1 glass of wine per night at home.

Family history is noncontributory.

PHYSICAL EXAMINATION

Vital signs: HR 112, BP 90/60, RR 25, SpO_2 95% on room air, temp. 35.8°C, weight 70 kg.

Examination reveals a frail female. Head and neck exam shows very dry mucous membranes, and the jugular venous pulse is not visible. Neck is supple with no meningismus. The axillae are dry, and she is noted to have poor skin turgor. Lungs are clear bilaterally with good air entry. Cardiac sounds are normal with no murmurs or extra sounds heard. There is no peripheral edema. Abdominal exam is unremarkable. There is no costovertebral angle tenderness. Glasgow Coma Scale score is currently 9 (E2V3M4). Neurologic exam reveals no focal deficits.

DIFFERENTIAL DIAGNOSIS OF ALTERED MENTAL STATUS

1. D—drugs (anticholinergics, opiates, benzodiazepines).
2. I—infections (sepsis, pneumonia, urinary tract infections, skin and soft tissue infections).
3. M—metabolic (electrolyte abnormalities, hypo or hyperglycemia).
4. S—structural (stroke, subdural hematoma).

TESTS

Most recent laboratory investigations are from admission day 3, notable for a resolving leukocytosis. Her sodium was 135 mmol/L that day. Repeated values now show:

Complete blood count: normal white blood cell count, platelets, and hemoglobin.
Chemistry panel: sodium 109 mmol/L (135–145 mmol/L), chloride 80 mmol/L (96–106 mmol/L), creatinine 167 μmol/L (53–97 μmol/L).
Normal potassium, bicarbonate, and glucose
Urinalysis: no blood, nitrites, leukocyte esterase, or white blood cells.
Urine sodium: 15 mmol/L.
Urine osmolality: 200 mOsm/kg.
Serum osmolality: 260 mOsm/kg.
Chest X-ray: normal cardiac silhouette, clear lungs; no acute abnormality.
Computed tomography head: Nil acute.

CLINICAL COURSE

The patient was placed on nasal cannula oxygen and a cardiac monitor. Ringer's lactate solution was started at 1 L per hour. The patient was moved to the intermediate care unit, where she had another 2-minute seizure. Her labs returned shortly thereafter, and it was decided to correct her hyponatremia with 3% saline. She was given 150 mL of 3% saline over 20 minutes. Serum electrolytes were then drawn again 20 minutes following this infusion. Maintenance fluid of normal saline, based on a rate calculated to attain an increase of 6 mmol/L over 24 hours, was then initiated.

KEY MANAGEMENT STEPS

1. For patients with altered mental status and subsequent seizure, initial management is airway, breathing, and circulation (ABCs).
2. Consideration of a wide differential diagnosis is imperative in patients with altered mental status.
3. Evaluation of a patient with hyponatremia should include a serum and urine osmolality, urine sodium concentration, and a volume assessment.
4. Serum sodium should be corrected at a maximum rate of 8 to 10 mmol/L over 24 hours or 18 mmol/L over 48 hours to avoid cerebral pontine myelinolysis.
5. Hyponatremia should be corrected more acutely with hypertonic saline in patients who are seizing or in a coma.

DEBRIEF

This patient presented with altered mental status and subsequent seizures. The differential diagnosis for altered mental status is broad, but the DIMS mnemonic is helpful in directing the thought process. In terms of medications, dimenhydrinate was stopped days ago. New or worsening infection seemed less likely. Computer tomography head ruled out a structural cause. As seen from her laboratory investigations, her sodium was critically low.

The first step in evaluation of hyponatremia is to measure serum osmolality and determine if the patient has serum:

- Hyperosmolality with a resultant dilution effect (e.g., hyperglycemia or mannitol use).
- Iso-osmolality leading to pseudohyponatremia (secondary to elevated serum lipids or protein).
- Hypo-osmolality.

When serum hypo-osmolality is present, the next steps are measuring a urine osmolality and urine sodium while assessing volume status to aid in determination of etiology and subsequent treatment (see Figure 47.1).

In this case, the patient's serum shows hypo-osmolality, and she is hypovolemic on clinical examination. She has a urine sodium consistent with hypovolemic hyponatremia. The etiology is likely her recent vomiting and diarrhea. Based on history, our patient most likely has chronic hyponatremia (hyponatremia lasting for more than 48 hours).

Treatment of hypovolemic hyponatremia requires removal or amelioration of the underlying cause with fluid and sodium repletion. Normal saline is often the treatment of choice, unless there is an indication to raise the sodium level very quickly with 3% saline. The sodium

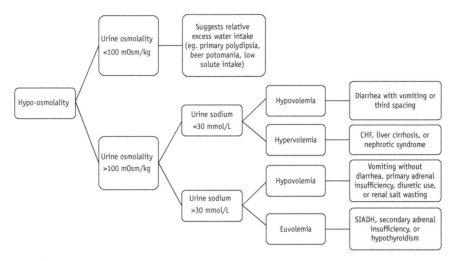

FIGURE 47.1 Hypo-osmolar hyponatremia flow chart.

CHF = congestive heart failure; SIADH = syndrome of inappropriate antidiuretic hormone.

deficit can be calculated and the rate of fluid adjusted to achieve a safe rate of sodium correction (Adrogué and Madias formula).

In patients who are acutely seizing or have severe neurologic symptoms, the sodium level may be increased by 4 to 6 mmol/L over 1 to 2 hours. Increases in sodium should not exceed a maximum of 8 to 10 mmol/L in 24 hours or 18 mmol/L in 48 hours due to the risk of osmotic pontine demyelination; ideally, this would be 4 to 6 mmol/L in 24 hours. Serum sodium should be monitored every 2 to 6 hours during replacement to avoid overcorrection.

Indications for 3% saline replacement in hyponatremia include seizures, severe confusion, coma, or signs of brainstem herniation. While an infusion of the fluid can be used, bolus dosing is also safe and has been endorsed in expert consensus guidelines.[1] This entails a 100 to 150 mL bolus of 3% saline over 10 to 20 minutes, which should raise serum sodium concentration by 2 to 3 mmol/L. Serum sodium should be checked again 20 minutes after the infusion. The 3% saline bolus may be repeated if required.

REFERENCE

1. Moritz ML, Ayus JC. 100 cc 3% sodium chloride bolus: a novel treatment for hyponatremic encephalopathy. *Metab Brain Dis.* 2010;25:91–96.

FURTHER READING

Mount D. Fluid and electrolyte disturbances. In: Kasper D, Fauci A, Hauser S, Longo D, Jameson JL, Loscalzo J, eds. *Harrison's Principles of Internal Medicine.* 19th ed. New York, NY: McGraw Hill; 2015. http://accessmedicine.mhmedical.com/content.aspx?bookid=1130&sectionid=79726591. Accessed July 09, 2018.

Spasovski G, Vanholder R, Allolio B, et al. Clinical practice guideline on diagnosis and treatment of hyponatraemia. *Nephrol Dial Transplant.* 2014;29(Suppl 2):i1–i39.

Verbalis JG, Goldsmith SR, Greenberg A, et al. Diagnosis, evaluation, and treatment of hyponatremia: expert panel recommendations. *Am J Med.* 2013;126:S1–S42.

LOW BLOOD PRESSURE

SCOTT LEE

SETTING

Inpatient Medicine Ward

CHIEF COMPLAINT

Dizziness

HISTORY

A 47-year-old male is admitted to hospital overnight with a suspected upper gastrointestinal bleed (UGIB). He complains of a 2-day history of black tarry stool. He admits to taking nonsteroidal anti-inflammatory drugs multiple times per day for the last 2 weeks due to worsening knee pain. He describes feeling tired but denies shortness of breath, chest pain, presyncope, or syncope. The gastroenterology (GI) service is consulted, and it is felt that endoscopy could wait until the next morning. The patient is started on a pantoprazole infusion.

Early the next morning, he feels dizzy and is noted to be hypotensive. He then begins to pass hematochezia and has an episode of hematemesis.

He has a past medical history of dyslipidemia, hypertension, transient ischemic attack, and osteoarthritis. He is managed on a statin, angiotensin converting enzyme-inhibitor, and aspirin. He does not take iron, bismuth, or Pepto-Bismol.

He is an active smoker with a 20 pack-year history and drinks 15 beer per week.

He denies family history of bowel or liver disease.

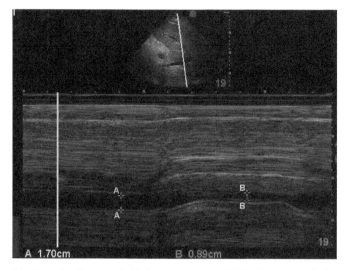

FIGURE 48.1 Bedside M-mode ultrasound of inferior vena cava (IVC). Note the variation in diameter of the IVC on respiration. It is greater than 40%, suggesting that the hypotensive patient is fluid responsive. Ideally, the IVC diameter should be assessed 2 to 3 cm caudal to the right atrial junction when using M-mode to ensure that the same area of the IVC is being measured during inspiration and expiration. If movement hinders this, simply follow the IVC through a respiratory cycle in 2D mode and measure the smallest and largest diameters for comparison.

PHYSICAL EXAMINATION

Vital signs: HR 128, BP 85/57, RR 27, SpO_2 95% on room air, temp. 37.2°C.

Examination reveals a well-nourished, but diaphoretic male in obvious distress. He is alert, oriented, and responds appropriately. There is no asterixis. Examination of his head and neck reveals pallor with no evidence of parotid gland enlargement or scleral icterus. He has palpable, rapid radial pulses bilaterally. His jugular venous pressure is flat. Heart sounds are normal. His chest is clear bilaterally to the bases. There is no evidence of nailbed changes, palmar erythema, thenar or hypothenar atrophy, or spider angiomas. On inspection of his abdomen, it is not distended, and there is no fluid wave or shifting dullness. There is no organomegaly, and it is soft diffusely. Digital rectal exam reveals melena.

Figure 48.1 shows bedside M-mode ultrasound of inferior vena cava.

DIFFERENTIAL DIAGNOSIS

1. UGIB
   a. Variceal
   b. Nonvariceal
      i.   Peptic ulcer disease
      ii. Nonsteroidal anti-inflammatory drugs gastritis
      iii. Duodenitis
      iv. Dieulafoy lesion

2. Lower GI bleed
    a. Diverticular
    b. Polyp
    c. Angiodysplasia

TESTS

Complete blood count: hemoglobin 68 g/L (110 g/L on admission), white blood cell count normal, platelets 175×10^9/L.

Chemistry panel: normal sodium, potassium, chloride, bicarbonate. Urea 18 mmol/L (2.5–7.0 mmol/L), creatinine 88 µmol/L (50–90 µmol/L).

Coagulation: normal international normalized ratio and partial thromboplastin time.

Type and screen completed.

CLINICAL COURSE

The patient has 2 large-bore intravenous (IV) lines placed in his antecubital fossae. He was placed on a cardiac monitor. Two liters of Ringer's lactate solution and 2 units of packed red blood cells were administered. Additionally, he was given a bolus of 80 mg IV pantoprazole and started on an infusion again at 8 mg/hr. Due to his alcohol history and possible cirrhosis, he received a bolus of octreotide followed by an infusion and ceftriaxone. Given his rapid clinical deterioration, the intensive care unit was consulted for assistance in management. He required ongoing hemodynamic support and a massive transfusion protocol was activated. Ultimately, the patient stabilized and underwent gastroscopy, which revealed a large duodenal ulcer with visible oozing of blood. This was treated endoscopically. The octreotide drip was stopped as there were no varices. The pantoprazole drip was continued for 72 hours postintervention, and he was transitioned to oral pantoprazole.

KEY MANAGEMENT STEPS

1. Obtain at least 2 large-bore IVs early with prompt initiation of fluids and blood products in a bleeding patient.
2. Prompt administration of pantoprazole and early investigations including blood type, cross match, and coagulation studies.
3. Consider empiric treatment with octreotide in those patients at risk of having varices.
4. Appropriate early consultation of intensive care unit and GI in patients with brisk GI bleeds.

DEBRIEF

This patient was experiencing a brisk UGIB, caused by a duodenal ulcer and an oozing vessel. Typical symptoms of UGIB include shortness of breath, presyncope, syncope, hematemesis, melena, and bright red blood per rectum.

Initial management includes rapidly assessing the differential diagnosis of hypotension. A broad approach to this is to evaluate for cardiogenic (e.g., acute ventricular or valvular dysfunction), hypovolemic (e.g., dehydration, bleeding), obstructive (e.g., massive pulmonary embolism, tension pneumothorax, cardiac tamponade), and distributive (e.g., sepsis, spinal shock) causes. In our case, the diagnosis is hypovolemic shock secondary to active GI bleeding. This patient's bedside ultrasound of his inferior vena cava demonstrated collapsibility of more than 40%, suggesting fluid responsiveness.[1] Therapy involves stabilization of hemodynamics with IV fluids, blood, pantoprazole, and possibly vasopressors. If liver disease is suspected, it is reasonable to initiate therapy with octreotide in case of a variceal bleed and a third-generation cephalosporin for infectious prophylaxis.

To help differentiate an UGIB from a lower GI bleed, there are pertinent clues both on laboratory investigations and physical exam.[2] The presence of melena on physical exam is associated with a positive likelihood ratio (LR) of 25 for an upper gastrointestinal bleed (UGIB). Other helpful signs are nasogastric lavage for blood or coffee emesis, previous UGIB, and a serum blood urea nitrogen (mg/dL): creatinine (mg/dL) ratio >30. Clots in the patient's stool significantly decrease the likelihood of an UGIB.

There are various scoring systems to grade the severity of a GI bleed. One common scoring system is the Glasgow-Blatchford Bleeding score. A patient with a score greater than 0 should be considered high risk and warrants medical intervention with endoscopy. Severe UGIBs are considered those that require transfusion or intervention endoscopically, radiologically, or surgically. A history of cirrhosis, malignancy, or syncope, and findings of tachycardia, hypotension, nasogastric lavage of red blood, shock, and a hemoglobin of less than 80 g/L increase the likelihood of a severe UGIB.[2]

When considering blood transfusions in actively bleeding patients, it is important to note that the initial hemoglobin may be an overestimate, and the severity may not become apparent until fluid resuscitation has begun. In choosing a transfusion threshold, a restrictive strategy of using a hemoglobin threshold of 70 g/L versus a more liberal 90 g/L has been studied.[3] A restrictive transfusion threshold in patients with an acute UGIB significantly improved survival over a liberal threshold. Patients experiencing massive exsanguinating bleeds were excluded, however. There is a paucity of data in this group of patients, and clinical judgement regarding transfusion is required.

REFERENCES

1. Bentzer P, Griesdale DE, Boyd J, MacLean K, Sirounis D, Ayas NT. Will this hemodynamically unstable patient respond to a bolus of intravenous fluids? *J Am Med Assoc*. 2016;316(12):1298–1309.
2. Srygley, D, Gerardo CJ, Tran T, Fisher DA. Does this patient have a severe upper gastrointestinal bleed? *J Am Med Assoc*. 2012;307(10):1072–1079.
3. Villanueva C, Colomo A, Bosch A, et al. Transfusion strategies for acute upper gastrointestinal bleeding. *New Eng J Med*. 2013;368(1):11–21.

FURTHER READING

Del Valle J. Peptic ulcer disease and related disorders. In: Kasper D, Fauci A, Hauser S, Longo D, Jameson J, Loscalzo J, eds. *Harrison's Principles of Internal Medicine.* 19th ed. New York, NY: McGraw-Hill; 2014.

Laine L, Jense DM. Management of patients with ulcer bleeding. *Am J Gastroenterol.* 2012;107:345–360.

BLISTERING RASH

ASHLEY SUTHERLAND

SETTING

Internal Medicine Ward

CHIEF COMPLAINT

Painful Rash

HISTORY

An 80-year-old male was admitted to the internal medicine ward with a 4-day history of diarrhea. On admission 1 week ago, he was dehydrated and hypotensive, but this resolved with intravenous fluids. He remains admitted to the hospital for rehabilitation with physiotherapy to return him to his normal functional baseline.

The patient now has a 4-day history of a burning and tingling sensation across one side of his back. A blistering rash, localizing to his back where he was complaining of pain, began 2 days ago. He otherwise has been feeling systemically well with no fevers or chills. The rash is extremely painful, and he has not found anything that improves the pain. It has not been spreading anywhere else on his body.

He has no history of significant skin disease other than chicken pox as a young child.

He takes no medications regularly and has no known medication allergies, and there is no family history of skin disease.

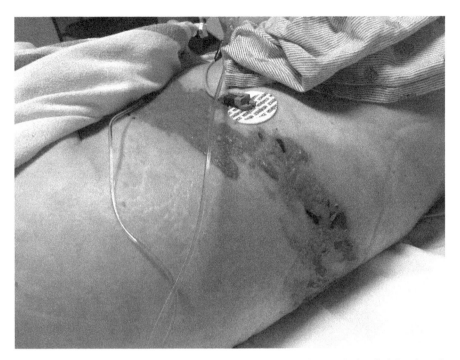

FIGURE 49.1 Skin eruption. Painful vesiculobullous eruption on a background of well-defined erythema that is confined to a single dermatome on the left back and flank.

PHYSICAL EXAMINATION

Vital signs: HR 75, BP 134/78, RR 18, SpO$_2$ 97% on room air, temp. 36.9°C.

Examination reveals a healthy-appearing elderly male in no significant distress. Head and neck exam is unremarkable. Cardiovascular exam reveals normal S$_1$ and S$_2$ heart sounds with no murmurs or extra heart sounds. Respiratory exam demonstrates normal breath sounds bilaterally with no crackles or wheezes. Abdomen is soft and nontender. Skin exam reveals well-defined erythema with overlying intact vesicles filled with cloudy fluid. There is also serous, purulent, and hemorrhagic crusting present on some of the lesions. The eruption is confined to the skin overlying the left T10 dermatome and stops abruptly at the midline. There are similar coalescing vesicles extending over the left flank on to the abdomen, also along the T10 dermatome distribution. It does not cross midline. The skin is tender to palpation over this eruption. Mucosal membranes are not involved.

Figure 49.1 shows skin eruption.

DIFFERENTIAL DIAGNOSIS

1. Herpes zoster
2. Varicella zoster
3. Herpes simplex virus (HSV)

4. Drug eruption such as Stevens Johnson syndrome/toxic epidermal necrolysis (SJS/TEN)

TESTS

Complete blood count: normal white blood cell count, hemoglobin, and platelets.
Chemistry panel: normal sodium, potassium, bicarbonate, blood urea nitrogen, creatinine, and glucose.

A vesicle was deroofed and swabs were sent:

HSV polymerase chain reaction (PCR): negative for HSV-1 and HSV-2.
Varicella zoster virus PCR: positive.

CLINICAL COURSE

Based on the clinical examination, the patient was empirically started on oral valacyclovir prior to the results of the PCR being available. As the patient is not immunocompromised, airborne and contact precautions were not needed. The lesions were completely covered with nonadherent dressings until they became dry and crusted. The burning pain and associated skin eruption improved over the next week.

KEY MANAGEMENT STEPS

1. Recognition of herpes zoster as the cause of a painful vesiculobullous eruption occurring in a dermatomal distribution.
2. Rule out severe drug reaction, such as SJS/TEN in any bullous condition, especially in the context of painful skin.
3. Initiation of antiviral treatment in patients within 72 hours of the onset of the cutaneous eruption to prevent postherpetic neuralgia. Also consider starting antivirals in those with ongoing new vesicle formation even if it is greater than 72 hours since onset of eruption.
4. Institute airborne and contact precautions in an immunocompromised patient with herpes zoster until disseminated disease is ruled out.

DEBRIEF

This patient presented with an acute onset, painful vesiculobullous eruption in a dermatomal distribution. The diagnosis of herpes zoster (shingles) was made by the clinical presentation of a generally systemically well patient with painful erythema, vesicles, and crusting along a single dermatome in the setting of prior exposure to varicella zoster virus as a child.

Apart from herpes zoster, the differential diagnosis of a painful vesiculobullous eruption includes SJS/TEN. These conditions are classically caused by exposure to a medication rather than infection. Patients with SJS/TEN will typically be systemically unwell with widespread erythema, painful skin, and mucosal membrane involvement. HSV can present with similar clinical features to varicella zoster virus but would be unusual to be localized to a dermatomal distribution. Varicella zoster (chicken pox) is also not typically seen in a dermatomal distribution and presents as widespread pruritic vesicles on an erythematous base ("dew drops on a rose petal"). Dissemination of cutaneous herpes zoster may present in immunocompromised patients, such as those with hematologic malignancy or a solid organ transplant. These patients may present with a generalized painful vesicular eruption involving multiple dermatomes and crossing the midline. Patients with disseminated cutaneous zoster may also be at risk of developing visceral involvement of herpes zoster.

Airborne and contact precautions are required in the setting of disseminated herpes zoster infection until all lesions are dry and crusted. In localized herpes zoster, these precautions are only required in immunocompromised patients until disseminated zoster has been ruled out. The lesions should be completely covered, though, in localized herpes zoster.

Varicella zoster virus is the cause of both varicella zoster (chicken pox), as well as herpes zoster (shingles). Once a patient is exposed to varicella zoster virus, either through primary infection or varicella zoster vaccination, he or she is at risk of developing herpes zoster. Following exposure, the virus travels to the dorsal root ganglion where it becomes dormant. Reactivation of the virus can occur in the setting of stress, fever, radiation therapy, local trauma, or immunosuppression. The incidence of herpes zoster is believed to be 2.5 in 1,000 patients aged 20 to 50 years old, 5 in 1,000 in those 51 to 79 years old, and 10 in 1,000 patients over 80 years of age.

Herpes zoster occurring on the face can potentially lead to significant complications. Approximately 50% of patients with involvement of the ophthalmic branch of the trigeminal nerve (V1) with will have ocular involvement, which could result in scarring and visual loss. Lesions of herpes zoster on the nasal tip, also known as Hutchinson's sign, can indicate involvement of the V1 branch and warrants urgent ophthalmology consultation.

Treatment of uncomplicated herpes zoster with systemic antiviral medications is initiated with the goal of decreasing the duration and severity of the eruption. Antivirals can also reduce the risk of postherpetic neuralgia, which is the most common complication. Initiating treatment within 72 hours of the development of skin lesions is believed to be most effective in reducing postherpetic neuralgia; however, treating within 7 days has also shown beneficial effects. Postherpetic neuralgia is characterized by pain such as burning, stinging, or a stabbing sensation after the skin lesions have healed and can persist chronically.

FURTHER READING

Mendoza N, Madkan V, Sra K, Willison B, Morrison LK, Tyring S. Human herpesviruses. In: Bolognia J, ed. *Dermatology*. 3rd ed. Philadelphia, PA. Elsevier; 2012: 1321–1343.

Preventing varicella-zoster virus (VSV): transmission from zoster in healthcare settings. Centers for Disease Control and Prevention. May 1, 2014. https://www.cdc.gov/shingles/hcp/hc-settings.html

Tremaine AM, Bartlett B, Gewirtzman A, Tyring S. Herpes zoster. In: Lebwohl M, ed. *Treatment of Skin Disease Comprehensive Therapeutic Strategies*. 3rd ed. Philadelphia, PA. Saunders; 2010: 306–308.

CHAPTER 50

AGITATION

CHRISTOPHER J. M. GREEN

SETTING

Inpatient Medicine Floor

CHIEF COMPLAINT

Agitation

HISTORY

A 72-year-old male was found down in a public park early this morning. He was taken to the hospital and admitted with a right middle lobe pneumonia. Throughout the day, he was started on antibiotics and given intravenous fluids. He had recovered entirely from a cognitive standpoint, and his supplemental oxygen has been weaned from 4 to 2 L/min by nasal cannula.

His past medical history includes only anxiety. He is on no home medications. He is a current smoker and drinks 16 ounces of liquor per day.

Approximately 20 hours after being found, he becomes acutely agitated. For the past hour, the patient has been trying to get out of bed and leave the hospital. He is very angry and yelling at hospital staff. He states that he does not want to be in the hospital anymore and that his bed is infested with bed bugs, which are making it impossible for him to sleep.

PHYSICAL EXAMINATION

Vital signs: HR 95, BP 160/80, RR 18, SpO$_2$ 94% on 2 L/min oxygen, temp. 37.4°C.

He is sitting on the edge of the hospital bed with his sneakers on and a jacket on over his hospital gown. A nurse is at his side. He appears slightly under weight, fidgety, restless, and markedly diaphoretic. He often scratches at "bed bugs," which you are not able to see. When he speaks, he raises his voice and appears angry. He is oriented to the year and place but does not seem to understand the consequences of leaving hospital.

His pupils are slightly dilated. There is no ophthalmoplegia. He demonstrates grossly normal strength, sensation, reflexes, and tone in all extremities. A postural tremor is noted. Gait and balance appear normal.

Examination of cardiovascular system, lungs, and abdomen is consistent with a right middle lobe pneumonia but otherwise unremarkable.

DIFFERENTIAL DIAGNOSIS

1. Alcohol withdrawal (or other substance intoxication/withdrawal)
2. Delirium
3. Hepatic encephalopathy
4. Hypo/hyperglycemia
5. Dementia
6. Primary psychiatric illness
7. Central nervous system Infection

TESTS

Other than a point-of-care glucose test (glucose = 6.5 mmol/L) and an electrocardiogram (ECG; normal with no signs of ischemia), the patient refuses any additional testing. His admission investigations show the following:

Complete blood count: hemoglobin 105 g/L (120–160 g/L), mean corpuscular volume 110 fL (80–100 fL), white blood cells 14.1 × 10^9/L (4.0–12.0 × 10^9/L), platelets 150 × 10^9/L (150–350 × 10^9/L).

Chemistry panel: normal electrolytes, creatinine, urea, troponin, creatine kinase and glucose. Gamma-glutamyl transferase 60 U/L (0–49 U/L); alanine aminotransferase, aspartate aminotransferase, and alkaline phosphatase: normal. Albumin 30 g/L (35–50 g/L). International normalized ratio and bilirubin are normal.

ECG: normal.

Chest X-ray: right middle lobe pneumonia.

Computed tomography head: Figure 50.1.

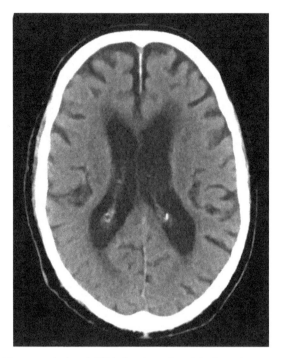

FIGURE 50.1 Computed tomography head. Mild atrophy and ventricular enlargement; otherwise, unremarkable.

CLINICAL COURSE

The patient's nurse convinced him to take a stat dose of sublingual lorazepam. The Clinical Institute Withdrawal Assessment for Alcohol (CIWA-Ar) scale was done every 2 hours, and additional lorazepam was given when the CIWA-Ar score was above 10. He was started on thiamine, a multivitamin, and intravenous fluids. Within a few hours, the patient's symptoms had markedly improved. Over the next 2 days, he was weaned off oxygen. He declined an offer for a supervised benzodiazepine taper or referral for further addiction management and was discharged home.

KEY MANAGEMENT STEPS

1. Considering the etiology of acute agitation before ordering sedatives.
2. Recognition of the signs and symptoms of alcohol withdrawal.
3. Administration of benzodiazepines using a symptom-triggered protocol in the setting of alcohol withdrawal.
4. Early administration of thiamine—ideally, prior to any glucose, but concurrently if there is symptomatic hypoglycemia.
5. Avoidance of medications that lower seizure threshold (e.g., antipsychotics).

DEBRIEF

This acutely agitated inpatient was experiencing symptoms of severe alcohol withdrawal. Acute agitation is a common problem seen on medical and surgical wards and has a broad differential diagnosis.[1] The key to identifying alcohol withdrawal is recognizing the distinct clinical syndrome occurring within the appropriate time frame and ruling out other potential diagnoses.

Alcohol withdrawal typically presents as a sympathomimetic toxidrome: patients may experience minor symptoms that include anxiety, tremor, diaphoresis, palpitations, headache, and nausea. Severe symptoms of withdrawal, which can occur in isolation, are hallucinations (typically visual, auditory, and tactile), withdrawal seizures, and delirium tremens. This constellation of symptoms is less common for other etiologies of inpatient delirium. In this patient, minor withdrawal symptoms combined with visual and tactile hallucinations raise the suspicion of alcohol withdrawal.

Most symptoms of withdrawal typically begin 6 to 48 hours after the patient's last alcoholic drink. An exception is the life-threatening syndrome of delirium tremens, which manifests in the 48- to 96-hour time frame. Symptoms beginning after these time frames are not consistent with a diagnosis of alcohol withdrawal. The patient in this case can be reasonably inferred to fall into this time frame.

A workup for other causes of delirium should be performed; however, treatment of alcohol withdrawal should not be delayed if suspicion is strong. Important considerations in the short-term include life-threatening causes of delirium such as hypo- or hyperglycemia, myocardial infarction, severe infection, and hepatic encephalopathy. In this case, normal blood glucose, ECG, and liver function tests make these alternative diagnoses less likely. The patient's pneumonia may be a contributing factor; however, the patient is not showing other signs of worsening infection (e.g., worsening hypoxemia, fever).

The cornerstone of alcohol withdrawal management is administration of benzodiazepines. Treatment protocols that trigger benzodiazepine dosing based on symptom severity (assessed using a tool such as the CIWA-Ar scale[2]) result in shorter hospital stays and lower cumulative benzodiazepine doses compared to a fixed dosing schedule with otherwise similar clinical outcomes. For this reason, symptom-triggered therapy is generally preferred. If symptoms continue to worsen on therapy, it is important to consider increasing the dose of benzodiazepine used. Refractory seizures or progression to delirium tremens should trigger transfer to an intensive care unit.[3-5]

Medications that lower the seizure threshold, most notably atypical antipsychotics (e.g., haloperidol), should be avoided in agitated patients when there is suspicion for alcohol withdrawal due to the elevated risk of seizures in this state.

Patients being treated for alcohol withdrawal are often nutritionally deficient. Due to a possible risk of iatrogenic Wernicke encephalopathy, patients should ideally receive parenteral thiamine before or concurrent to glucose administration. However, correction with glucose should not be delayed in the event of symptomatic hypoglycemic. General nutritional supplementation with a multivitamin, intravenous fluid repletion, and electrolyte replacement is advisable.

REFERENCES

1. Kalish VB, Gillham JE, Unwin BK. Delirium in older persons: evaluation and management. *Am Fam Physician*. 2014;90(3):150–158.

2. Sullivan JT, Sykora K, Schneiderman J, Naranjo CA, Sellers EM. Assessment of alcohol with-drawal: the revised clinical institute withdrawal assessment for alcohol scale (CIWA-Ar). *Addiction*. 1989;84(11):1353–1357.
3. Kosten TR, O'Connor PG. Management of drug and alcohol withdrawal. *New Engl J Med*. 2003;348(18):1786–1795.
4. Schuckit MA. Recognition and management of withdrawal delirium (delirium tremens). *New Engl J Med*. 2014;371(22):2109–2113.
5. Bernstein E, Bernstein JA, Weiner SG, D'Onofrio G. Substance use disorders. In: Tintinalli JE, Stapczynski J, Ma O, Yealy DM, Meckler GD, Cline DM, eds. *Tintinalli's Emergency Medicine: A Comprehensive Study Guide*. 8th ed. New York, NY: McGraw-Hill; 2016: 1976–1982.

DYSPNEA

MARKO BALAN

SETTING

Inpatient Medicine Ward

CHIEF COMPLAINT

Shortness of Breath

HISTORY

A 78-year-old female is admitted to the hospital inpatient unit with dehydration and weakness secondary to a urinary tract infection. She is treated with antibiotics and intravenous crystalloids at 200 mL/hour. On post-admission day 2, she develops increasing shortness of breath and orthopnea requiring urgent assessment. Currently, she denies chest pain, fever, cough, or recent vomiting. She does not report a previous history of shortness of breath occurring at rest.

The patient's medical history is significant for obesity, hypertension, diabetes mellitus type 2, and osteoarthritis of the knees.

She has never smoked and does not consume alcohol.

PHYSICAL EXAMINATION

Vital signs: HR 104 BPM, BP 166/88, RR 28, SpO_2 95% on FiO_2 35% by facemask, temp. 37.2°C.

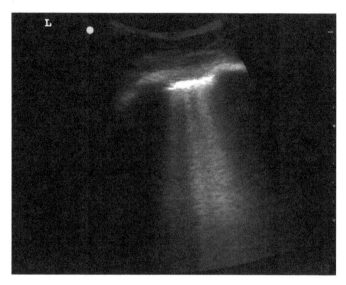

FIGURE 51.1 Lung ultrasound. Note hyperechoic B lines that extend from the pleural surface to the bottom of the image and obliterate A lines.

On examination, the patient is obese and appears unwell, in respiratory distress, and only able to answer in two- to three-word phrases. She is leaning forward, with increased work of breathing and using accessory muscles. Jugular venous pulsation is 6 cm above the sternal angle, and the central pulse is regular with normal volume and contour. Auscultation of the precordium reveals a normal first and second heart sound. A third heart sound is heard. There are no murmurs. Auscultation of the chest reveals bibasilar crackles. There is no wheeze. The abdomen is obese, soft, and nontender. There is no palpable organomegaly or lymphadenopathy. The extremities feel warm and pedal edema is noted extending up to both knees equally.

Point-of-care ultrasound examination of the lungs is seen in Figure 51.1. This figure is representative of the findings seen throughout both hemithoraces. Bedside echocardiography shows grossly normal left ventricular systolic function with no pericardial effusion. The inferior vena cava was 2.6 cm in diameter and did not show respiratory variation.

Lung ultrasound: Figure 51.1.

DIFFERENTIAL DIAGNOSIS

1. Congestive heart failure
2. Myocardial ischemia/acute coronary syndrome
3. Acute respiratory distress syndrome
4. Pulmonary embolism
5. Pulmonary aspiration
6. Allergic reaction/anaphylaxis

TESTS

Complete blood count: white blood cells 12.5×10^9/L ($4.5–11.0 \times 10^9$/L). Normal hemoglobin and platelet count.

Chemistry panel: normal sodium, potassium, chloride, and bicarbonate. Creatinine 115 µmol/L (49–90 µmol/L). Normal thyroid stimulating hormone.

Arterial blood gas: pH 7.42, PCO_2 34 mm Hg, PaO_2 63 mm Hg, and HCO_3 24 mmol/L.

Troponin I: 0.1 ng/mL (0–0.04 ng/mL).

N-terminal pro-brain natriuretic peptide (NT pro-BNP): 12,000 pg/mL (<300 pg/mL; 300–1,800 pg/mL consider age-stratified cut-points)

Electrocardiogram: Sinus rhythm with tachycardia.

Chest X-ray: normal cardiac silhouette, increased interstitial markings bilaterally, blunted costophrenic angles bilaterally.

CLINICAL COURSE

Based on her respiratory distress and need for cardiopulmonary monitoring, the patient was moved to an intermediate care unit while therapy was concurrently initiated. Noninvasive positive pressure ventilation was started to improve oxygenation and support the patient's increased work of breathing.

The intravenous fluid was stopped. Nitroglycerin intravenous infusion was initiated with close monitoring of the patient's blood pressure and for the development of side effects (hypotension, headache, and dizziness). Intravenous furosemide was administered, and a urinary catheter was inserted to monitor for a response.

Over the subsequent 12 hours, the patient was regularly reassessed and was found to have responded appropriately to the interventions. Her oxygen requirements decreased, allowing her to transition to nasal prongs. An additional furosemide intravenous dose was ordered and the nitroglycerin infusion was transitioned to a transdermal patch. Troponin I levels decreased on subsequent blood work. An echocardiogram was ordered to be completed prior to discharge from hospital.

KEY MANAGEMENT STEPS

1. Recognition of a patient's unstable and deteriorating respiratory status necessitating transfer to a monitored unit.
2. Urgent institution of pharmacologic therapies including diuresis and afterload reduction.
3. Rapid initiation of noninvasive ventilation to support patients with acute heart failure in respiratory distress.
4. Completion of workup to determine cause of acute heart failure (history, physical examination, thyroid stimulating hormone, serial electrocardiograms/troponin, echocardiogram).

5. Re-evaluation of patient to assess for response to therapies and consideration for need for further diuresis, afterload reduction, inotropic support, intubation, or urgent cardiology consultation.

DEBRIEF

In this case, the patient's dyspnea and orthopnea were most likely due to congestive heart failure, but it is important for the clinician to consider and evaluate patients for other common and life-threatening causes of dyspnea. This patient has several risk factors for heart failure, including diabetes, hypertension, obesity, and increased age. Other common risk factors for the development of heart failure are history of coronary artery disease, smoking, and valvular heart disease. The patient's concurrent infection and aggressive intravenous fluid resuscitation earlier in the admission may also have contributed to the patient developing congestive heart failure.

B lines on point-of-care ultrasound are thought to be due to increased lung density from interstitial edema, causing a distinct reverberation artifact. B lines are identified by the following characteristics[1,2]:

1. Discrete vertical hyperechoic reverberation artifacts.
2. Arise at the pleural line.
3. Continue to bottom of ultrasound screen without fading.
4. Obliterate A lines.
5. Move with the pleural line.

The presence of three or more B lines per longitudinal plane between two ribs is considered pathologic. Although a diffuse bilateral B line pattern can occur in pulmonary edema from congestive heart failure, it can also occur due to other diseases. These include pneumonia, pulmonary hemorrhage, atelectasis, pulmonary fibrosis, and acute respiratory distress syndrome. Thus, clinicians need to apply clinical judgement when interpreting their presence to determine their most likely etiology. Protocols have been developed in the assessment of acutely dyspneic patients using point-of-care ultrasound and have shown promise in their ability to determine the cause of respiratory failure (e.g., Bedside Lung Ultrasound in Emergency [BLUE] protocol).[3]

Although this patient's bloodwork is consistent with a presentation of congestive heart failure (increased BNP and troponin), one must also consider other causes of dyspnea that have similar biochemical abnormalities. For instance, advanced age, kidney disease, acute coronary syndrome, pulmonary embolism, and right heart failure can all cause elevations in BNP. Similarly, due to this patient's troponin elevation, one must be careful to rule out myocardial ischemia secondary to acute coronary syndrome as a precipitant or consequence of congestive heart failure since this would require additional treatment and potentially urgent invasive cardiology management.

Once the clinical diagnosis of congestive heart failure has been made, therapy should be initiated urgently. Diuresis, afterload reduction (particularly in hypertensive patients), respiratory support (supplemental oxygen and/or noninvasive positive pressure ventilation), and symptomatic treatments are the mainstays in therapy for patients with acute congestive heart failure. Early diuresis in patients with acute heart failure can lead to decreased mortality rates.[4] If patients are critically ill, they should be monitored closely for response to therapy as they may require mechanical ventilation, inotropic agents, or mechanical support.

REFERENCES

1. Volpicelli G, Elbarbary M, Blaivas M, et al. International evidence-based recommendations for point-of-care lung ultrasound. *Intensive Care Med.* 2012;38(4):577–591.
2. Dietrich CF, Mathis G, Blaivas M, et al. Lung B-line artefacts and their use. *J Thorac Dis.* 2016;8(6):1356–1365.
3. Lichtenstein DA. Lung ultrasound in the critically ill. *Ann Intensive Care.* 2014;9(4):1.
4. Matsue Y, Damman K, Voors AA, et al. Time-to-furosemide treatment and mortality in patients hospitalized with acute heart failure. *J Am Coll Cardiol.* 2017;69(25):3042–3051.

FURTHER READING

Lichtenstein DA, Mezière GA. Relevance of lung ultrasound in the diagnosis of acute respiratory failure. *Chest.* 2008;134(1):117–125.

Mehra MR. Heart failure: management. In: Kasper D, Fauci A, Hauser S, Longo D, Jameson J, Loscalzo J, eds. *Harrison's Principles of Internal Medicine.* 19th ed. New York, NY: McGraw-Hill; 2014. http://accessmedicine.mhmedical.com.ezproxy.library.dal.ca/content.aspx?bookid=1130&sectionid=79742558. Accessed July 03, 2018.

Wang CS, FitzGerald JM, Schulzer M, Mak E, Ayas NT. Does this dyspneic patient in the emergency department have congestive heart failure? *J Am Med Assoc.* 2005;294(15):1944–1956.

SECTION VI

PEDIATRIC CLINIC

JENNIFER SANDERS

RULE OUT SEPSIS IN INFANT

TEMIMA WALTUCH

SETTING

Pediatric Emergency Department

CHIEF COMPLAINT

Fever in Infant

HISTORY

A 7-week-old full-term girl presents to the emergency department with 2 days of subjective fevers. The infant was in her normal state of health until 2 days ago when her mother noticed she felt warm to the touch and was crying more than usual. The mother notes that she also has some nasal congestion but no cough or difficulty breathing. She has continued to tolerate breastfeeding well and has had 5 to 6 wet diapers/day. There is no associated vomiting, diarrhea, conjunctivitis, or rash. She has been receiving Tylenol every 6 hours for the past 24 hours. She has no recent travel or sick contacts, but she does attend daycare.

She was born full term by spontaneous vaginal delivery without complications. Maternal prenatal labs (group B *Streptococcus*, syphilis, rubella, HIV, chlamydia, and gonorrhea) were negative.

Newborn screen: normal.

PHYSICAL EXAMINATION

Vital signs:, HR 132, RR 26, BP 90/60, SpO$_2$ 99% on room air, temp. 38.4°C.

Examination reveals a well-appearing female sleeping comfortably in her mother's arms. Her anterior fontanelle is open, soft, and flat. Her lungs are clear bilaterally with good air movement, and her cardiac rate and rhythm are normal. No murmurs, rubs, or gallops are appreciated. Her abdomen is soft, nontender, and nondistended. She has good peripheral pulses, and her extremities are warm and well-perfused. Skin exam is normal without rashes or bruising. Neurologic examination reveals normal reflexes including Moro, suck, and Babinski. When awoken, she is comfortable in her mother's arms and is moving all 4 extremities spontaneously.

DIFFERENTIAL DIAGNOSIS

1. Viral illness
2. Urinary tract infection (UTI)
3. Bacteremia
4. Viral meningitis
5. Bacterial meningitis
6. Pneumonia
7. Nonaccidental trauma

TESTS

Complete blood count: hemoglobin: 14 g/L, hematocrit: 42%, platelets: 250 × 10^9/L, white blood cell count: 16.5 × 10^9/L.

Chemistry panel: sodium 141 mEq/L, potassium 4.2 mEq/L, chloride 102 mmol/L, bicarbonate 21 mmol/L, blood urea nitrogen 6 mg/dL, creatinine 0.3 mg/dL, and glucose 95 mg/dL.

Urinalysis: positive for leukocyte esterase and nitrites, >10 white blood cell count (WBC)/high power field (hpf), 5 red blood cell count/hpf; many bacteria.

Cerebrospinal fluid (CSF) studies: appearance, clear, WBC 2 cells/μL, red blood cell count 0 cells/μL, glucose 50 mg/dL, and protein 58 mg/dL.

Blood culture: pending.

Urine culture: pending.

CSF culture: pending.

CLINICAL COURSE

Based on the patient's age (>28 days) and history and physical exam suggestive of an overall well-appearing infant, the patient initially had a partial sepsis workup performed, including a complete blood count, blood culture, urinalysis, and urine culture. The results of this initial laboratory workup help determine whether to perform a lumbar puncture and start the infant on antibiotics or to closely observe the infant without antibiotics.

Given that the urinalysis was strongly suggestive of a UTI and the peripheral WBC > 5, a lumbar puncture was performed, and spinal fluid was tested for cell count, glucose, protein, and bacterial culture. The cell count, glucose, and protein were all normal. She was started on broad-spectrum antibiotics with ceftriaxone to treat the UTI, as well as any other coexisting bacterial infections for 48 hours. The urine culture grew >100,000 CFU/mL of *Escherichia coli*, while the blood and CSF culture remained without any growth. After 48 hours of intravenous (IV) antibiotics, she was afebrile and transitioned to cefixime to complete a 14-day course of antibiotics. She subsequently had a normal renal ultrasound performed and required no additional follow-up.[1]

KEY MANAGEMENT STEPS

1. Febrile infants (rectal temperature of >38°C) <28 days require a full sepsis workup and admission to the hospital for monitoring and parenteral empiric antibiotic treatment.
2. Workup and management of febrile infants between 29 and 90 days present more of a controversy in the literature. At minimum, infants 1 to 2 months of age should have blood and urine cultures performed, while the lumbar puncture is dependent on their individual risk stratification based on age, history, physical and laboratory results (in this case, positive urinalysis and elevated WBC count). Workup for infants 2 to 3 months of age will be completely dependent on risk stratification.
3. Treatment of fever in infants is directed toward the most common bacterial and viral organisms infants are susceptible to, based on their age and clinical presentation.
4. Self-limited viral illness is the most common cause of fever in infants, while UTI in the most common bacterial cause of fever in infants.
5. Indications for inpatient management of a UTI include age <2 months, clinical urosepsis, and immunocompromised patients.[2]

DEBRIEF

Febrile infants <3 months are a unique population as their immune systems are immature, placing them at increased risk for serious bacterial infections. Most febrile infants have self-limited viral illnesses; however, it is important to identify those that have a coexisting or isolated bacterial illness. In the first 28 days of life, the most common bacterial pathogens infants are susceptible to are *Escherichia coli*, group B *Streptococcus* and *Listeria monocytogenes*. From 1 to 3 months of life, infants are additionally at risk for *Streptococcus pneumoniae, Neisseria meningococcemia, Salmonella,* and *Haemophilus influenza*. Aside from bacterial pathogens, infants are also at increased risk for herpes simplex virus and enterovirus meningitis.[3,4]

Febrile infants < 28 days are managed with a full sepsis workup, broad-spectrum IV antibiotics and hospitalization. Infants 1 to 3 months of age, however, provide more of a diagnostic and therapeutic dilemma. The Boston, Philadelphia, and Rochester criteria provide clinicians with evidence-based strategies for evaluation and management of this population. Although, the design and results of each study vary slightly, they all aim to identify which infants are least likely to develop severe bacterial infection (SBI), based on age, history, physical, and laboratory results.

The study in Boston aimed to identify febrile infants, at low risk for SBI, who can be safely managed as outpatients. They recruited 503 febrile infants 28 to 89 days of age who were well appearing, had no source of fever detected on physical exam, had a peripheral WBC <20,000, had a CSF WBC < 10, had negative urinary leukocyte esterase and had a caretaker available by phone. These infants were labeled as low risk febrile infants. After blood, urine and CSF cultures were obtained, the infants were given a dose of ceftriaxone and discharged home with instructions to return 24 hours later for evaluation and a second dose of ceftriaxone. On follow-up, 5.4% of infants were identified as having a SBI (UTI, bacteremia or bacterial gastroenteritis). Although screening did not identify these infants, all infants were clinically well appearing on follow-up, received appropriate treatment, and had no complications attributable to their initial outpatient management. This study therefore concluded that following full sepsis workup and ceftriaxone, outpatient treatment with close follow-up for re-examination and antibiotics is a safe alternative to hospitalization for low-risk febrile infants.[5]

The study in Philadelphia aimed to identify febrile infants at low risk for SBI, who can be managed without antibiotics. They conducted a prospective study of 747 febrile infants, 29 to 56 days of age, who were all screened for the presence of SBI with a thorough history, physical, and full sepsis workup; 460/747 infants were identified as having clinical or laboratory evidence suggestive of SBI and were given antibiotics and hospitalized. The remaining 287 low-risk infants had no signs of bacterial infection, no known immune deficiency, peripheral WBC <15,000, band/neutropil ratio <0.2, urinalysis with <10 WBC/hpf and no bacteria and CSF with <8 WBC and a negative gram stain. These infants were randomized to inpatient observation without antibiotics or outpatient care without antibiotics. The inpatient group was observed for 48 hours, and the outpatient group returned at 24 and 48 hours for evaluation. Of the initial 747 infants, 8.7% were found to have SBI; however, only 1/287 low-risk infants assigned to observation with no antibiotics was found to have a SBI. The Philadelphia study concluded that with the use of strict screening criteria, many low-risk febrile infants 1 to 2 months of age can be safely monitored as outpatients without antibiotics.[6]

The Rochester study aimed to develop strict criteria to identify which febrile infants were at low risk of developing SBI. They recruited 233 febrile infants from birth through 3 months of age and screened them for likelihood of SBI. They categorized 144 infants as low risk based on history (>37 weeks, never hospitalized, no chronic or underlying illness, no unexplained hyperbilirubinemia, no previous antibiotics), physical exam (showing a well appearing infant) and labs (peripheral WBC between 5,000–15,000, band count <1500, and urinalysis showing WBC <10/hpf). Only 1/144 infants labeled as low risk, based on the criteria, developed a SBI, compared to 22/89 in the high-risk group. The Rochester study, therefore, concluded that previously healthy febrile infants <3 months of age are unlikely to have SBI if they meet the low-risk criteria. They suggest that it would likely be safe to hospitalize and observe these low-risk patients without administering antibiotics; however, this study did not directly address criteria for hospitalization and antibiotic administration as the Boston and Philadelphia studies did.[7]

These 3 studies suggest that, based on history, physical exam, and laboratory studies, febrile infants can be stratified into low- and high-risk groups to predict their individual risk of developing a SBI. This risk stratification helps guide the clinician in determining the infant's diagnostic workup and treatment plan (Figure 52.1). All infants <28 days are labeled as high risk and so require that a full sepsis workup be performed, including lumbar puncture, blood culture, and urine culture. For infants 1 to 2 months of age, blood and urine cultures at minimum are recommended, while the lumbar puncture is dependent on risk stratification. Proposed

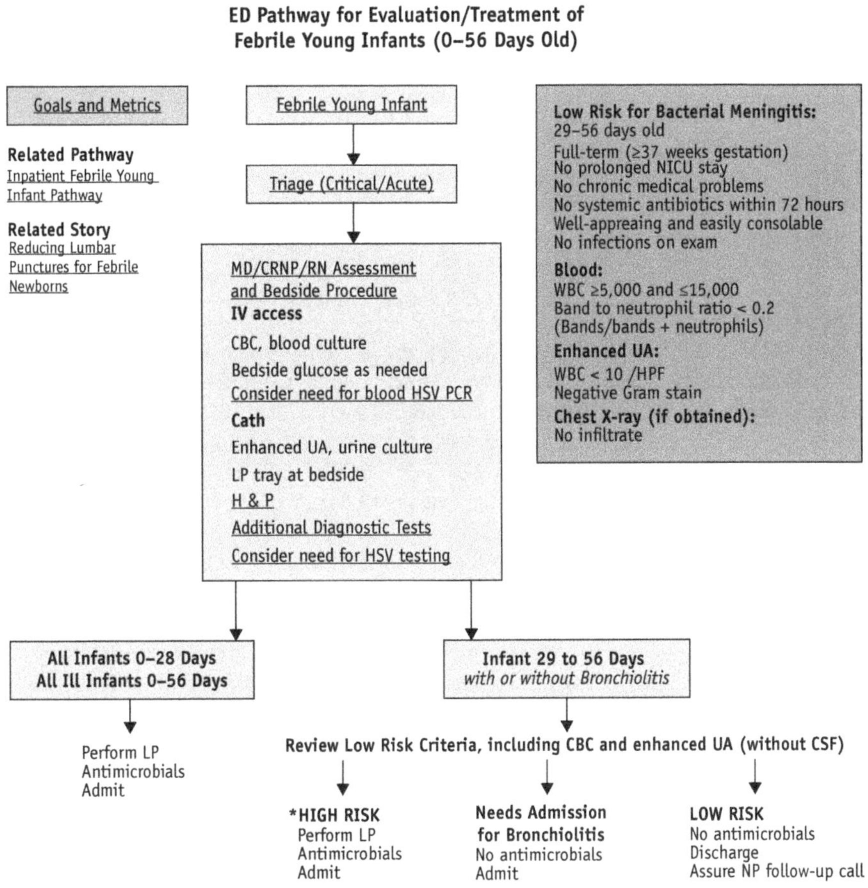

ED Pathway for Evaluation/Treatment of
Febrile Young Infants (0–56 Days Old)

| Goals and Metrics | Febrile Young Infant | Low Risk for Bacterial Meningitis: |

Goals and Metrics

Related Pathway
Inpatient Febrile Young
Infant Pathway

Related Story
Reducing Lumbar
Punctures for Febrile
Newborns

Febrile Young Infant

Triage (Critical/Acute)

**MD/CRNP/RN Assessment
and Bedside Procedure**
IV access

CBC, blood culture

Bedside glucose as needed
Consider need for blood HSV PCR
Cath

Enhanced UA, urine culture

LP tray at bedside
H & P
Additional Diagnostic Tests
Consider need for HSV testing

Low Risk for Bacterial Meningitis:
29–56 days old
Full-term (≥37 weeks gestation)
No prolonged NICU stay
No chronic medical problems
No systemic antibiotics within 72 hours
Well-appreaing and easily consolable
No infections on exam

Blood:
WBC ≥5,000 and ≤15,000
Band to neutrophil ratio < 0.2
(Bands/bands + neutrophils)
Enhanced UA:
WBC < 10 /HPF
Negative Gram stain

Chest X-ray (if obtained):
No infiltrate

**All Infants 0–28 Days
All Ill Infants 0–56 Days**

Perform LP
Antimicrobials
Admit

Infant 29 to 56 Days
with or without Bronchiolitis

Review Low Risk Criteria, including CBC and enhanced UA (without CSF)

*HIGH RISK
Perform LP
Antimicrobials
Admit

**Needs Admission
for Bronchiolitis**
No antimicrobials
Admit

LOW RISK
No antimicrobials
Discharge
Assure NP follow-up call

FIGURE 52.1 Children's Hospital of Philidelphia proposed fever evaluation algorithm for infants based on age.

IV = intravenous; CBC = complete blood count; HSV = herpes simplex virus; PCR = polymerase chain reaction; UA = urinalysis; LP = lumbar puncture; H & P = history and physical; WBC = white blood cell; HPF = high power field; CSF = cerebral spinal fluid; NP = nurse practitioner.

http://www.chop.edu/clinical-pathway/febrile-infant-emergent-evaluation-clinical-pathway

algorithm for infants based on age is shown in Figure 52.1. Workup for infants 2 to 3 months of age will be completely dependent on risk stratification. Febrile infants who are at increased risk for SBI are treated with a third-generation cephalosporin, ampicillin (if concerned for Listeria), and acyclovir (if concerned for herpes simplex virus meningitis). In an ill-appearing infant, antibiotics should not be delayed for diagnostic purposes. However, correctly identifying the low-risk infants reduces exposure to superfluous antibiotics, eliminates unnecessary hospital stays, and overall reduces costs to the individual and the health system.[3]

Our patient was managed inpatient with a full sepsis workup as she did not meet the Boston, Philadelphia, or Rochester low-risk criteria for SBI. Although, she was >1 month, well appearing with no significant past medical history, her laboratory studies placed her in the high-risk category; she had a WBC of 16.5×10^9/L and had > 10 WBC/hpf and many bacteria noted on urinalysis. She was ultimately diagnosed with an *Escherichia coli* UTI. UTIs are the most common bacterial illness in a well-appearing febrile infants <8 weeks old, occurring in 7.5% of these infants. Given her age, she was hospitalized for IV antibiotics, and after 48 hours of antibiotics and >24 hours of being afebrile she was transitioned to outpatient management.[2,8,9]

REFERENCES

1. Hoberman A, Wald ER, Hickey RW, et al. Oral versus initial intravenous therapy for urinary tract infections in young febrile children. *Pediatrics.* 1999;104(1):79–86.
2. Chang SL, Shortliffe LD. Pediatric urinary tract infections. *Pediatr Clin North Am.* 2006;53(3):379–400.
3. Williams K, Jaffe D. Fever in the well-appearing young infant, *Pediatr Emerg Med.,* 2008; 291–298.
4. Baskin M. The prevalence of serious bacterial infections by age in febrile infants during the first 3 months of life. *Pediatr Ann.* 1993;22(8):462–466.
5. Baskin M, O'Rourke E, Fleisher G. Outpatient treatment of febrile infants 28–89 days of age with intramuscular administration of ceftriaxone. *J Pediatr.* 1992;120(1):22–27.
6. Baker M, Bell L, Avner J. Outpatient management without antibiotics of fever in selected patients. *N Engl J Med.* 1993;32 (20):1437–1441.
7. Dagan R, Powell K, Hall C, et al. Identification of infants unlikely to have serious bacterial infection although hospitalized for suspected sepsis. *J Pediatr.* 1985;107(6):855–860.
8. Neuhaus TJ, Berger C, Buechner K, et al. Randomised trial of oral versus sequential intravenous/oral cephalosporins in children with pyelonephritis. *Eur J Pediatr.* 2008;167(9):1037–1047.
9. Crain E, Shelov S. Febrile infants: predictors of bacteremia. *J Pediatr.* 1982;101(5):686–689.

CHAPTER 53

DROWNING

ELYSHA PIFKO

SETTING

Pediatric Emergency Department

CHIEF COMPLAINT

Drowning

HISTORY

An 8-year-old male presents via emergency medical services (EMS) after being found unresponsive at the bottom of a swimming pool. His mom stated that patient was playing in the pool when she noticed he had become quiet, and she saw him at the bottom of the pool. She immediately pulled him out of the water and estimated that he was under water for approximately 1 minute. Mom noted full-body shaking with associated peri-oral cyanosis. Shaking continued for 2 minutes and then resolved spontaneously. A bystander called EMS and upon their arrival patient was sleepy but aroused with stimulation. He was then brought to the pediatric emergency department (ED) for evaluation. Mom denies any recent fevers, cough, congestion, known head trauma, altered mental status, headaches, or vomiting. Prior to drowning, patient was at his neurologic baseline.

He has a past medical history of mild allergies. He has had normal development.

He is currently in the third grade.

Maternal history of epilepsy.

PHYSICAL EXAMINATION

Vital signs: HR 105, BP 105/60, RR 25, SpO_2 98 on room air, temp. 37°C.

Examination reveals a well-developed and well-nourished male in no acute distress who appears tired. Answers all questions appropriately but prefers to keep eyes closed. Exam of head is nontraumatic. No C-spine tenderness. His lungs are clear to auscultation with good air movement. His cardiac rate and rhythm are normal; no murmurs, rubs, or gallops. He has normal central and distal pulses. His abdomen is soft, nontender, and nondistended. Neurologic examination reveals normal cranial nerves 2 to 12. Normal 5/5 strength bilaterally in all extremities and normal sensation. Glasgow Coma Scale score 14 (E3V5M6). Normal coordination and normal gait.

DIFFERENTIAL DIAGNOSIS

1. Head trauma
2. Seizure
3. Cardiac arrhythmia
4. Dehydration

TESTS

Blood glucose: 130 mg/dL.
Arterial blood gas: pH 7.39, pCO_2 41, pO_2 94, HCO_3 22, base excess −1.
Electrocardiogram: normal sinus rhythm.
Chest X-ray: normal cardiac silhouette, clear lungs. No acute abnormality.

CLINICAL COURSE

Patient presented to the ED via EMS on a non-rebreather oxygen mask. He appeared sleepy on arrival but following all commands. He was weaned to room air soon after arrival to ED. After 30 minutes of observation, he became more awake and alert. Mom states that he was back to his neurologic baseline after 1 hour of observation in the ED. There was no evidence of trauma or injury on exam. Pediatric neurology was consulted, who recommended an outpatient electroencephalogram (EEG). He remained stable on room air after a 6-hour period of observation without any increased work of breathing. He was not started on antiepileptic drugs (AEDs). He was then discharged home with scheduled outpatient follow-up with pediatric neurology and an outpatient EEG scheduled.

KEY MANAGEMENT STEPS

1. Recognize seizure in a patient found unresponsive, especially with history of noted shaking.
2. Consider chest imaging to evaluate for evidence of pulmonary edema or effusions in patients presenting after an episode of drowning.
3. Limited laboratory tests needed in stable patients with new-onset unprovoked seizure.
4. Defer head imaging and EEG in patients with new-onset seizure that quickly return to neurologic baseline.
5. Defer initiation of outpatient AEDs in patients who present after unprovoked new-onset seizure in stable patient.

DEBRIEF

This patient was found unresponsive at the bottom of a pool after likely having a new-onset seizure. The diagnosis of seizure was presumed due to witnessed tonic-clonic shaking after he was removed from the pool and an apparent postictal period with a complete return to neurologic baseline after a period of observation. This case addresses two separate problems: drowning and new-onset seizures.

Per the World Health Organization, "Drowning is the process of experiencing respiratory impairment from submersion/immersion in liquid." The majority of people who have drowned recover spontaneously without the need for medical intervention. In cases of cardiac arrest, the primary cause is a lack of oxygen and as such resuscitation should start with 5 initial rescue breaths and then followed by 30 compressions, which is a departure from traditional cardiopulmonary resuscitation.

In the ED, immediate attention should be given to the ABCs (airway, breathing, and circulation) in patients that present after drowning. Attention should also be given to rewarming the patient. After stabilization, chest X-ray and an evaluation of blood gas should be obtained. Patients with a normal physical exam (including the absence of any rales) and lab evaluation can be safely discharged home. Any patient who presents with significant rales in all lung fields, hypotension, unresponsiveness, or ventilatory failure will require admission to the intensive care unit.

The evaluation of an unprovoked first nonfebrile seizure in the ED should be catered to each individual patient. Per the American Academy of Neurology guidelines, emergent laboratory tests and radiologic imaging should not be obtained unless there is a concerning significant history such as persistent vomiting or head trauma. An EEG should be a part of the evaluation for these patients, but there is no evidence that supports this study needs to be performed prior to discharge home.

The American Academy of Neurology does not recommend treatment with an AED in children and adolescents who experience a first seizure. However, the guidelines do state that the initiation of an AED may be considered based on an individual circumstance when the benefits of reducing the risk of subsequent seizures outweigh the risks of the medication. Our patient did not have any significant past medical history with significant risk factors and so an AED would not be indicated at this time.

People with epilepsy have a 15- to 19-fold increased risk for drowning compared to the general population. As such, prevention is incredibly important in this population of patients to reduce the risk of drowning, including complete avoidance of swimming alone and showering instead of bathing unless supervised.

FURTHER READING

Bell GS, Gaitatzis A, Bell CL, et al. Drowning in people with epilepsy: how great is the risk? *Neurology.* 2008;71(8):578–582.

Hirtz D, Ashwal S, Berg A, et al. Practice parameter: evaluating a first nonfebrile seizure in children: report of the Quality Standards Subcommittee of the American Academy of Neurology and the Practice Committee of the Child Neurology Society. *Neurology.* 2000;55:616–623.

Hirtz D, Berg A, Bettis D, et al. Practice parameter: treatment of the child with a first unprovoked seizure: report of the Quality Standards Subcommittee of the American Academy of Neurology and the Practice Committee of the Child Neurology Society. *Neurology.* 2003;60:166–175.

Szpilman D, Bierens JJLM, Handley AJ, Orlowski JP. Drowning. *New Engl J Med.* 2012; 366:2102–2110.

Zuccarelli BD, Hall AS. Utility of obtaining a serum basic metabolic panel in the setting of a first-time nonfebrile seizure. *Clin Pediatr (Phila).* 2016;55(7):650–653.

CRYING INFANT

CAROLINE BLACK

SETTING

Pediatric Emergency Department

CHIEF COMPLAINT

Crying

HISTORY

A 3-month-old female presents to the pediatric emergency department with parental concern of fussiness for the past 24 hours. Parents state that the infant was intermittently fussy initially but now continuously crying throughout the day and is minimally consolable. The fussiness associated with poor formula intake, decreased wet diapers, and intermittent increased belly breathing. Parents deny fever, cough, congestion, and rash. She has had 1 episode of a small amount of nonbilious, nonbloody spit up. Parents state that she has had no diarrhea, but she has had no stools since fussiness began. They do note a decrease in energy level and pallor.

She has no past medical history. She is an ex-full-term infant, with an uncomplicated spontaneous vaginal delivery.

Mom and dad are the primary caregivers. She has 2 older siblings, both of whom are in good health.

Mom and dad deny history of congenital diseases in the family. The maternal grandfather has atrial flutter and a prior myocardial infarction at the age of 68 years.

PHYSICAL EXAMINATION

Vital signs: HR 232, BP 78/40, RR 38, SpO_2 98% on room air, temp. 37.2°C.

Examination of the infant reveals a fussy, pale, and distressed infant who is otherwise well-developed and well-nourished. Her anterior fontanelle is open and flat with moist mucous membranes. Her lung exam reveals equal and symmetric air movement bilaterally with mild subcostal retractions. There are no crackles, wheezing, or rhonchi. Her cardiac exam is significant for tachycardia but normal rhythm with S_1 and S_2 present, no murmurs, rubs, or gallops appreciated. Her abdomen is soft, nontender, and without distention. A small umbilical hernia is present and reducible on exam. Her extremities are warm, well-perfused with palpable and symmetric femoral pulses. There is no edema or erythema of fingers and toes. Her neurological exam is grossly normal reflexes for age, strength, and sensation.

DIFFERENTIAL DIAGNOSIS

1. Supraventricular tachycardia (SVT)
2. Congenital heart defect
3. Intussusception
4. Hair tourniquet
5. Colic
6. Corneal abrasion
7. Sepsis

TESTS

Venous blood gas: normal pH, pCO_2, HCO_3, base excess +1, lactate 0.8.
Chemistry panel: normal sodium, potassium, chloride, bicarbonate, blood urea nitrogen, creatinine, and glucose.
Electrocardiogram (ECG), 12-lead: Figure 54.1.

CLINICAL COURSE

Following history and clinical findings, the infant was placed on cardiac and O_2 sat probe monitoring with intravenous (IV) access established in antecubital fossa. After blood work and 12-lead ECG were evaluated, the infant was placed on continuous ECG monitoring as well as defibrillation pads (should she suddenly deteriorate) during initiation of therapeutic maneuvers. She was deemed stable and vagal maneuvers were attempted by applying a bag of ice to the face above nose for 15 to 30 seconds, which was unsuccessful. This was followed by knee to chest positioning with no decrease in heart rate. Adenosine was then administered at an initial dose of 0.1 mg/kg IV rapid push followed by a normal saline flush using a 3-way stopcock. There was a brief pause on the cardiac monitor, and then the patient returned to a narrow complex tachycardia. A secondary adenosine dose of 0.2 mg/kg was provided. The rhythm converted within

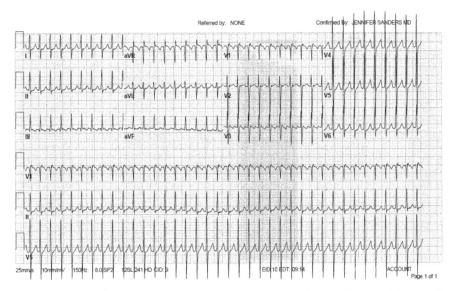

FIGURE 54.1 Electrocardiogram. Note narrow QRS complex tachycardia and absence of discrete P waves in all leads. No RR interval variability. Heart rate is not variable and greater than 220 beats/min.

30 seconds of the second adenosine dose with normalizing heart rate of 110 beats/min, stable blood pressure, and good perfusion. Cardiology was consulted, and the infant was admitted for telemetry monitoring. Repeat ECG showed continued sinus rhythm in the pediatric intensive care unit. Echocardiogram showed no structural heart abnormalities and normal ventricular function.

KEY MANAGEMENT STEPS

1. Assessment of hemodynamic stability and early placement on cardiac monitors.
2. Obtaining ECG in a patient with tachycardia and suspected arrhythmia.
3. Recognition and differentiation of narrow-complex tachycardia without P waves on ECG suggestive of SVT versus sinus tachycardia.
4. Appropriate early intervention of synchronized cardioversion in hemodynamically unstable patient versus vagal maneuvers and/or antiarrhythmic therapy in stable patient.
5. Appropriate consultation with cardiology based on ECG findings.

DEBRIEF

This infant was experiencing fussiness from likely increased heart rate and precordial discomfort. Typical symptoms include awareness of rapid heart rate, chest pain, and palpitations in older patients able to verbalize complaints. Infants often present with signs and symptoms of cardiac failure such as pallor, restlessness/ irritability, tachypnea, cough, poor feeding, and weak pulse. Duration may vary between a few seconds to persistent tachycardia lasting hours and be conveyed as "intermittent fussiness" confused for intussusception and colic.

SVT is the most common arrhythmia in the pediatric population.[1] Diagnostic criteria for defining SVT is defined as follows by American Heart Association guidelines for cardiopulmonary resuscitation and emergency cardiovascular care science[2]:

- Vague history
- Abrupt onset of tachycardia
- P waves are absent; usually hidden in QRS interval or ST segment
- No heart rate variability with activity
- Heart rate >220 beats/min in infants; heart rate >180 beats/min in children

When SVT is recognized, it is important obtain IV access, place on cardiac monitor with continuous ECG, and place defibrillation pads on patient in case of acute hemodynamic deterioration. Of note, peripheral access should be placed as close as possible to the central circulation (such as the antecubital fossa) for quick delivery of antiarrhythmic drugs to the heart.

In this case, the ECG revealed changes concerning for narrow complex tachyarrhythmia, SVT. The infant was stable with no signs of shock, lethargy, or decompensation. Vagal maneuvers may be initiated in children with stable SVT who are unlikely to decompensate. The goal of such maneuvers is to stimulate vagal nerve center (increase vagal tone) leading to a reflex bradycardia and thereby terminating the arrhythmia and converting SVT to sinus rhythm.[3] Of note, vagal maneuvers should be appropriate for age and performed for at least 15 to 30 seconds for conversion to occur.[4]

In infants, maneuvers such as diving reflex, knee to chest position, and rectal stimulation are appropriate measures. In children and adolescents who can follow directions, Valsalva ("bear down") maneuver or knee to chest may be attempted. Carotid sinus massage and orbital pressure are maneuvers not recommended for children.

In patients with stable SVT who do not covert with vagal maneuvers, pharmaceutical cardioversion with adenosine is first-line therapy. Treatment should be given as a "fast push" followed by saline flush for immediate effect. The choice of either pharmaceutical cardioversion and/or synchronized cardioversion is based on stability of the patient according to the following American Heart Association algorithm:

- In cases of hemodynamic instability without change in mental status, adenosine may be administered if there is no delay in synchronized cardioversion.
- Immediate synchronized cardioversion should not be delayed if both hemodynamically unstable with altered mental status or inability to obtain access.

Cardiology should be consulted as soon as SVT is recognized or suspected as evaluation for underlying cause needs to be assessed once the acute episode of SVT is terminated. A 12-lead ECG should be obtained postcardioversion to assess for underlying arrhythmic cause. An echocardiogram should be obtained to rule out structural cardiac abnormalities, as SVT has been associated with congenital cardiac defects for which ablation therapy may be required. Chronic therapy with an antiarrhythmic agent may not be necessary following one episode of SVT with minimal symptoms and responsive to acute therapy. However, in cases of refractory and/or symptomatic episodes of SVT, prophylactic therapy may be warranted.

REFERENCES

1. Lewis J, Gaurav A, Tudorascu D, Hickey RW, Saladino RA, Manole M. Acute management of re-fractory and unstable pediatric supraventricular tachycardia. *J Pediatrics*. 2017;181:177–182.
2. Kleinman ME, Chameides L, Schexnayder SM, et al. Part 14: pediatric advanced life support: 2010 American Heart Association guidelines for cardiopulmonary resuscitation and emergency cardio-vascular care. *Circulation*. 2010;122: S876.
3. Manole M, Saladino R. Emergency department management of the pediatric patient with supraventricular tachycardia. *Pediatr Emerg Care*. 2007;23(3):176–185.
4. Quiñones C, Bubolz B. Cardiac emergencies. In: Bachur RG, Shaw KN, Chamberlain, J, Lavelle, J, Nagler, J, Shook, J., eds. *Fleischer & Ludwig's Textbook of Pediatric Emergency Medicine*. 7th ed. Philadelphia, PA: Lippincott Williams & Wilkins; 2016; 627–656.

FURTHER READING

Van Hare GF. Disturbances of rate and rhythm of the heart. In Kliegman RM, Stanton BF, St. Geme, J, Schor, N., eds. *Nelson's Textbook of Pediatrics*. 20th ed. Philadelphia, PA: Elsevier; 2016; 2251–2261.

LIMP

SARAH YALE AND DAVID MILLS

SETTING

Pediatric Clinic

CHIEF COMPLAINT

Limp

HISTORY

A 3-year-old previously healthy male presents to the pediatric outpatient clinic with concern for new onset limp. His mother reports that over the past day he has seemed less active, and this morning was complaining that his "leg hurt." She noted that he has been hesitant to put weight on his left leg and has been walking with a limp since yesterday. She also noticed that he felt warm but did not take his temperature. He is still eating and drinking at baseline and has had no changes in his urination or bowel movements. His mother knows of no specific trauma that occurred but says he is a "very active toddler." He has no current cough, rhinorrhea, emesis, or diarrhea, but his mother reports that the whole family, including the patient, had "a bad cold" 2 weeks ago.

Past Medical History: The patient was born at 39 weeks via spontaneous vaginal delivery without complications. He has had no prior surgeries. He does not take any medications except for a daily pediatric multivitamin. He has no known drug allergies.

Social History: He lives at home with his parents and older sister. There are no pets in the home and no recent travel. He attends daycare during the week.

Family history: There is no history of arthritis or neurologic diseases.

PHYSICAL EXAMINATION

Vital signs: HR 110, BP 84/62, RR 18, SpO$_2$ 100% on room air, temp. 38.1°C.

Examination reveals a well-nourished child in no acute distress. Examination of head is normocephalic and atraumatic. He has full range of motion of the neck and no lymphadenopathy. Skin exam reveals no rashes, ecchymoses, or lesions. His cardiac rate and rhythm are normal with no murmur, and his capillary refill is 2 seconds. His lungs are clear bilaterally with no increased work of breathing. His abdomen is soft, nontender, nondistended, and with no hepatosplenomegaly. There is no tenderness noted with palpation of the spine or paraspinal musculature. Neurologic exam is without focal cranial nerve deficits. He has normal patellar reflexes, and normal strength and sensation in the bilateral upper extremities. His left lower extremity is held mildly abducted, flexed, and externally rotated at the hip. There is mild tenderness to palpation over the left anterior thigh, but no other areas of point tenderness. There are no obvious deformities of the lower extremities and no left hip or knee edema, warmth, or erythema noted. The patient tolerates passive adduction, full flexion and extension, and both internal and external rotation of the left hip. He is hesitant but is able to bear weight and walks to his mother with encouragement with an antalgic gait.

DIFFERENTIAL DIAGNOSIS

1. Toxic synovitis
2. Septic arthritis of the hip or knee
3. Fracture (toddler's fracture, nonaccidental trauma)
4. Osteomyelitis
5. Mass (osteochondroma, osteoid osteoma, malignancy)
6. Legg-Calvé-Perthes disease
7. Developmental dysplasia of the hip

TESTS

Complete blood count with differential: white blood cell count (WBC) 10×10^9/L (normal: 5–11×10^9/L), hemoglobin 12 g/dL (11–15 g/dL), platelets 260×10^9/L ($140–440 \times 10^9$/L), differential 52% lymphocytes, 46% neutrophils, no bands.

Erythrocyte sedimentation rate (ESR): 18 mm/h (3–13 mm/h).

C-reactive protein (CRP): 1.0 mg/L (<0.7 mg/L).

Hip radiograph: within normal limits—no osseous abnormalities or widening of the hip space.

CLINICAL COURSE

Based on the patient's history, physical examination, and laboratory review, there was a low suspicion for septic arthritis, fracture, or osteomyelitis. The Kocher criteria were applied, with the patient found to be at low risk of septic arthritis given his temperature <38.5°C, WBC count <12 × 10^9/L, ESR <40 mm/h, and his ability to bear weight. As such, no further radiologic workup or testing was deemed necessary. He was diagnosed with toxic synovitis and was started on nonsteroidal anti-inflammatory drug treatment (ibuprofen 10 mg/kg every 6 hours). His gait improved after administration of ibuprofen in the clinic, and he was continued on therapy for the next 48 hours. His mother was instructed to monitor for fevers and ability to walk at home, as symptomatic improvement over the next 24 hours should be expected. The following day, his mother noted that he was afebrile and that his limp continued to improve. She called back 1 week later, stating that he was back to his normal active self and that his gait had returned completely to normal. No further workup or treatment was initiated.

KEY MANAGEMENT STEPS

1. Obtaining a complete history is essential, including eliciting the timeline of presentation (acute vs. chronic) as well as any pertinent preceding events such as recent viral illness or trauma.
2. Creating a focused yet appropriately broad differential diagnosis of limp relative to patient's age is important.
3. Recognizing features of septic arthritis, the urgent nature of diagnosis and treatment, and the consequences of delayed intervention is vital.
4. Appropriate use of the Kocher criteria to assess whether further workup such as ultrasound, joint aspiration, or orthopedic consultation is warranted.
5. Counseling regarding supportive care, expected timeline of improvement, and appropriate follow-up with toxic synovitis.

DEBRIEF

The patient presented with unilateral leg pain and limp that was the result of transient inflammation of the hip, referred to as toxic (or transient) synovitis. Toxic synovitis is the most common cause of nontraumatic hip pain in children, most commonly affecting patients between 3 and 8 years of age with the male-to-female ratio greater than 2:1. Hip symptoms are usually unilateral (though up to 5% of cases may be bilateral) and are commonly preceded by a viral upper respiratory infection (often 2–4 weeks prior to onset). Typical symptoms of toxic synovitis include low-grade fever, pain, potentially decreased range of motion of the affected hip, and a notable limp.

To help distinguish between toxic synovitis and more emergent infectious diagnoses such as septic arthritis, laboratory studies should be considered for children who present with both limp and fever. When obtained in patients with toxic synovitis, laboratory studies such as the WBC and inflammatory markers usually remain within normal limits or are only mildly elevated. While not clinically indicated in patients with toxic synovitis, if obtained, radiographs appear normal while ultrasound may reveal a small effusion of the hip joint. Treatment of toxic synovitis is supportive and focuses on pain management with nonsteroidal anti-inflammatory drugs and activity modification with return to full activity as tolerated. Full recovery is expected over 7 to 10 days, and the long-term prognosis is excellent, with only rare cases of subsequent avascular necrosis reported.

Differentiating between a self-limited illness such as toxic synovitis and an emergent diagnosis such as septic arthritis of the hip can be challenging but is critically important in the assessment of a limping child. Failure to identify septic arthritis could result in diminished blood flow to the affected hip within 6 to 12 hours and irreversible damage within 1 to 2 days of symptom onset. To help determine if a child is at higher risk of septic arthritis, application of the Kocher criteria is recommended.[1] Risk factors include:

1. WBC >12,000
2. Fever >38.5°C
3. ESR >40
4. Refusal to bear weight

One point is given per risk factor, and the more criteria met, the higher the likelihood of septic arthritis (0 criteria met = 0.2% risk, 1 = 3% risk, 2 = 40% risk, 3 = 93.1% risk and 4 = 99.6% risk). Another helpful predictor is the addition of a CRP, as patients with a CRP >2.0 are also more likely to have septic arthritis.[2]

If the clinical suspicion of septic arthritis is high, urgent radiographic evaluation is recommended. An ultrasound of a septic hip may reveal joint space widening and the presence of an effusion, and joint aspiration for synovial fluid analysis is recommended. Joint fluid analysis with septic arthritis usually demonstrates WBC >50,000 with a predominance of polymorphonuclear leukocytes and may reveal a positive gram stain. Conversely, joint fluid analysis from a patient with toxic synovitis typically reveals a WBC count ranging from 5,000 to 15,000 with a negative gram stain. Again, early identification and treatment of septic arthritis with open drainage of the affected joint and empiric antibiotics are of the utmost importance, as damage to the vascular structures and cartilage of the joint can occur abruptly and may be irreversible.

Of note, differentiation of toxic synovitis from septic arthritis can be more difficult with the hip joint than other joints (knee, ankle), as the hip joint is deeper and therefore may mask symptoms such as overlying edema and erythema. In younger children it is imperative to fully assess the joints adjacent to the suspected joint, as they often cannot localize or verbalize pain well.

The initial differential diagnosis for limp in the pediatric population is broad and varies based on patient age, but a thorough history with symptom timeline and a systematic physical exam can help to appropriately narrow the differential. Red flag features necessitating further workup include fatigue, weight loss, and hepatosplenomegaly (oncologic process), refusal to bear weight, high fever (T >38.5°C), holding the extremity in a fixed position (septic joint, osteomyelitis), prolonged limp (Legg-Calvé-Perthes, developmental dysplasia of the hip, leg length discrepancy), fractures or injuries that do not match developmental stage (nonaccidental trauma), and association with rashes (Lyme disease, juvenile idiopathic arthritis). In summary, toxic synovitis is a self-limited joint inflammatory process, but other more serious etiologies of limp must be excluded prior to making this diagnosis of exclusion.

REFERENCES

1. Kocher MS, Zurakowski D, and Kasser JR, et al. Differentiating between septic arthritis and transient synovitis of the hip: an evidence based clinic prediction algorithm. *J Bone Joint Surg Am.* 1999;81(12):1662–1670.
2. Caird MS, Flynn JM, Leung YL, et al. Factors distinguishing septic arthritis from transient synovitis of the hip in children. *J Bone Joint Surg Am.* 2006;88(6):1251–1257.

FURTHER READING

Herman MJ, Martinek M. The limping child. *Pediatr Rev.* 2015;36(5):184–196.

Sankar WN, Horn D, Wells L, and Dormans JP. The Hip. In: Kliegman RM, Stanton BF, St Geme III JW, Schor NF, Behrman RE, eds. *Nelson Textbook of Pediatrics.* 20th ed. Philadelphia, PA: Elsevier. 2015:3274–3283.

FEVER IN A CHILD

SHANNON DROHAN

A cute otitis media (AOM) is a common cause of fever especially in the first 2 years of life. This condition can be easily diagnosed in a child with an acute illness by presence of middle ear effusion on exam in addition to signs of inflammation revealed by intense erythema or report of otalgia. Recent guidelines recommend a "watchful waiting" approach to treatment in certain patients to help reduce antibiotic usage as most cases of AOM resolve spontaneously. This strategy can be used in children >6 months old with nonsevere symptoms, as long as follow-up is ensured to provide a rescue antibiotic if symptoms do not improve within 48 to 72 hours.

SETTING

Pediatric Office

CHIEF COMPLAINT

Fever

HISTORY

A 14-month old previously healthy female presented to her pediatrician's office due to a 1-day history of fever. The highest temperature recorded at home was 101.2°F. She has had a 3-day history of runny nose and mild cough. Parents deny any shortness of breath, wheezing, vomiting, diarrhea, or rash. She has been fussy over the last 2 days but is sleeping well and eating

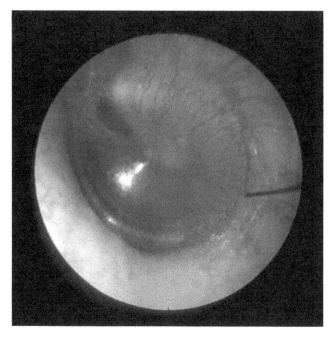

FIGURE 56.1 Erythematous tympanic membrane with an effusion and bulging.

at baseline. She has been treated with ibuprofen. There are no known sick contacts in the home. She has no chronic medical problems and is up to date on vaccinations.

PHYSICAL EXAMINATION

Vitals signs: HR 120, BP 88/64, RR 28, SpO_2 96%, temp. 37.6°C.

Examination reveals a nontoxic appearing child who is fussy but able to be consoled by her parents. She has nasal discharge present. There is no conjunctival erythema or discharge. Her oral exam reveals normal tonsils without hypertrophy, erythema, or exudate. Her right tympanic membrane (TM) is pearly white without erythema or effusion and has normal landmarks and mobility. Her left TM is bulging with a purulent effusion and intense erythema (see Figure 56.1). Pneumatic otoscopy reveals impaired mobility of her left TM. There is no mastoid tenderness or erythema. Her lungs are clear to auscultation bilaterally, and she has no retractions or nasal flaring. Cardiac exam reveals a regular rate and rhythm with no murmur, and her capillary refill is less than 2 seconds. Her abdomen is soft and nondistended without organomegaly. She has no rashes, and her skin is warm and well perfused.

DIFFERENTIAL DIAGNOSIS

1. AOM
2. Viral respiratory infection
3. Community acquired pneumonia

TESTS

No tests were performed.

CLINICAL COURSE

Due to her mild symptoms (fever <39°C and mild otalgia), the pediatrician discussed with the parents the benefits of "watchful waiting" in treating her AOM. The parents agreed to this plan and were instructed to call back if her fever or irritability continued past 48 to 72 hours as she may require antibiotic treatment. The pediatrician recommended continuing treating the child's fever and pain with ibuprofen. Her fever resolved, and her fussiness and poor sleep improved within 48 hours.

KEY MANAGEMENT STEPS

1. Accurate diagnosis of AOM and distinguishing between AOM and otitis media with effusion (OME).
2. "Watchful waiting" approach in certain cases of AOM after discussion with the parents, with ensured follow-up and rescue antibiotic if no improvement in symptoms in 48 to 72 hours.
3. High-dose amoxicillin is the initial antibiotic of choice for AOM. However, an antibiotic with β-lactamase coverage is recommended if the child has received amoxicillin in the last 30 days, has a history of recurrent AOM not responsive to amoxicillin, or has purulent conjunctivitis.

DEBRIEF

This patient with fever was found to have AOM in the setting of a viral respiratory infection. AOM is extremely common with 80% of all children experiencing at least one episode of AOM by 3 years old. It is the leading pediatric diagnosis for which antibiotics are prescribed. The most common pathogens include *S. pneumonia*, nontypeable *H. influenza*, and *Moraxella catarrhalis*. Nontypeable *H. influenza* is now the most common pathogen since the introduction of the pneumococcal vaccine.

The incidence of AOM peaks during the first 2 years of life, likely due to lower immunologic defenses and the structure and function of the eustachian tube. Factors that are protective against AOM include exclusive breastfeeding and vaccination against *S. pneumonia* and influenza. Risk factors include tobacco smoke exposure, low socioeconomic status, pacifier use, supine bottle feeding ("bottle propping"), exposure to other children such as in daycare, and congenital anomalies such as cleft palate.

Symptoms of AOM may include fever, irritability, change in sleeping habits, and evidence of ear pain such as tugging on the ear. The diagnosis of AOM requires:

1. Recent and acute onset of illness.
2. Presence of middle ear effusion, which includes TM bulging, impaired mobility, opacification and/or air fluid level, or otorrhea.
3. Evidence of middle ear inflammation shown by either intense erythema of the TM (mild erythema can be result of crying or vascular flushing) or otalgia (tugging or holding ear, poor sleep, etc.).

AOM must be differentiated from OME as antibiotics are not indicated for the treatment of OME. OME will have evidence of middle ear effusion on exam but without the marked erythema, bulging, and severe otalgia that supports a diagnosis of AOM.

Automatic antibiotic treatment of AOM has been questioned due to increasing rates of bacterial resistance. Antibiotics do allow more prompt improvement of symptoms and reduce the risk of suppurative complications such as mastoiditis; however, these complications are rare and most cases of AOM resolve spontaneously. The American Academy of Pediatrics recommends offering an observation, or "watchful waiting," approach to uncomplicated AOM, as long as follow-up is ensured if the child was to worsen or fail to improve within 48 to 72 hours. Patients eligible for observation include those with nonsevere symptoms (mild otalgia for <48 hours and temperature <39°C). Initial treatment with antibiotics is recommended for children with severe AOM (defined as moderate or severe otalgia or otalgia for >48 hours, or temp >39°C), children 6 to 23 months with bilateral AOM regardless of severity, and all children <6 months old.

If the child does not improve in 48 to 72 hours, then a rescue antibiotic should be prescribed. This can be done by giving the prescription to the parent with instructions to fill if needed or to instruct the parent to call or return to clinic. Studies have shown that only one third of children who were initially observed had persistent or worsening AOM that required a rescue antibiotic. This statistic suggests that the observation approach in eligible patients with AOM could potentially reduce antibiotic use by 65%.

High-dose amoxicillin (80–90 mg/kg/day) is the antibiotic of choice for treatment of AOM. If the child has received amoxicillin in the last 30 days, has a history of recurrent AOM not responsive to amoxicillin, or has purulent conjunctivitis, then an antibiotic with β-lactamase coverage needs to be selected instead. Parents should be instructed to have the child reevaluated if symptoms do not improve within 72 hours. Duration of treatment has historically been 10 days, but several studies show that a 7-day course is equally effective for children >2 years old with mild or moderate AOM.

FURTHER READING

Avner JR. Acute Fever. *Pediatr Rev*. 2009;30(1):5–13.

Lieberthal AS, Carroll AE, Chonmaitree T, et al. The diagnosis and management of acute otitis media. *Pediatrics*. 2013;131(3):e964–e999.

Nield LS, Kamat D. Fever without a focus. In: Kliegman RM, Nelson WE, eds. *Nelson Textbook of Pediatrics*. Philadelphia, PA: Elsevier, Saunders; 2011: 896–898.

———————————————

ALTERED MENTAL STATUS

MICHELLE N. MARIN

SETTING

Emergency Department

CHIEF COMPLAINT

Altered Mental Status

HISTORY

A 6-year-old boy presents with his parents to the pediatric emergency department with lethargy and abdominal pain. He has been complaining of diffuse abdominal pain for the past 2 days and noted by the parents to be lethargic since the morning of the emergency department visit. He is easily arousable and answers questions appropriately for his age. On the day of the emergency room visit, he had multiple episodes of nonbilious nonbloody emesis. Over the past week, the parents have noted he has been frequently asking them for apple juice and water, urinating more frequently with occasional daytime accidents, and wetting the bed nightly. The parents deny fever, diarrhea, rash, or cough. He also has no sick contacts or recent travel.

He has no past medical or surgical history.

His immunizations are up to date.

His mother has a past medical history of Grave's disease and his maternal grandmother has diabetes mellitus type I.

PHYSICAL EXAMINATION

Vital signs: HR 125, BP 100/65, RR 25, SpO_2 100% on room air, temp. 36.5°C, weight 20 kg.

Neurologic examination reveals a well-developed young boy who appears sleepy but responds appropriately to questions and noted to have a sweet-smelling breath. His head is normocephalic, atraumatic, and pupils are equal and reactive to light and accommodation. He appears to have a deep and labored breathing pattern although his lungs are clear to auscultation bilaterally with good air entry. On cardiac exam, he is tachycardic without no murmurs, rubs, or gallops. His abdomen is soft and nondistended with diffuse mild tenderness to palpation with no guarding or rebound. He has good peripheral pulses, and his extremities are warm and well perfused. He has normal strength, sensation, and a normal gait.

DIFFERENTIAL DIAGNOSIS

1. Diabetic ketoacidosis
2. Supratentorial or central brain tumor
3. Pyelonephritis
4. Ingestion

TESTS

Dextrose fingerstick: 350 mg/dL.

Venous blood gas: pH 7.20, pCO_2 25 mm Hg, pO_2 40 mm Hg, HCO_3 9 mEq/L, base deficit –30, venous O_2 saturation 80%, lactate 8.0 mEq/L.

Chemistry panel: sodium 133 mEq/L, potassium 6.0 mEq/L, chloride 100 mEq/L, bicarbonate 9 mEq/L, blood urea nitrogen 12 mg/dL, creatinine 0.1 mg/dL, glucose 355 mg/dL, magnesium 0.75 mEq/L, phosphate 1.7 mEq/L, anion gap 24 mEq/L.

Urinalysis: specific gravity 1.025, pH 6.5, urobilinogen negative, bilirubin negative, glucose 300 mg/dL, ketones 50 mg/dL, blood negative, protein negative, nitrite negative, leukocyte esterase negative, serum beta-hydroxybutyrate level 3.5 mmol/L (0.4–0.5 mmol/L).

Complete blood count: normal white blood cell count, hemoglobin, hematocrit, and platelets.

CLINICAL COURSE

Based on the history and clinical evaluation, there was a strong clinical suspicion for diabetic ketoacidosis in the setting of new-onset diabetes. The patient was placed on a cardiac monitor, had 2 large-bore peripheral intravenous lines placed, and additional new-onset diabetes labs were drawn. Secondary to the diabetic ketoacidosis, he was started on a bolus 10 mL/kg of normal saline to be run over an hour, and pediatric endocrinology was consulted. He had an hourly glucose checks as well as venous blood gas, basic metabolic panel with magnesium and phosphate, and urinalysis checked every 2 hours. Once the initial bolus finished, his repeat finger stick was 280 mg/dL. He was started on an insulin drip of 0.1 U/kg/hour, as well as on normal saline with 10 mEq of potassium acetate at a rate of 1.5 maintenance fluids. There was a second bag of intravenous fluid containing 10% dextrose normal saline and 10 mEq of potassium phosphate ready for titration with the first bag to 1.5 maintenance once the boy's blood glucose was below 250 mg/dL. He was admitted to the pediatric intensive care unit for close monitoring of his mental status and electrolyte levels. Within 2 hospital days, he was weaned off the insulin drip and transitioned to subcutaneous insulin once his ketoacidosis resolved and his beta-hydroxybutyrate levels normalized. He was sent home on hospital day 5 with an insulin regimen and close pediatric endocrine follow-up.

KEY MANAGEMENT STEPS

1. Obtain a fingerstick blood glucose, venous blood gas, basic metabolic panel, and urinalysis in a patient with suspected diabetic ketoacidosis.
2. Conservative intravascular repletion in patients with diabetic ketoacidosis to prevent cerebral edema.
3. After the initial normal saline bolus, an insulin drip should be started at a rate of 0.1U/kg/hr.
4. Closely monitor mental status and electrolytes in diabetic ketoacidosis.

DEBRIEF

The child in this case was exhibiting symptoms of diabetic ketoacidosis in the setting of a new diagnosis of type I diabetes. He was experiencing the typical symptoms of diabetic ketoacidosis that include polydipsia, polyuria, enuresis, abdominal pain, a change in mental status, ketosis breath, and an irregular breathing pattern known as Kussmaul breathing. Other symptoms of diabetic ketoacidosis, which the boy did not have, can include muscle pain and cramping from dehydration and electrolyte derangements.

The biochemical diagnostic criteria for diabetic ketoacidosis, as described by Olivieri et al.[1] include:

- Hyperglycemia with blood glucose concentration greater than 200 mg/dL.
- Venous pH less than 7.3 or a bicarbonate concentration less than 15 mmol/L.
- Ketonuria and ketonemia.

Diabetic ketoacidosis can be classified as mild, moderate, or severe. The classification is designated according to the patient's pH and bicarbonate value, as indicated in Table 57.1. In addition to the laboratory results, findings consistent with severe diabetic ketoacidosis include changes in mental status, Kussmaul respirations, and a sweet ketosis breath.

When there is a strong clinical concern for diabetic ketoacidosis, it is imperative to place 2 peripheral lines for management and draw labs prior to starting fluids. If it is a patient with known diabetes presenting with diabetic ketoacidosis, the following labs should be drawn: a fingerstick blood glucose, venous blood gas, basic metabolic panel, magnesium, phosphate, serum osmolality, amylase, lipase, preserved glucose, complete blood count, urinalysis, and hemoglobin

Table 57.1 Diabetic Ketoacidosis Classification

Severity	pH	Bicarbonate
Mild	<7.3	<15
Moderate	<7.2	<10
Severe	<7.1	<5

A1C. If it a patient presenting with new onset type I diabetes with diabetic ketoacidosis, these additional labs should be drawn: total insulin, C-peptide, anti-insulin antibodies, antigeneralized anxiety disorder antibodies, anti-islet cell antibody, thyroid stimulating hormone, thyroxine (T4), triiodothyronine (T3), thyroids stimulating immunoglobulin, and thyroid peroxidase antibody. Thyroid studies are important to obtain because type I diabetes is an autoimmune disorder and may be associated with other autoimmune disorders such as Hashimoto's thyroiditis or Grave's disease.

Diabetic ketoacidosis warrants close monitoring of fluids and electrolytes. Patient should have hourly fingerstick blood glucose and a venous blood gas, basic metabolic panel with magnesium and phosphate, and urinalysis checked every 2 hours. Fluids are required to improve tissue perfusion to facilitate euglycemia and improve the resultant metabolic acidosis from diabetic ketoacidosis. The osmotic diuresis in diabetic ketoacidosis leads to a whole body depletion of the electrolytes sodium, potassium, chloride, magnesium, and phosphate. All should be closely monitored. Sodium and potassium must be repleted through intravenous fluids and additives according to their serum levels. If with intravascular repletion there is no change or a decrease in serum sodium, there should be a clinical suspicion cerebral edema. There is no evidence showing benefit for the repletion of magnesium in diabetic ketoacidosis, it will normalize with the improvement of the patient's clinical status.

While awaiting the lab results, the patient can receive a bolus of normal saline over 1 hour. Patients older than 5 years of age and with a known diagnosis of type I diabetes may receive a bolus of 20 mL/kg. New-onset diabetics or children <5 years old presenting with diabetic ketoacidosis should receive a 10 mL/kg bolus to prevent cerebral edema as studies have shown these populations have rapid osmotic shifts into the central nervous system during management.

After the bolus, the patient will be started on the insulin drip and continuous fluids at a rate of 1.5 maintenance. If there is a concern for shock or severe dehydration, a patient may require fluids at a rate of 2 times maintenance. A common method of fluid management, known as the "two bag system" is often employed in patients with diabetic ketoacidosis. This system involves a bag of 0.9% normal saline plus 20 mEq of potassium chloride or acetate, while the other bag continues 10% dextrose in 0.9% normal saline plus 20 mEq of potassium chloride or acetate. Both bags of fluids contain potassium additives, a total of 40 mEq/L, to replete the total body potassium, which is driven intracellularly with the administration of insulin. Obtaining fluids with potassium additives may take time. Therefore, after the first bolus, a patient may be started on a continuous infusion of normal saline at a rate of 1.5 maintenance while waiting for the normal saline with potassium additives. When the bag of normal saline with potassium additive arrives, the patient should be placed on those fluids at a rate of 1.5 maintenance. Once the glucose is <300 mg/dL, the fluids will need to be titrated to avoid hypoglycemia and the need to hastily stop insulin therapy prior to ketoacidosis correction. At this point, the patient should be started on the bag of fluids containing dextrose and the rates of each bag should be adjusted for a total fluid volume of 1.5 maintenance. With each glucose check, the 2 bags should be titrated to avoid dropping the blood sugar too quickly. When the serum glucose is <150 mg/dL then the patient should receive fluids from the 10% dextrose normal saline bag alone to prevent hypoglycemia and continue the correction of ketoacidosis to prevent hypoglycemia and continue the correction of ketoacidosis.

The underlying lipolysis and ketogenesis of diabetic ketoacidosis cannot be stopped unless insulin is administered. The insulin infusion may be started at a rate of 0.1 units/kg/hr. An insulin infusion can be titrated down to 0.05 units/kg/hr and then transitioned to subcutaneous insulin once ketoacidosis resolves.

A patient's disposition will depend on his or her degree of diabetic ketoacidosis. Patients with mild diabetic ketoacidosis may have a resolution of the underlying acidosis and hyperglycemia in the pediatric emergency department and may be able to go home with close endocrine follow-up. Patients with moderate diabetic ketoacidosis may be managed on a floor capable of frequent finger sticks and blood draws. Intensive care is reserved for patients with severe diabetic ketoacidosis or with signs of altered mental status concerning for possible cerebral edema.

REFERENCE

1. Olivieri L, Chasm R. Diabetic ketoacidosis in the pediatric emergency department. *Emerg Med Clin North Am.* 2013;31(3):755–773.

FURTHER READING

Chansky ME, Lubkin CL. Diabetic ketoacidosis. In: Tintinalli JE, Stapczynski JS, Ma OJ, Yealy DM, Meckler GD, Cline DM. *Tintinalli's Emergency Medicine: A Comprehensive Study Guide.* 8th ed. New York, NY: McGraw-Hill; 2016. http://accessmedicine.mhmedical.com.elibrary.einstein.yu.edu/content.aspx?bookid=1658&sectionid=109443771.

Kim SY. Endocrine and metabolic emergencies in children: hypocalcemia, hypoglycemia, adrenal insufficiency, and metabolic acidosis including diabetic ketoacidosis. *Ann Pediatr Endocrinol Metab.* 2015;20(4):179–186.

Lavoie ME. Management of a patient with diabetic ketoacidosis in the emergency department. *Pediatr Emerg Care.* 2015;31(5):376–380; quiz 381–383.

Wiener E. Diabetic ketoacidosis. In: Mojica MA, ed. *PEM Guides.* New York, NY: New York University Langone Medical Center; 2015; 104–110.

CHAPTER 58

SWOLLEN EYES

JEFF MEYER

SETTING

Pediatric Clinic

CHIEF COMPLAINT

Swollen Eyes

HISTORY

A 3-year-old male presents with a 3-day history of "swollen eyes," and his mother is concerned that his face now appears swollen as well. His mother reports that this swelling seems worst when he wakes up in the morning and gradually improves as the day goes on, though it does not fully resolve. She also reports that he has complained of a stomach ache during the last 18 hours. He seemed fussier than normal as well, though he consoles readily with mom's efforts. He is still taking fluids normally, but his appetite has decreased somewhat. He has been urinating 4 to 5 times a day without complaint. He has been afebrile, with no cough, coryza, vomiting, diarrhea, or rash reported. He has not been exposed to any new soaps, lotions, or detergents, nor has he eaten any new foods.

He has been previously well aside from occasional symptoms of allergic rhinitis.

He has no recent sick contacts. He is on no medications, and no allergies are reported.

He has no significant family history aside from mild hypertension reported in his grandparents.

Further review of systems is negative except as previously stated.

PHYSICAL EXAMINATION

Vital signs: HR 102, BP 98/64, RR 14, SpO$_2$ 97% on room air, temp. 37.1°C.

Physical exam reveals a well-nourished and developed male in no acute distress. He prefers to be held by his mother and is fussy during his examination. The head and neck exam is unremarkable aside from bilateral periorbital and palpebral swelling. Examination of the ears, nose, throat, and neck is normal. Cardiovascular examination reveals regular rate and rhythm with good capillary refill of the extremities and normal pulses. Pulmonary exam discloses easy work of breathing and clear auscultation in all lung fields. The abdomen is soft and nondistended, with normal bowel sounds and no hepatosplenomegaly. The skin shows no rashes; however, both feet appear swollen, with decreased skin lines and slight pitting of the skin from the distal third of the tibia onto the dorsum of the foot. His scrotum appears swollen as well, with decreased rugae; the testicles are descended bilaterally and are otherwise unremarkable.

DIFFERENTIAL DIAGNOSIS

1. Nephrotic syndrome from minimal change disease
2. Food allergy
3. Bee sting
4. Focal segmental glomerulosclerosis
5. Membranous nephropathy

TESTS

Dipstick urinalysis: yellow, clear urine with foam; 4+ protein and negative blood; normal pH, specific gravity, glucose, ketones, leukocyte esterase, nitrites, and urobilinogen.

Spot urine protein and urine creatinine were obtained, showing U$_P$:U$_{Cr}$ elevated at 3.6.

Lipid panel: total cholesterol elevated at 240 mg/dL (normal <200 mg/dL); triglycerides elevated at 320 mg/dL (normal <150 mg/dL).

Complete blood count: normal hemoglobin, hematocrit, white blood cells, platelets, and mean corpuscular volume.

Complete metabolic panel: sodium low-normal at 135; normal potassium, chloride, bicarbonate, blood urea nitrogen, creatinine, alanine aminotransferase, aspartate aminotransferase, alkaline phosphatase, and bilirubin; total protein is decreased (normal: 6–8 g/dL) and albumin is decreased to 1.8 g/dL (normal: 3.5–5 g/dL).

Serum C3 and C4 levels are normal.

CLINICAL COURSE

Nephrology was consulted via telephone due to concern for a diagnosis of nephrotic syndrome, likely from underlying minimal change disease. Given the absence of both gross hematuria and hypertension, along with a normal creatinine level, a course of corticosteroids was recommended. After a tuberculosis test was placed and read as negative, prednisone was started at 2 mg/kg/d × 4 weeks. This was followed by an additional 6 weeks of tapering, alternating-day prednisone starting at 1.5 mg/kg/d. The patient's edema resolved gradually over the following weeks. Follow-up in clinic revealed complete resolution of proteinuria and clinical edema. He completed the steroid taper. He experienced a single relapse nearly 6 months later, which was treated with an identical steroid regimen; again, he recovered promptly.

KEY MANAGEMENT STEPS

1. Recognize the clinical presentation of nephrotic syndrome in a child with facial swelling and edema.
2. Obtain urinalysis and recognize nephrotic-range proteinuria is present.
3. Recognize the pertinent absence of hypertension, gross hematuria, and renal insufficiency.
4. Further laboratory evaluation can help confirm the diagnosis (i.e., hypoproteinemia and hypoalbuminemia) and exclude alternate diagnoses (i.e., normal serum complement levels help preclude lupus nephropathy).
5. Initiation of appropriate corticosteroid therapy will lead to remission in the vast majority of patients, though relapse is possible.

DEBRIEF

This patient presented with facial swelling and edema of gradual onset and was found to have significant proteinuria, without evidence of renal insufficiency, nephritis, or hypertension—all consistent with a diagnosis of nephrotic syndrome. In children, nephrotic syndrome is most likely secondary to minimal change disease, also known as lipoid nephrosis. This is most commonly diagnosed in children between ages 2 and 6 years; presentation after age 10 is atypical and merits high suspicion for an alternate diagnosis or an underlying primary illness precipitating a secondary nephrotic syndrome. Nephrotic syndrome can be a paraneoplastic process, sometimes associated with Hodgkin's lymphoma.

Clinical suspicion, coupled with appropriate history, physical, and laboratory evaluations, is sufficient to make the initial diagnosis, and renal biopsy may be avoided if the patient conforms to a typical presentation. Exclusion of atypical features is vital, however, as other clinical syndromes can also present with proteinuria and/or edema. Glomerulonephritis, lupus, and even frank renal failure could present with proteinuria or edema. Nonnephrogenic etiologies of edema such as heart failure, allergic reactions, envenomations and nutritional deficiencies should also be excluded by history and physical examination before nephrotic syndrome is diagnosed.

The mainstay of therapy for first-episode nephrotic syndrome is corticosteroid therapy, and nearly 90% of children with nephrotic syndrome will respond to steroids. Relapse is common, however, with most patients experiencing at least one relapse within their first year of diagnosis. Home monitoring of both weight and urine protein can be helpful in early detection of relapse. Small populations of nephrotic syndrome patients may have steroid-dependent illness, characterized by frequent relapses when off steroid therapy (>4×/year). Even rarer are steroid resistant cases; often related to genetic mutations, these patients may require stronger immuno-suppression regimens, or even renal transplantation.

While nephrotic syndrome is often benign, it can have significant complications. Urinary protein losses include immunoglobulins and complement; fluid accumulations such as ascites can predispose bacterial growth; immunosuppression from therapies can further increase such risk. As such, patients are more likely to develop a variety of infections, such as spontaneous bacterial peritonitis. Furthermore, loss of anticoagulant factors such as antithrombin III can predispose for thromboembolic events like renal vein thrombosis. This risk is further increased when coupled with hemoconcentration and immobility. A high index of suspicion for secondary complications is critical when managing nephrotic syndrome patients.

FURTHER READING

Ellis, D. Pathophysiology, evaluation, and management of edema in childhood nephrotic syndrome. *Front Pediatr.* 2015;3(111). doi: 10.3389/fped.2015.00111.

Kerlin BA, Ayoob R, Smoyer EW. Epidemiology and pathophysiology of nephrotic syndrome–associated thromboembolic disease. *Clin J Am Soc Nephrol.* 2012;7(3):513–520.

Pais P, Avner ED. Conditions particularly associated with proteinuria. In: Kliegman RM, Stanton BF, St. Geme J, Schor N, eds. *Nelson Textbook of Pediatrics.* 20th ed. Philadelphia, PA: Elsevier/Saunders; 2016; 2517–2527.

CHEST PAIN

JENNIFER BELLIS

SETTING

Pediatric Emergency Department

CHIEF COMPLAINT

Chest Pain

HISTORY

A 14-year-old male, who is otherwise healthy, presents in the emergency department with left-sided chest pain for 2 days. The pain is slightly lateral to his mid-sternum. He had an upper respiratory tract infection about 2 weeks ago with congestion and coughing, which has mostly resolved, but he has continued to have a dry cough. He denies any trauma. He has been able to do his usual activity, including playing basketball with his friends yesterday without difficulty. The pain is intermittent and is worse with coughing and taking a deep breath. The pain is not positional or associated with eating. He has not taken any medication for the pain. He has no shortness of breath or dyspnea on exertion. He has been afebrile. He is tolerating fluids with no vomiting or diarrhea. He has never had any similar episodes in the past and has no history of syncopal episodes.

He has no past medical history. His vaccines are up to date.

He denies smoking, alcohol, or drug use. He plays basketball and baseball regularly.

He has no family history of cardiac disease, sudden cardiac death, or unexplained childhood deaths.

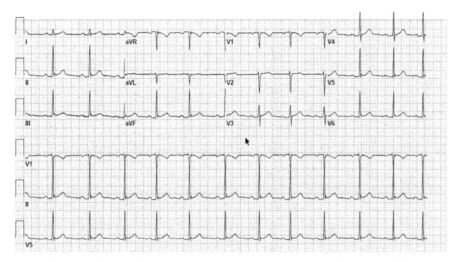

FIGURE 59.1 Electrocardiogram. The patient is in normal sinus rhythm and there are no ST elevations or depressions.

PHYSICAL EXAMINATION

Vital signs: HR 78, BP 114/62, RR 18, SpO$_2$ 100% on room air, temp. 36.7°C.

Examination reveals a well-developed, well-nourished male in no acute distress. Head and neck examination is normal, including no lymphadenopathy and a normal oropharynx. His lungs are clear to auscultation bilaterally with good air entry and without wheezes, crackles, or retractions. Cardiovascular exam reveals regular rate and rhythm, with no murmurs, rubs, or gallops appreciated. Examination of his chest wall reveals point tenderness over the third and fourth costochondral joint on the left side. His abdomen is soft, nontender, and nondistended. Examination of his extremities is normal without peripheral edema. He has 2+ distal pulses and extremities are warm and well perfused. His neurologic examination is grossly normal without focal deficits.

DIFFERENTIAL DIAGNOSIS

1. Costochondritis
2. Gastro-esophageal reflux
3. Reactive airway disease
4. Pneumonia
5. Pneumothorax
6. Pericarditis

TESTS

Electrocardiogram (ECG): Figure 59.1.
Chest radiograph: normal cardiac silhouette, no focal infiltrate, no pneumothorax.

CLINICAL COURSE

The patient had an ECG that showed normal sinus rhythm, normal intervals, and normal ST segments. Chest X-ray was negative for pneumonia or pneumothorax. He was given ibuprofen with improvement in the pain. He was discharged home with a diagnosis of costochondritis. He was discharged with instructions for rest and to continue ibuprofen as needed. The pain and cough had resolved on follow-up with his primary physician.

KEY MANAGEMENT STEPS

1. Identify any concerning chest pain features warranting further investigation through careful history and physical examination, including a thorough review of systems, family history, and social history.
2. Identify other potential noncardiac causes of chest pain.
3. Recognize that most children with chest pain have benign etiology and require minimal workup.

DEBRIEF

The patient in this scenario presented with classic symptoms of costochondritis, including reproducible intermittent focal chest pain that is worse with palpation, deep inspiration, or coughing. For this patient, the continued cough likely precipitated the musculoskeletal chest pain. In addition to cough, strain from physical activity or carrying a heavy back pack over one shoulder are other common causes of costochondritis in children. The reproducible nature of the chest pain is highly suggestive of a musculoskeletal cause. The patient also has been able to complete his normal activity, and exercise does not worsen his chest pain. He otherwise has a negative history and normal exam, which is also reassuring for a benign cause of chest pain.

Chest pain in children can cause a significant amount of anxiety for patients and their parents. In a small study of 100 adolescents, 50% of parents attributed the pain to a cardiac cause and 12% to cancer, though the actual number of children in the study with a cardiac or life-threatening cause was very rare.[1] Musculoskeletal causes of chest pain are one of the most common causes of pediatric chest pain accounting for approximately 30% of cases.[2] Other common noncardiac causes include anxiety/stress, hyperventilation, breast pain, gastrointestinal, and respiratory causes including asthma/reactive airway disease, pneumonia, and pneumothorax.

While most children will need minimal to no workup for their chest pain, clinicians need to be aware of red flags from the history or physical examination that could indicate a more serious or potentially life-threatening cause in the otherwise stable child. Concerning features on history are shown in Table 59.1.[3] Persistently abnormal vital signs, abnormal heart or lung sounds, or other abnormalities on exam are also indications for further workup and possible consultation with a subspecialist. Hemodynamically unstable patients will always require a more extensive workup.

Table 59.1 Concerning Features ("Red Flags") on History that
May Require Further Work Up for Pediatric Patients Presenting
with Chest Pain

Concerning Features on History

History of Presenting illness	*Past Medical History*
Exertional chest pain	Cardiac disease or surgery
Exercise intolerance	Kawasaki disease
Syncope with chest pain	Rheumatologic disorder
Dyspnea or orthopnea	Connective tissue disease
Palpitations	Malignancy
Fever	Renal failure
Symptoms of heart failure	Sickle Cell disease
Possible foreign body	Recent surgery
Prolonged immobilization	
Family History	*Social History*
Arrythmia	Cocaine use
Cardiac lesions in childhood	Sympathomimetic drug use
Early cardiac death	Oral contraceptive use
Hypercoagulability	Pregnancy
Marfan's Syndrome	Smoking

The workup of a patient with a history and exam consistent with costochondritis, such as our patient, is generally limited. An ECG can be an effective screening tool for cardiac etiologies in most settings. ECG evaluation can also help to allay parental and patient anxiety, though in some cases testing may worsen anxiety by indicating to parents that there is a concern for a more serious pathology. Clinicians must evaluate the utility of an ECG for patient or parental reassurance only on a case-by-case basis.

Similarly, a chest X-ray can be used to rule out other causes of chest pain but are indicated only in select cases based on history or physical examination. In our case, a chest X-ray is reasonable given the prolonged cough in a teenage boy to evaluate for a pneumonia or pneumothorax. For patients with a negative workup, reassurance and close follow-up with the primary doctor are the mainstays of treatment in both the emergency department or clinic. Costochondritis typically responds well to rest and treatment with non-steroidal anti-inflammatories.

REFERENCES

1. Pantell RH, Goodman GW Jr. Adolescent chest pain: a prospective study. *Pediatrics.* 1983;71(6):881–887.
2. Son MBF, Sundel R. Musculoskeletal causes of pediatric chest pain. *Pediatr Clin N Am.* 2010;57(6):1385–1395.
3. Byer, R. Pain—chest. In: Fleisher G, Ludwig S, eds. *Textbook of Pediatric Emergency Medicine.* 6th ed. New York, NY: Lippincott, Wiliams and Wilkins; 2010.

FURTHER READING

Friedman K, Alexander M. Chest pain and syncope in children: a practical approach to the diagnosis of cardiac disease. *J Pediatr*. 2013;163(3):896–901.

ABDOMINAL PAIN

PETER GUTIERREZ

SETTING

Pediatric Emergency Department

CHIEF COMPLAINT

Abdominal Pain

HISTORY

A 9-year-old male is brought to the emergency department by his parents for 12 hours of constant, progressive, moderate to severe periumbilical abdominal pain. He was awoken from sleep early this morning with the pain. Since the onset of pain, he has had 4 episodes of nonbloody, nonbilious emesis and has not wanted to take anything by mouth. His parents report that he had a mild fever this morning to 100.6°F, which improved with ibuprofen. He has not had any diarrhea, hematuria, dysuria, or testicular pain. They also report that he would cry out in pain whenever their car hit a pothole on the drive to the hospital.

He has no past significant past medical history.

He attends elementary school with up to date immunizations.

Parents deny any significant past medical history, including inflammatory bowel disease or renal issues.

PHYSICAL EXAMINATION

Vital signs: HR 112, BP 101/68, RR 22, SpO$_2$ 99% on room air, temp. 38°C.

On physical exam, he is awake and alert but holding his abdomen in obvious pain. Examination of his head and neck are normal. He is tachycardic but with a regular rate and rhythm with no murmurs, rubs, or gallops. His lungs are clear to auscultation bilaterally. His abdominal exam shows mild diffuse tenderness, but significant tenderness in the right lower quadrant (RLQ). He has localized rebound tenderness and tenderness to percussion in the RLQ as well. There is reported pain in the RLQ with deep palpation of the left lower quadrant, as well as with internal rotation of the right hip. The patient is asked to stand and jump, which also elicits abdominal pain. His extremities are warm and well perfused with a capillary refill that is less than 2 seconds. He had a normal testicular exam with intact cremasteric reflexes bilaterally. His neurologic exam is grossly normal.

DIFFERENTIAL DIAGNOSIS

1. Appendicitis
2. Constipation
3. Testicular torsion
4. Iliopsoas abscess
5. Nephrolithiasis

TESTS

Complete blood count: white blood cell count of 11,200/mm^3 with 80% polymorphonucleocytes. Hemoglobin and platelet counts were normal.

Comprehensive metabolic panel: normal electrolytes, bicarbonate, and liver function tests.

C-reactive protein: 7.3 mg/L.

Abdominal ultrasound: Figure 60.1.

CLINICAL COURSE

Intravenous access was obtained, and he was given a dose of morphine for pain control and a 20 mL/kg normal saline fluid bolus. His exam was unchanged after the morphine and fluid bolus. Once the labs and imaging returned, the pediatric surgery service was consulted for evaluation. Since the diagnosis of appendicitis had been confirmed, he was taken to the operating room without further labs or imaging for appendectomy.

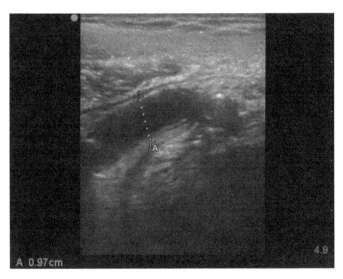

FIGURE 60.1 Ultrasound image. Enlarged blind-ended tubular structure that is noncompressible and has no observable peristalsis.

KEY MANAGEMENT STEPS

1. RLQ tenderness with signs of localized peritonitis should be very suspicious for the diagnosis of appendicitis.
2. Red flag signs/symptoms for potentially serious causes of abdominal pain include report of colicky pain; focal, nonperiumbilical pain/tenderness; presence of peritoneal signs; or if the tenderness is associated with mass palpated on exam.
3. Patients with a recent history of trauma or abdominal surgery, those who are pregnant, and postmenarchal females are at higher risk of serious causes of abdominal pain.
4. For any male with abdominal pain, the diagnosis of testicular torsion should be considered.
5. The Pediatric Appendicitis Score can be a useful tool in predicting the likelihood that appendicitis is present, which includes physical exam and lab findings.
6. Ultrasonography, including point-of-care studies, can be useful in the diagnosis of appendicitis without the need for computed tomography (CT).
7. Once the diagnosis is established, a surgical specialist should be consulted for further management.
8. When abdominal pain is associated with toxic appearance, peritoneal signs, trauma, or a rapid worsening in clinical condition, consider early surgical consultation even if all labs or imaging are not resulted.

DEBRIEF

This patient is having abdominal pain with localized peritoneal signs in the RLQ, suspicious for appendicitis. The classic presentation of appendicitis is a progressive periumbilical pain that migrates the RLQ as the inflamed appendix comes in contact with the parietal peritoneum.

These patients will also present with vomiting, usually starting after the abdominal pain begins. They can also have anorexia and fever. Pain is typically elicited with anything that jars the abdominal viscera, including walking, jumping, hitting the bottom of the feet, or shaking the bed. Patients may report abdominal pain en route to the emergency department when going over speed bumps or hitting potholes.

There are many nonclassic presentations for appendicitis. One reason for this is that the appendix can be located in different areas of the RLQ, including in the retrocecal area, in the pelvis, or anywhere around the ileum. These variable positions may make eliciting peritoneal signs from the anterior abdomen more difficult. More specialized physical exam maneuvers may be needed, including eliciting a Rovsing sign (pain in the RLQ with deep palpation of the left lower quadrant), an obturator sign (pain with internal rotation of the right hip; indicates the possibility of a pelvic appendix), or a psoas sign (pain with passive hyperextension of the right hip; indicates the possibility of a retrocecal appendix).

The Pediatric Appendicitis Score is a validated scoring system for the risk stratification of patients with abdominal pain.[1] These include

- Anorexia (1 point)
- Nausea or emesis (1 point)
- Migration of pain (1 point)
- Fever >38°C (1 point)
- Pain with cough, percussion, or hopping (2 points)
- RLQ tenderness (2 points)
- White blood cell >10,000/mm3 (1 point)
- Absolute band count >7,500/mm3 (1 point)

A score of <3 is low risk, 3 to 6 is medium risk, and 7 to 10 is high risk. Further management may vary from institution to institution depending on the resulting score. In general, medium-risk patients should undergo further evaluation (likely imaging), and high-risk patients may be taken directly to the operating room for appendectomy.

The imaging for appendicitis has been shifting away from CT with intravenous contrast to formal or bedside ultrasound studies. Focal CT of the abdomen has a sensitivity of 95% and specificity of 96% for the diagnosis of appendicitis. Conversely, ultrasound has a sensitivity of 80% to 92% and a specificity of 86% to 98%, with added benefit of no radiation exposure. Ultrasound studies can be of limited usefulness if the patient is uncooperative or has a large body habitus. Figure 60.2 is a labeled bedside ultrasound image of a normal appendix with the typical surrounding anatomy.

Recently, there are been trials evaluating conservative management of appendicitis with antibiotics, instead of appendectomy. In a recent retrospective study,[2] patients who were managed nonoperatively and followed in the preceding 12 months were more likely to have one or more hospitalizations (49.8%) or require more imaging studies, including CT or magnetic resonance imaging. Fourteen percent of these patients developed perforated appendicitis, and 46% eventually had an appendectomy performed. The overall utility and target population for nonoperative treatment is still being investigated.

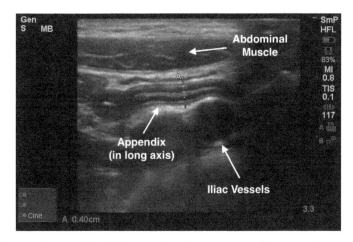

FIGURE 60.2 Ultrasound image. Labeled image of similar structure to Figure 60.1, but in a normal patient.

REFERENCES

1. Samuel M. Pediatric Appendicitis Score. *J Pediatr Surg.* 2002;37(6):877–881.
2. Bachur R, Lipsett S, Monuteaux M. Outcomes of nonoperative management of uncomplicated appendicitis. *Pediatrics.* 2017;140(1).

FURTHER READING

Bachur R. Abdominal emergencies. In: Shaw KN, Bachur R, eds. *Fleischer and Ludwig's Textbook of Pediatric Emergency Medicine.* 7th ed. Philadelphia, PA: Wolters Kluwer; 2016: 1313–1333.

Doniger S, ed. *Pediatric Emergency and Critical Care Ultrasound.* 1st ed. Cambridge, UK: Cambridge; 2013.

SHORTNESS OF BREATH

SYLVIA E. GARCIA

SETTING

Pediatric Clinic

CHIEF COMPLAINT

Shortness of Breath

HISTORY

A 10-month-old male presents to the clinic with cough, decreased oral intake, and noisy breathing that has worsened over the past 3 days. The mother thought she heard wheezing and became concerned. She reports that the patient has had a fever, with a maximum temperature of 38.7°C today for which he was given a subtherapeutic dose of acetaminophen. Prior to arrival to the clinic, he had an episode of post-tussive emesis. He was eating and drinking well until this morning, when he did not want to take his bottle. He has had 3 wet diapers so far today.

He has no significant past medical history. He was born full term, via vaginal delivery. All his immunizations are up to date.

There is no family history of asthma. There is a sister at home who is ill with an upper respiratory infection.

PHYSICAL EXAMINATION

Vital signs: HR 150, BP 80/60, RR 63, SpO_2 89% on room air, temp. 38.7°C.

On arrival, he is alert and active, is noted to be in respiratory distress, and has audible wheezing. Examination of his head and neck shows copious nasal congestion, with nasal flaring and serous fluid behind both tympanic membranes. He is tachypneic with scattered intermittent wheezing with fair aeration, and he has abdominal muscle use, as well as supraclavicular retractions and head bobbing. On cardiac exam, he is tachycardic, with no murmurs, thrills, or rubs, and his capillary refill is 2 seconds. His abdominal exam reveals a soft, nontender and nondistended abdomen, with no hepatosplenomegaly or masses palpated. His extremities have full range of motion and reveal no swelling or tenderness. There are no rashes noted on his skin.

DIFFERENTIAL DIAGNOSIS

1. Bronchiolitis
2. Pneumonia
3. Reactive airways disease
4. Upper respiratory tract infection
5. Aspirated foreign body

TESTS

No tests were ordered.

CLINICAL COURSE

Based on the history and presentation, the patient was presumed to have bronchiolitis, normal saline was instilled in his nares, and he was suctioned with a bulb syringe. He was placed on 2 L O_2 via nasal cannula to maintain his oxygenation at 94%. Ibuprofen 10 mg/kg was given orally for his fever. No steroids, albuterol, or racemic epinephrine were given. Because he remained tachypneic, he was transferred to the local pediatric emergency department via emergency medical services. In the emergency department, the patient had repeat vital signs, with a HR 150, BP 80/60, RR 72, SpO_2 94% on 2 L of O_2 via nasal cannula, and a temperature of 38°C. Examination revealed an active infant in respiratory distress, with continued scattered intermittent wheezing with fair aeration, abdominal muscle use, supraclavicular retractions, and head bobbing. Due to increased work of breathing, respiratory therapy was consulted, and the patient was started on high-flow nasal cannula. His repeat respiratory rate was 55, and his work of breathing improved, with no head bobbing or retractions noted, and mild wheezing heard on lung exam. Because of the severity of his disease, a portable chest X-ray was obtained, which showed no infiltrate. A respiratory panel for reactive airways disease and influenza viruses was obtained, and an intravenous (IV) fluid bolus was given to correct for dehydration from insensible loss. The patient was admitted to the hospital for severe bronchiolitis and dehydration.

KEY MANAGEMENT STEPS

1. Recognizing that this patient is exhibiting signs of respiratory distress, evidenced by head bobbing, retractions, and abdominal muscle use.
2. Providing supportive care via upper airway suctioning and supplemental oxygen.
3. Transferring the patient to a facility that can offer a higher level of management care.
4. Addressing the issue of dehydration by obtaining IV access and providing rehydration.

DEBRIEF

This patient had a first-time event of wheezing, preceded by an upper respiratory infection, and presented in respiratory distress, as evidenced by his nasal flaring, abdominal use, and supraclavicular retractions. He was diagnosed with bronchiolitis, which occurs in children between the ages of 1 to 23 months of age. Bronchiolitis is caused by primary infection or reinfection by a viral pathogen affecting the lower respiratory airways. The most common viral pathogen is respiratory syncytial virus. Bronchiolitis is a clinical diagnosis, and intervention depends on the severity of presentation. Children who are less than 3 months of age, were born prematurely, or have significant cardiopulmonary disease or immunodeficiency are at risk for more severe presentations. Though there are no set criteria that define severity of disease, persistent respiratory distress (tachypnea, retractions, nasal flaring, grunting, accessory muscle use), hypoxemia in association with respiratory distress, apnea, or acute respiratory failure indicate severe disease.

The most recent American Academy of Pediatrics clinical practice guideline on bronchiolitis outlined recommendations for the diagnosis, management, and prevention of the disease. The treatment of bronchiolitis is focused on supportive care and requires serial examinations to determine severity. Suctioning the nares after instillation of normal saline with a bulb syringe can alleviate upper airway obstruction from mucus, is helpful in most presentations, and may be all that is needed in less severe cases. The use of bulb suctioning at regular intervals has shown benefit in the management of these patients. Supplemental oxygen is recommended if oxyhemoglobin concentration is below 90%, and the use of continuous pulse oximetry may be optional, as patients with bronchiolitis may have occasional short episodes of desaturation that are not indicative of worsening disease. In those patients with severe disease, heated humidified high-flow nasal cannula and/or continuous positive airway pressure may prevent the need for intubation and mechanical ventilation. Hydration status should be closely monitored, with fluids delivered either intravenously or through a nasogastric tube in patients who are unable to effectively orally hydrate.

Certain interventions have shown inconsistent or no benefit. Bronchodilators, such as albuterol, have shown no consistent benefit and should not be routinely administered. Though a small subset of affected patients may have reversible airway obstruction from decreasing smooth muscle constriction, no study has defined which patients would consistently benefit from bronchodilator administration. Nebulized epinephrine, used for both upper and lower respiratory tract illnesses, has shown no benefit in the inpatient setting, and no consistent benefit in the outpatient setting. Nebulized hypertonic saline, though shown to be effective in improving mild to moderate symptoms after 24 hours of use, should not be administered in the emergency department as it does not reduce the rate of hospitalization after short-term administration. It may be considered in the hospitalized setting, where it has been shown to reduce hospital length of stay when the hospitalization is longer than 3 days. Corticosteroids are not recommended, and their use may prolong viral shedding. The combination of corticosteroids and bronchodilators or nebulized epinephrine has not been shown in current studies to offer any consistent benefit. Routine use of antibacterial medications is not recommended, unless there is a concurrent bacterial infection or a suspected infection, such as in children who require intubation and mechanical ventilation. In addition, chest physiotherapy is not recommended.

Chest X-ray may be considered in those patients with severe disease, who require heated humidified high-flow nasal cannula and/or continuous positive airway pressure, intubation and mechanical ventilation, or those who do not improve as expected, to rule out other causes of wheezing, such as a foreign body, heart failure, or vascular ring. It is not necessary to obtain a chest X-ray in every single case of first-time wheeze if there are no other concerning components of the case. A respiratory panel to identify the viral cause is not routinely required to confirm the diagnosis but may be useful for cohorting purposes or in determining the cause of severe presentations requiring ventilatory support. Those patients who do not require hospitalization should be followed by their pediatricians within 1 to 2 days. In addition, consideration should be given to those families who cannot provided care at home, as these patients may require hospitalization for supportive care.

The prevention of bronchiolitis is multifocal. In those patients with significant heart disease or chronic lung disease of prematurity, palivizumab prophylaxis should be administered in the first year of life during respiratory syncytial virus season, which is usually November or December through March or April. Disinfection of hands, preferably with alcohol-based rubs, before and after direct contact with patients and inanimate objects in direct contact with patients, and before and after removal of gloves, can reduce the spread of disease in hospitalized patients. Caregivers should be educated on the impact of tobacco smoke exposure on increasing the risk and severity of bronchiolitis. Breastfeeding during the first 6 months of infancy significantly reduces respiratory infections and the risk of hospitalization for respiratory complaints.

FURTHER READING

Cunningham S, Rodriguez A, Adams T, et al. Oxygen saturation targets in infants with bronchiolitis (BIDS): a double-blind, randomized, equivalence trial. *Lancet.* 2015;386:1041–1048.

Fernandes RM, Bialy LM, Vandermeer B, et al. Glucocorticoids for acute viral bronchiolitis in infants and young children. *Cochrane Database Sys Rev.* 2013;10:CD004878.

Mansbach JM, Clark S, Piedra PA, et al. Hospital course and discharge criteria for children hospitalized with bronchiolitis. *J Hosp Med.* 2015:10:205-211.

Ralston SL, Lieberthal AS, Meissner HC, et al. Clinical practice guidelines: the diagnosis, management and prevention of bronchiolitis. *Pediatrics.* 2014;134(5):e1474–e1502.

Sinha PI, McBride AK, Smith R, Fernandes RM. CPAP and high-flow nasal cannula oxygen in bronchiolitis. *Chest.* 2015;148:810–823.

Wing R, James C, Maranda LS, Armsby CC. Use of high-flow nasal cannula support in the emergency department reduces the need for intubation in pediatric acute respiratory insufficiency. *Pediatr Emerg Care.* 2012;28:1117–23.

RASH

KARA COCKRUM AND DAVID MILLS

SETTING

Pediatric Inpatient Wards

CHIEF COMPLAINT

Rash

HISTORY

A 12-year-old previously healthy female was admitted to the inpatient ward last night due to dehydration after developing a rash that began early yesterday morning. The rash started on the back of her hands and subsequently spread to her palms, soles, forearms, neck, lips, and inside the mouth. Her mother states that it initially manifested as small, red bumps that now appear to be blisters surrounded by red rings. The rash is nonpruritic, and they have not noticed any pus or drainage. The patient reports the rash on her body is not uncomfortable except for the areas inside her mouth, which are painful, making it difficult to eat or drink. She denies fatigue, cough, congestion, or sick contacts. She denies any fevers, myalgias, gastrointestinal symptoms, vision changes, redness of the eyes, or neurologic changes. The remainder of the review of systems is negative, and her mother denies giving her any medications in the last week. On admission, the patient reported decreased oral intake from pain due to ulcers in her mouth and only urinated twice in the 24 hours prior to her hospitalization. She received a normal saline bolus in the emergency department and was admitted to the hospital for ongoing intravenous (IV) hydration and pain control.

Past Medical History: She has no significant past medical history other than one "fever blister" on her lip about 10 days ago that self-resolved. She does not take any medications. She has no known drug allergies.

Social History: She lives at home with her mother, father, and two younger siblings.

Family History: Her mother has hypercholesterolemia, and her father has hypertension. There is no family history of rashes or skin infections.

PHYSICAL EXAMINATION

Vital signs: HR 114, BP 105/68, RR 18, SpO$_2$ 100% on room air, temp. 37.2°C.

Examination reveals a well-developed adolescent female in no acute distress. Her head and neck exam is normal, with no cervical lymphadenopathy noted. Eye exam reveals no scleral icterus or conjunctival injection. She has dry mucous membranes with erosions, erythema, and crusting noted on the vermilion border of her lips, tongue, and buccal mucosa. Her posterior pharynx is without erythema, ulcerations, or exudate. Her lungs are clear to auscultation with no wheezes, rales, or increased work of breathing. The cardiac exam reveals tachycardia but regular rhythm, normal S$_1$ and S$_2$, and no murmurs, rubs, or gallops. Her abdomen is soft, nondistended, and nontender with no hepatosplenomegaly noted. She can move all extremities freely, and her bilateral strength is intact. The neurologic exam reveals no gross motor or sensory deficits. Her skin exam is significant for a rash affecting just under 10% of her body surface area (BSA), with multiple lesions of various sizes (ranging from 0.5–2.0 cm) that are well-demarcated, doughnut-shaped, papular lesions with dusky centers. Numerous centers have appreciable blisters, and all of the interiors are encircled by inner pale rings with darker erythematous borders. The rash is prominently located on the bilateral extensor surfaces of her hands and forearms, palms and soles, anterior neck, and upper chest (see Figures 62.1 and 62.2). Her external genitourinary and anal exam are normal.

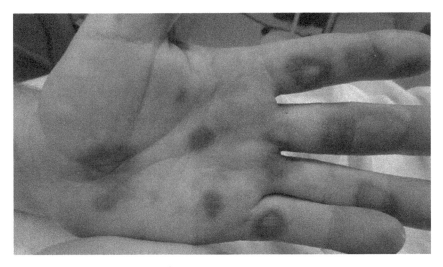

FIGURE 62.1 Erythematous lesions on palm.

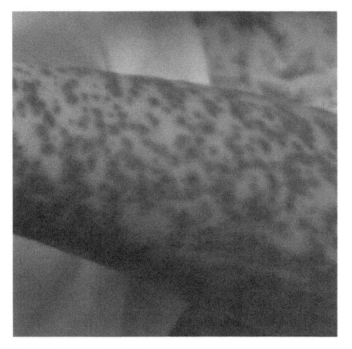

FIGURE 62.2 Papular erythematous rash on forearm.

DIFFERENTIAL DIAGNOSIS

Erythema multiforme (EM)
Stevens-Johnson syndrome (SJS)/toxic epidermal necrolysis (TEN)
Urticaria multiforme
Urticaria
Bullous pemphigoid
Viral exanthem/enanthem
Polymorphous/bullous drug eruption
Hand, foot, and mouth disease

TESTS

A basic metabolic panel was obtained given concerns for dehydration, and all electrolytes were within normal limits.

CLINICAL COURSE

The patient was admitted to the pediatric inpatient wards for IV fluid rehydration secondary to poor oral intake due to discomfort from her oral lesions. Her clinical picture was deemed to be a classic clinical presentation of EM given the pathognomonic target lesions and oral involvement. Acetaminophen and a combination mouthwash (diphenhydramine, lidocaine, and antacid) were provided as needed for pain management and to encourage oral intake. It was felt that the episode was triggered by a recent herpes simplex virus (HSV) infection given her "fever blister" history, and no additional testing was deemed necessary. She required 1 day of IV hydration and pain control and, after improved oral intake, was documented she was discharged home with a principal discharge diagnosis of EM.

KEY MANAGEMENT STEPS

1. Recognize the classic clinical presentation of EM.
2. Identify concerning features of a life-threatening disease process like SJS/TEN.
3. Provide supportive care including hydration, pain management, and pruritus relief.
4. Understand that EM is self-limiting and does not progress to SJS/TEN.

DEBRIEF

The patient in the vignette presented with a classic clinical presentation of EM. EM is an acute, immune-mediated condition defined by the pathognomonic presentation of target-like lesions on the skin. The associated rash may be polymorphic, ranging from erythematous macules, papules, urticarial-appearing plaques, vesicles, or bullae, often with confluent areas of erythema.

The classic appearance is the target lesion, which includes three components:

1. A dusky central area that may blister
2. A dark red inflammatory zone surrounded by a pale ring of edema
3. An outer erythematous ring on the periphery of the lesion

Lesions typically appear abruptly, beginning on the extensor surfaces of the upper extremities with progression to the palms, soles, neck, and mucosal surfaces (most commonly the vermilion border of the lips and buccal mucosa). While often asymptomatic, some patients experience associated pruritus and pain. Similar to the patient in the vignette, prodromal symptoms such as fever, upper respiratory symptoms, myalgias, and malaise are uncommon with EM.

EM involves less than 10% of the BSA and can be further differentiated into two main categories—EM minor and EM major—based on the extent of mucosal involvement. EM minor is defined by no or limited mucosal involvement (limited to one site, usually the mouth), while EM major includes mucosal involvement of two or more mucosal sites, with more severe oral involvement. Given that the patient had less than 10% of her BSA involved and mucous membrane involvement of her mouth only, her diagnosis would be classified as EM minor.

Many factors have been implicated in the development of EM, but infectious causes are responsible for nearly 90% of cases. HSV infection is responsible for 60% to 70% of episodes of EM and is believed to be a precipitating factor in nearly all cases of recurrent EM. Similar to the patient's history in the vignette, target lesions typically present within 10 days of oral or genital HSV reactivation. *Mycoplasma pneumoniae* is another important infectious trigger of EM that should be considered. Less than 10% of EM cases are drug-induced, with nonsteroidal anti-inflammatory drugs (NSAIDs), sulfonamides, antiepileptics, and other antibiotics as known etiologic agents. As such, obtaining a history including symptoms of recent HSV or *Mycoplasma* infection and a detailed medication recall is important in eliciting the precipitant of EM.

As EM is primarily a clinical diagnosis, laboratory testing and imaging are generally not indicated. When the diagnosis is in question, additional testing such as a skin biopsy may be warranted. With lesions that appear consistent with active HSV infection, viral culture or polymerase chain reaction testing may be considered. In patients with concurrent respiratory symptoms, serologic or polymerase chain reaction testing for *Mycoplasma* may help to confirm the diagnosis.

Treatment of EM depends on the severity of disease. Most cases of EM are self-limited and require no treatment, as lesions typically appear over the course of 3 to 5 days and resolve within 2 weeks without long-term sequelae. For mild cases of EM, supportive care is the mainstay of treatment. Pain management should include treatment with acetaminophen or NSAIDs, while oral lesions can be treated topically with a high potency corticosteroid gel and combination mouthwashes that include a mixture of lidocaine, antacids, and diphenhydramine. Pruritus control can be accomplished with oral antihistamines or topical corticosteroids. For extensive oral mucosal involvement that results in the inability to take fluids or nutrition by mouth, systemic corticosteroids may be considered. However, there is a lack of high-quality studies supporting the efficacy of steroids in severe cases of EM, with some data suggesting that steroids may increase the risk for disease chronicity and prolonged duration of acute illness.

While infectious causes are the primary precipitants of EM, research is lacking on whether acutely treating the inciting infection has an effect on the severity or duration of EM. As EM associated with HSV infections typically occurs about 10 days after the acute infection, treatment with oral antiviral therapy at the time of target lesion development is not indicated and has not been shown to alter the clinical course. However, patients who experience frequent recurrence (greater than 6 episodes per year or fewer but more debilitating attacks) may benefit from chronic suppressive antiviral prophylaxis. If drug-induced EM is suspected, the offending agent should be discontinued immediately.

In synthesizing the differential diagnosis, recognizing key features of SJS and TEN is of paramount importance (see Table 62.1). SJS and TEN are potential life-threatening dermatologic diseases primarily caused by drug-mediated reactions, with a typical latency of 4 days to 4 weeks after starting the offending drug. Sulfonamides, NSAIDs, antibiotics, and antiepileptics are the most common precipitating agents. SJS and TEN are associated with extensive epidermal necrosis and detachment, with mucocutaneous complications occurring in ~90% of patients. SJS and TEN differ only based on the percentage of BSA involvement, with <10% BSA affected in SJS, 10% to 30% BSA affected in SJS/TEN overlap, and >30% BSA affected with TEN.

While prodromal symptoms with EM are rare, initial systemic manifestations of SJS/TEN are common and include fever, skin tenderness, and flu-like symptoms/signs of early mucosal involvement (malaise, myalgias, dysphagia, conjunctival itching/burning). Progression to skin and mucosal involvement in SJS/TEN typically occurs 1 to 3 days later. Skin involvement begins with erythematous macules that rapidly and variably develop central necrosis to form vesicles, bullae, and sloughing that results in large areas of denuded skin. Pain is typically pronounced and often out of proportion to the cutaneous findings. Patients commonly have a positive Nikolsky sign, in which lateral pressure with the examiner's finger at an apparently uninvolved site induces epidermal detachment and sloughing of the skin. In addition, two or more mucosal surfaces are involved with SJS/TEN, namely, the eyes, oral cavity, upper airway, gastrointestinal tract, or anogenital mucosa. SJS/TEN carry high morbidity and mortality rates and should be managed in an intensive care unit or burn center. Of note, EM is self-limiting and does not progress to SJS/TEN, an important fact to consider in patient prognosis and management.

Table 62.1 Distinguishing Features of Erythema Multiforme Minor, Erythema Multiforme Major, Stevens-Johnson Syndrome, and Toxic Epidermal Necrolysis

	Precipitating Factors	Skin Findings	Distribution	Mucosal Involvement	Systemic Symptoms
Erythema Multiforme Minor	Infectious most common HSV (60%–70%) Mycoplasma Drugs (<10%)	Typical target lesions Possible papular atypical target lesions	Extensor surfaces of upper extremities, neck/face, palms, and soles <10% BSA	None or limited to 1 site Most commonly lips/ buccal mucosa	Usually absent
Erythema Multiforme Major	Infectious most common HSV (60%–70%) Mycoplasma Drugs (<10%)	Typical target lesions Possible papular atypical target lesions Occasional bullous lesions	Extensor surfaces of upper extremities, neck/face, palms and soles <10% BSA	Two or more mucosal sites More severe oral involvement	Usually present
Stevens-Johnson Syndrome	Drugs most common Occasionally infectious Mycoplasma	Erythematous or violaceous patches Atypical targetoid lesions Bullous lesions Positive Nikolsky sign Minimal tenderness	Trunk, face, neck <10% BSA	Two or more mucosal sites Severe	Usually present
Toxic Epidermal Necrolysis	Drugs most common Occasionally infectious Mycoplasma	Erythematous or violaceous patches Atypical targetoid lesions Bullous lesions Positive Nikolsky sign Severe tenderness	Trunk, face, neck, limbs >30% BSA	Two or more mucosal sites Severe	Usually present

Notes: HSV = herpes simplex virus. BSA = body surface area. Stevens-Johnson syndrome/toxic epidermal necrolysis overlap is for patients with between 10% and 30% involvement.

Recognizing the clinical features associated with EM and developing a focused differential diagnosis for the corresponding target lesions are essential skills for any clinician. Awareness of infectious precipitating factors, that it is typically a self-limited diagnosis, and that supportive care is the hallmark of management are key features of caring for patients with EM.

FURTHER READING

Alerhand S, Cassella C, Koyfman A. Stevens-Johnson syndrome and toxic epidermal necrolysis in the pediatric population: a review. *Pediatr Emerg Care*. 2016;32(7):472–476.

Roujeau JC, et al. Re-evaluation of drug-induced erythema multiforme in the medical literature. *Br J Dermatol*. 2016;175(3):650–651.

Keller N, Gilad O, Marom D, Marcus N, Garty BZ. Nonbullous erythema multiforme in hospitalized children: a ten-year survey. *Pediatr Dermatol*. 2015;32:701–703.

Sokumbi O, Wetter DA. Clinical features, diagnosis, and treatment of erythema multiforme: a review for the practicing dermatologist. *Int J Dermatol*. 2012;51:889–902.

Wetter DA, Davis MD Recurrent erythema multiforme: clinical characteristics, etiologic associations, and treatment in a series of 48 patients at Mayo Clinic, 2000 to 2007. *J Am Acad Dermatol*. 2010;62:45–53.

Joyce JC. Vesiculobullous Disorders In: Schor NF, Behrman RE, eds. *Nelson Textbook of Pediatrics*. 20th ed. Philadelphia, PA: Elsevier Saunders; 2015: 3140–3150.

SECTION VII

MILITARY/TACTICAL

LESLIE V. SIMON

CHAPTER 63

PRIMARY BLAST INJURY

LESLIE V. SIMON

SETTING

Surgical Shock Trauma Platoon, Camp Fallujah, Iraq

CHIEF COMPLAINT

Improvised Explosive Device Blast, Arm Amputation

HISTORY

A 20-year-old male was brought in after his unarmored vehicle drove over an improvised explosive device. The patient was helmeted and wearing a Kevlar vest with small arms protective insert plates. He was the sole survivor of the crash and has an obvious amputation to his right upper arm (Figure 63.1) A combat action tourniquet was applied by first responders and an intraosseous needle was placed in his left humerus.

He has no significant past medical or surgical history; last meal was 2 hours ago.

He is an active duty marine and denies tobacco abuse.

He has no relevant family history.

PHYSICAL EXAMINATION

Vital signs: HR 99, BP 90/70, RR 26, SpO$_2$ 98% on room air, temp 36.8°C.

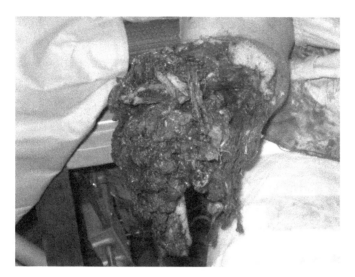

FIGURE 63.1 Right upper extremity amputation.

Primary survey reveals an anxious alert male in obvious distress due to pain. A tourniquet is in place proximal to a complete right arm amputation at the elbow, and there is no obvious external bleeding. He has a Glasgow Coma Scale score of 15. Airway is patent, breath sounds are equal with no obvious injury to the chest, and capillary refill is delayed in the remaining extremities with weak palpable distal pulses. Pelvis is stable, and abdomen is tender. Exam of the back is unremarkable. No apparent neurologic deficit with grossly normal range of motion and strength in the left upper and both lower extremities. Secondary survey reveals bilateral tympanic membrane rupture.

DIFFERENTIAL DIAGNOSIS

1. Traumatic amputation
2. Ruptured tympanic membrane
3. Intra-abdominal injury
4. Pulmonary blast injury
5. Occult injury

TESTS

Complete blood count: hemoglobin 11.2, hematocrit 33.8, white blood cell count 18,000 and platelets 117.

Chemistry panel: normal sodium, potassium, chloride, bicarbonate, blood urea nitrogen, creatinine, and glucose.

Extended Focused Assessment with Sonography for Trauma (eFAST) exam: right upper quadrant view shown in Figure 63.2. The reminder of the examination was negative for pneumothorax, pleural, or pericardial fluid.

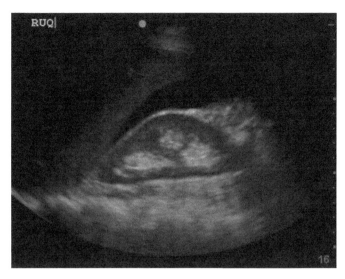

FIGURE 63.2 Right upper quadrant, eFAST exam. Note the hypoechoic (black) area of blood pooling between the liver (screen left) and kidney (center of screen).

Chest X-ray: no acute abnormality.
Pelvis X-ray: normal.
Cervical spine X-rays: normal.

CLINICAL COURSE

The air conditioner was turned off, and patient was exposed and then covered with thermal blankets. Additional large-bore intravenous (IV) access was obtained. Ketamine 20 mg IV was given for pain control. Tranexamic acid (TXA) 1 g IV was given and transfusion with packed red blood cells, fresh frozen plasma, and platelets in a 1:1:1 ratio was initiated. Antibiotic therapy with cefazolin and gentamycin was given for treatment of open fracture and tetanus status was confirmed. After volume resuscitation the patient was intubated and taken emergently for a laparotomy based on the positive eFAST exam.

KEY MANAGEMENT STEPS

1. A thorough, methodical, primary, and secondary survey is critical in managing blast injuries. Impressive soft tissue wounds may easily distract from more serious occult injuries.
2. A tourniquet should be placed immediately in the setting of a complete traumatic amputation. This is often placed by first responders. If not placed correctly, bleeding will increase as the resuscitation progresses and vital signs improve.
3. Obtaining a prompt eFAST exam. Plain X-rays are of limited use and computed tomography scanning is rarely available in forward-deployed settings.

4. Recognition of hemorrhagic shock and treatment with TXA. Blood products (plasma, platelets, and red blood cells) should be administered in a 1:1:1 ratio.
5. Prevention of hypothermia.
6. A screening chest X-ray should be obtained to assess for pulmonary blast injury. Effects may be delayed and exacerbated by positive pressure ventilation in intubated patients.

DEBRIEF

This patient presented with an obvious traumatic upper extremity amputation due to primary blast injury. After placement of a tourniquet for hemorrhage control, methodical primary and secondary surveys are critical to uncover less obvious but more lethal associated injuries. Vital signs and initial hematocrit may be deceptively normal in young healthy victims despite severe injuries. In this case, the patient had a positive eFAST exam, indicating hemoperitoneum. In the absence of a computer tomography scan availability to further assess the injuries, he was taken for an exploratory laparotomy prior to medevac. Damage control resuscitation with judicious use of fluids and blood products is the mainstay of field management of combat casualties.[1] TXA, when administered within the first 3 hours after injury, may decrease all-cause mortality in severely injured trauma patients.[2] Even with very high ambient temperatures, trauma patients may easily become hypothermic.

Blast injuries due to high-order explosives are described as primary, secondary, tertiary, and quaternary. Primary injuries are due to the blast wave itself. Secondary injuries are due to objects accelerated by the blast wind and are the most common injuries encountered.. Tertiary blast injuries are incurred when the victim's body is propelled into another object by the blast wind. Quaternary blast injuries, also referred to as miscellaneous blast effects, can include burns, inhalational injuries, toxic and radiation exposures, and crush injuries due to structural collapse. Many victims of blast injury will have elements of all 4 presenting with a complicated combination of blunt and penetrating injury with burns and inhalational exposure.

Primary blast injury is unique to high-order explosives and is due to the sheering effects of the blast wave on tissue. Severity is directly proportional to proximity to the blast and is most pronounced in enclosed spaces, which provide an interface for reverberation of the blast wave. Tissue damage is greatest in regions of air–tissue interface, the ear, lungs, and the gastrointestinal tract. Barotrauma to the ear is the most common, and pulmonary injury is the most lethal.[3] The presence of a ruptured tympanic membrane may indicate brain damage.[4] A high index of suspicion for pulmonary injury must be maintained as presentation may be delayed and is not excluded by an initially normal chest X-ray. Pulmonary injury can range for pulmonary contusions to pneumothorax to bronchopulmonary fistula, which may cause air embolism. Air embolism is a difficult diagnosis and may present as circulatory collapse after initiation of positive pressure ventilation. Abdominal barotrauma may present as pneumo- or hemoperitoneum due to bowel or solid organ rupture and a negative eFAST exam does not exclude intra-abdominal injury. The colon is the most common site of injury. Solid organs may rupture or tear at fixed points, and testicular rupture is also common. Extremity injury and amputation may occur in all categories of blast injury and may commonly be due to the blast wave itself. Traumatic amputations from primary blast injury were extremely rare in survivors prior to Operation Iraqi and Enduring Freedom but are now common among injured veterans. The blast wave's energy causes primary bone failure at predictable locations—usually the proximal third of the tibia, the proximal third of the arm or forearm, or the or distal third of the femur.

Early use of tourniquets has increased the likelihood of survival. Body armor is designed to protect against secondary blast injury but is not protective against primary injury and may even exacerbate the effects of the blast wave by providing an interface.

REFERENCES

1. Ball CG. Damage control resuscitation: history, theory and technique. *Can J Surg*. 2014;57(1):55–60.
2. Ker K, Kiriya J, Perel P, Edwards P, Shakur H, Roberts I. Avoidable mortality from giving tranexamic acid to bleeding trauma patients: an estimation based on WHO mortality data, a systematic literature review and data from the CRASH-2 trial. *BMC Emerg Med*. 2012;12:3.
3. Stewart C. Blast injuries: preparing for the inevitable. *Emerg Med Pract*. 2006;8(4):1–27.
4. Wolf SJ, Bebarta VS, Bonnett CJ, et al. Blast injuries. *Lancet*. 2009;374:405–415.

FURTHER READING

Centers for Disease Control and Prevention. *CDC blast injury*. Version 1.1. Atlanta, GA: CDC; 2015.

CHAPTER 64

SECONDARY BLAST INJURY

LESLIE V. SIMON

SETTING

Expeditionary Medical Facility, Kuwait

CHIEF COMPLAINT

Improvised Explosive Device Blast, Hand Trauma

HISTORY

An 18-year-old, right-handed male presents for evaluation of hand pain 7 hours after exposure to an improvised explosive device blast involving a suicide bomber in an open area. He is unable to flex his right index finger and has severe pain in the thenar web space. He denies other injury and specifically denies headache, tinnitus, neck pain, chest pain, shortness of breath, and abdominal pain.

He has no significant past medical or surgical history and is fully immunized.

He is an active duty marine and denies tobacco abuse.

He has no relevant family history.

PHYSICAL EXAMINATION

Vital signs: HR 60, BP 120/72, RR 12, SpO_2 100% on room air, temp. 37°C.

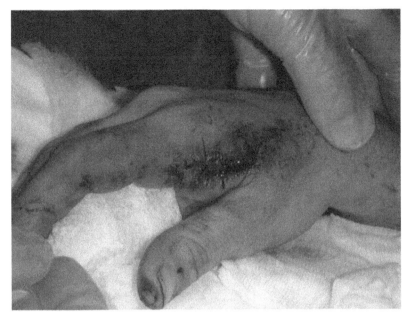

FIGURE 64.1 Right hand demonstrating burn injury, open wound.

Alert, well appearing male in no distress. Head and neck exam are normal; tympanic membranes are intact; and cardiac, pulmonary and abdominal exams are normal. Examination of the right hand (Figure 64.1) reveals noncircumferential, second-degree burns to the thumb and index finger, with multiple deep, foreign body containing lacerations without active bleeding. Two-point tactile discrimination is absent in the thumb and index finger. Radial, median, and ulnar nerve function is otherwise intact. Radial and ulnar pulses are palpable, and capillary refill time is 3 to 4 seconds. The joint capsule of the proximal interphalangeal (PIP) joint of the index finger is exposed, and he is unable to flex the PIP or distal interphalangeal joints.

DIFFERENTIAL DIAGNOSIS

1. Retained foreign body
2. Fracture
3. Flexor tendon injury
4. Open joint
5. Neuro-vascular injury
6. Dislocation
7. Burn
8. Biologic exposure

TESTS

X-ray right hand: Figure 64.2.

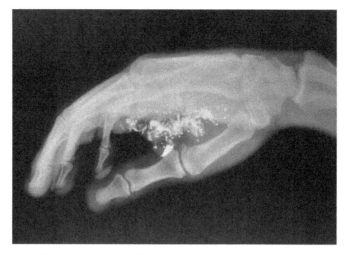

FIGURE 64.2 Right hand X-ray confirming radiopaque foreign bodies beyond what can be seen at the surface.

CLINICAL COURSE

A complete physical exam confirmed isolated hand injury. Wounds were copiously irrigated, anesthetized, and explored. Exam was consistent with flexor tendon laceration and open PIP joint. Tetanus and hepatitis B immunization status were confirmed and prophylactic antibiotics initiated. X-ray showed multiple retained foreign bodies, and obvious superficial debris was removed. Deeper foreign bodies were left in place to avoid further damage. Lacerations were left open. Topical antibiotic ointment was applied to the burns, which were then dressed with a nonadhesive bandage. The hand was splinted in the position of function, and medevac for hand specialist consultation was arranged.

KEY MANAGEMENT STEPS

1. Exclude associated occult injury/evidence of primary blast injury.
2. Copiously irrigate wounds, remove superficial foreign bodies, and debride obvious contamination.
3. Ensure immunization status and consider postexposure prophylaxis.
4. Initiate antibiotics for tendon laceration and open joint and topical burn care.
5. Splint in position of function.
6. Refer for hand specialist evaluation.

DEBRIEF

Secondary blast injury is caused by objects propelled by the energy release of an explosion and is the most common type of blast injury.[1] Depending on the size of the fragments, trauma may be blunt or penetrating, and most patients present with multiple injuries. Improvised explosive devices often contain objects, such as nails or bolts, deliberately added to increase the lethality of the device. Glass from surrounding structures is the most commonly encountered foreign body and may travel great distances causing injury remote from the blast site. Biological fragments, from suicide bombers or other victims, such as bone or teeth are often found in wounds.[2] Postexposure prophylaxis for tetanus, the human immunodeficiency virus, and hepatitis B may be indicated in some settings. Military personnel are immunized against tetanus and hepatitis B prior to deployment, but testing and treatment should be addressed in vulnerable patients. Small, innocuous-appearing lacerations may overlie large foreign bodies and deep, penetrating wounds. Secondary blast injury is usually associated with other categories of blast injury. In this case, the patient also had associated burns (a quaternary injury; see Chapter 63 for information on primary blast injury). Body armor is designed to protect military personnel from secondary blast injury. Since the head and torso are usually covered by armor, most secondary blast wounds are seen in the face, neck, and extremities. This is a major difference from injury patterns typically seen in unprotected civilians.

Blast injuries to the hand require careful evaluation for neurovascular injury, tendon injury, open joints, and retained foreign bodies. In this case, all were present including second-degree burns. Basic decontamination, wound and burn care, tetanus and antibiotic prophylaxis, and splinting in the position of function may be all that is appropriate in the forward-deployed setting. These complex injuries require management by a hand specialist to avoid significant morbidity and loss of function. Attempting to remove deeply embedded foreign bodies in anatomically complex areas such as the hand should not be attempted in the acute setting to avoid inflicting further damage.

REFERENCES

1. Wolf SJ, Bebarta VS, Bonnett CJ, et al. Blast injuries. *Lancet*. 2009;374:405–415.
2. Stewart C. Blast injuries: preparing for the inevitable. *Emerg Med Pract*. 2006;8(4):1–27.

FURTHER READING

Bono MJ, Halpern P. Bomb, blast, and crush injuries. In: Tintinalli JE, Stapczynski J, Ma O, Yealy DM, Meckler GD, Cline DM, eds. *Tintinalli's Emergency Medicine: A Comprehensive Study Guide*, 8th ed. New York, NY: McGraw-Hill; 2016: 34–38.

Centers for Disease Control and Prevention. *CDC blast injury*. Version 1.1. Atlanta, GA: CDC; 2015.

CHAPTER 65

CRUSH INJURY

CHRISTOPHER M. PERRY

SETTING

Military Aid Station, Combat Zone, No Surgical Support

CHIEF COMPLAINT

Bilateral Lower Leg Pain

HISTORY

A 22-year-old male paratrooper presents to the military aide station after a difficult landing parachuting. He presents with an inability to ambulate, bilateral lower extremity edema, and excruciating, deep pain. He was given fentanyl by medics in route that has done little to ease his pain. Additionally, he states that his feet are starting to feel numb. He denies back or neck pain.

He has no significant past medical history.

He is a current every day smoker and drinks several days a week when not in combat operations.

He denies significant family medical history.

PHYSICAL EXAMINATION

Vital signs: HR 120, BP 105/70, RR 26, SpO_2 99% on room air, temp. 36.8°C.

Examination reveals a well-developed, well-nourished male in moderate distress. The lower legs are swollen and tender to touch. The patient has palpable pulses in the bilateral dorsalis pedis and posterior tibialis. The pain is worse with passive dorsiflexion of the bilateral feet, and the patient refuses to move his left foot when asked. The patient's lower legs are relatively stiff when compared to his upper thighs. He states that his left foot is starting to become numb, and his skin is sensitive to touch.

His head, neck, heart, lungs, abdomen, and remaining neurological exams are all normal, with no other remarkable physical exam findings.

DIFFERENTIAL DIAGNOSIS

1. Fractures
2. Peripheral nerve injury
3. Achilles tendon rupture
4. Compartment syndrome
5. Vascular injury
6. Crush syndrome
7. Rhabdomyolysis

TESTS

Complete blood count: hemoglobin 12.6, hematocrit 38.4. White blood cell count and platelets are normal.

Chemistry panel: normal sodium, potassium, chloride, bicarbonate, blood urea nitrogen, creatinine, and glucose.

Total creatine kinase: normal.

Urinalysis: normal.

Lower extremity X-ray: Figure 65.1.

CLINICAL COURSE

Based on history and initial physical examination, the patient was placed on a cardiac monitor, and intravenous access was established with two large bore lines. The patient's pain was controlled with ketamine. X-ray (Figure 65.1) demonstrates bilateral comminuted tibial fractures. The patient's compartments were analyzed with a commercial intracompartmental pressure device. His right lower extremity compartments are measured 0 mm Hg while his left

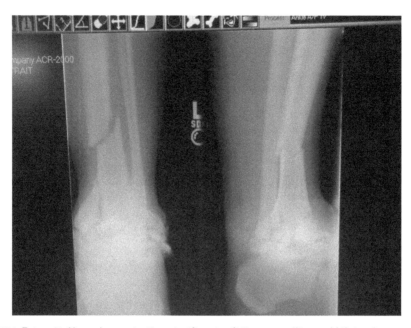

FIGURE 65.1 Extremity X-ray demonstrating significant soft tissue swelling and bilateral compound tibia and fibula fractures.

Courtesy of John Love, MD.

lower extremity anterior compartment measured 45 mm Hg. Other left lower compartments were 0 mm Hg. A 4-compartment fasciotomy is performed. The patient was transferred to a higher level of care, and the wounds were left open for 48 hours to reduce edema. After that time, the patient was taken back to the operating room for debridement, and the wounds were temporarily closed. His wounds were closed permanently after 7 days.

KEY MANAGEMENT STEPS

1. Early recognition of the signs, symptoms, and historical risk factors of compartment syndrome.
2. Resuscitation, blood pressure support, adequate oxygenation, and pain control.
3. Splinting as required.
4. Perform fasciotomy as soon as the clinical diagnosis of compartment syndrome is made.
5. If time permits, obtain X-ray for possible fractures (not required for diagnosis) and determine compartment pressures (if a device is available).
6. Do *not* elevate the limb above the heart or ice the extremity.

DEBRIEF

This patient was experiencing compartment syndrome after bilateral tibia and fibula fractures. The tibial fracture is the most common cause of compartment syndrome, but it may occur in a variety of compartments, with other fractures and several other mechanisms, including soft tissue injury. The discomfort is caused by hematoma or edema, which quickly overpressures a compartment with limited ability for expansion. In turn, this will cause nerve damage and muscle cell death if left untreated.

Historically, the 5 Ps of compartment syndrome were described as pain, pallor, paresthesia, pulselessness, and paralysis. However, these are actually typical findings associated with arterial disruption of a limb rather than compartment syndrome. In compartment syndrome, symptoms begin within a few hours of injury. The symptoms typically include deep, burning, and severe pain in the affected compartment that is difficult to localize and may be refractive to opioid pain medication. Pain with passive movement of muscles of an affected compartment is the most sensitive physical exam finding. Other symptoms may include firmness or stiffness of the compartment and extreme tenderness to palpitation. Of note, it is impossible for the compartment pressure to rise above systolic blood pressure. This allows for continued palpitation of peripheral pulses, normal skin color, and temperature even in the setting of compartment syndrome. If paralysis or pulselessness are present, consider arterial disruption.

If the circumstances allow, the evaluation may include measuring intracompartmental pressures of the extremity with any of several commercially available devices. For accurate results, the compartment should be measured within 5 cm of the injury. Normal compartment pressure is 0 mm Hg. Historically, levels of compartmental pressure <20 mm Hg were considered lower risk, with fasciotomy indicated with pressures between 30 and 50 mm Hg. In actuality, pathologic compartment pressure varies from patient to patient based on a variety of factors. However, recent texts recommend compartment syndrome be diagnosed and fasciotomy indicated when the "delta pressure," the pressure difference between diastolic blood pressure and the measured compartment pressure, is <30 mm Hg.

Performing fasciotomy as soon as possible is important when compartment syndrome is suspected. Irreversible muscle and nerve damage are nearly assured if compartment syndrome is not alleviated within 6 hours of onset. When performing a fasciotomy, ensure the incisions are long enough to completely reduce the compartment pressure. The muscle will often bulge from the compartment immediately after the procedure due to edema. Typically, wound closure can be scheduled 48 hours to 10 days after primary fasciotomy.

Initial labs are often unremarkable as in this case. However, hyperkalemia, rhabdomyolysis, lactic acidosis, and myoglobinuria do occur as sequelae of compartment syndrome and should be managed appropriately.

Treating with elevation and ice is not recommended. Elevating the limb substantially reduces relative arterial pressure and does not improve venous outflow. Additionally, ice causes microconstriction of the vessels with already limited perfusion.

If time permits and the equipment is available, measure compartment pressures:

- Normal pressure 0–10 mm Hg.
- Previously compartment pressure >30 mmHg requires intervention.
- Calculate the delta pressure
    Δ Pressure = (Diastolic Pressure) – (Compartment Pressure)
    Δ Pressure <30 mm Hg is suggestive of compartment syndrome.
- Measure within 5 cm of the injury for best accuracy.
- If initially uncertain, perform continuous or serial compartment pressures.

However, the diagnosis is clinical, and measurements are not required. Fasciotomy is indicated as soon as compartment syndrome is clinically diagnosed. Failure to promptly perform this procedure causes severe long-term nerve and tissue damage. Indications include:

- Clinical signs of compartment syndrome
- Δ Pressure <30 mm Hg
- Absolute pressure >30 mmHg

FURTHER READING

Elliott KG, Johnstone AJ. Diagnosing acute compartment syndrome. *J Bone Joint Surg Br.* 2003;85(5):625–32.

Geiderman JM, Katz D. General principles of orthopedic injuries. In: Marx JA, Rosen P, eds. *Rosen's Emergency Medicine: Concepts and Clinical Practice.* 8th ed. Philadelphia, PA: Elsevier/Saunders; 2014. 521–523.

Haller PR. Compartment syndrome. In: Tintinalli JE, Stapczynski JS, Ma OJ, Yealy DM, Meckler GD, Cline D, eds. *Tintinalli's Emergency Medicine: A Comprehensive Study Guide*, 8th ed. New York: McGraw-Hill Education; 2016. 1883–1886.

Newton EJ, Love J. Acute complications of extremity trauma. *Emerg Med Clin North Am.* 2007;25(3):751–761.

Perron AD, Brady WJ, Keats TE. Orthopedic pitfalls in the ED: acute compartment syndrome. *Am J Emerg Med.* 2001;19(5):413–416.

Shadgan B, Menon M, O'brien PJ, Reid WD. Diagnostic techniques in acute compartment syndrome of the leg. *J Orthop Trauma.* 2008;22(8):581–7.

CHAPTER 66

ABDOMINAL PAIN

ELIZABETH DEVOS

SETTING

USS Essex (Amphibious Assault Ship)

CHIEF COMPLAINT

Abdominal Pain

HISTORY

A 23-year-old male presents to the ship's medical department complaining of abdominal pain, which began suddenly at rest 12 hours ago. He first noticed the pain in the umbilical area, and throughout the day it has become worse in the right lower quadrant (RLQ). He reports nausea and vomiting and feels feverish. He denies diarrhea, dysuria, hematuria, flank pain, or shortness of breath. He has no recent illness or sick contacts. His discomfort increased with jarring movements onboard. His symptoms have been gradually worsening and are now constant.

He has a past medical history of asthma and no recent travel.

He is not a smoker, drinker, or illicit drug user.

He denies family history of Crohn's disease or ulcerative colitis.

PHYSICAL EXAMINATION

Vital signs: HR 118, BP 126/76, RR 18, SpO$_2$ 98%, temp. 38.8°C.

Examination reveals a well-developed, well-nourished male in pain. Examination of his head and neck is normal. His lungs are clear bilaterally with good air movement. He is tachycardic with a normal rhythm; no murmurs, rubs, or gallops are appreciated. His abdomen is soft, significantly tender in the RLQ over McBurney's point. He has voluntary and involuntary guarding as well as positive Rovsing's sign and positive psoas sign. Bowel sounds are normal in all quadrants. Genitourinary exam is normal. His extremities are warm and well-perfused, without edema. Neurologic examination reveals grossly normal strength and sensation in all extremities, normal gait, and coordination.

DIFFERENTIAL DIAGNOSIS

1. Appendicitis
2. Inguinal hernia
3. Renal colic
4. Right colon diverticulitis
5. Testicular torsion
6. Enteritis

TESTS

Complete blood count: white blood count 19,000 with 91% polymorphonuclear leukocytes (PMN) (4,000–12,000). Normal hemoglobin, hematocrit, and platelets.

Chemistry panel: normal sodium, potassium, chloride, bicarbonate, blood urea nitrogen, creatinine, and glucose.

RLQ ultrasound: (Figure 66.1).

CLINICAL COURSE

Intravenous (IV) access was established, and morphine and IV fluid boluses were administered. After the labs and ultrasound were obtained, the physician discussed diagnosis, treatment options, risks, and benefits at length with patient. Together, they decided upon an "antibiotics first" strategy as surgical care would require medevac. The patient received IV cefotaxime and metronidazole for 48 hours with serial abdominal exams. Tachycardia and fever resolved, symptoms improved, and the patient was discharged on oral antibiotics (cefdinir and metronidazole) when tolerated orally.

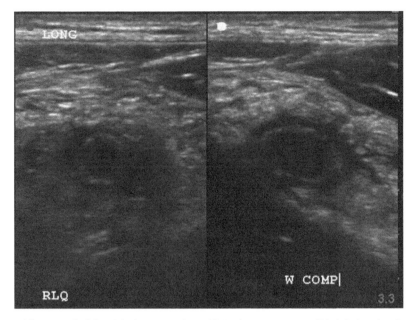

FIGURE 66.1 Ultrasound of the right lower quadrant. Note the noncompressible tubular structure, with a diameter over 6 mm, in right lower quadrant.

Courtesy of Michael Boniface, MD.

KEY MANAGEMENT STEPS

1. Consideration of appendicitis in the differential diagnosis of a patient with abdominal pain, fever, and vomiting.
2. Obtaining serum chemistry (including electrolytes and creatinine), complete blood count with differential, and abdominal imaging with ultrasound or computed tomography (CT) scan in a patient with suspected appendicitis where exam does not warrant immediate surgical consultation prior to imaging. Patients with classic findings may not warrant diagnostic imaging to confirm the diagnosis.
3. Recognition of patients who may be eligible for an "antibiotics first" approach to management of appendicitis: exclusions include pregnancy, immune compromise, clinical evidence of sepsis or peritonitis, and imaging-revealing perforation or abscess.
4. Appropriate early consultation with acute care surgery based on clinical, laboratory and imaging findings and shared decision-making with patient.

DEBRIEF

Appendicitis is believed to be related to a fecalith or other obstruction of the lumen of the vermiform appendix. Increasing pressure and appendiceal vascular insufficiency may lead to bacterial overgrowth, perforation, and abscess formation. Visceral irritation causes early, often vague symptoms. As inflammation increases, somatic innervation of the parietal peritoneum leads to localization of pain at McBurney's point, found one-third of the way between the umbilicus and the anterior superior iliac spine. Classic symptoms include abdominal pain migrating to the

RLQ, fever, and vomiting. Rebound tenderness and voluntary guarding clinically suggest peritonitis. Psoas and obturator signs are not specific but are classic indicators of peritoneal irritation.

Clinical scoring systems have better likelihood ratios than individual signs or symptoms but
cannot be used alone to definitively diagnose appendicitis. However, they can identify patients at
very low risk for appendicitis not requiring imaging or otherwise guide clinical management.[1,2]
Diagnosis is made with ultrasound, CT, or magnetic resonance imaging. Ultrasound has lower
sensitivity and specificity than CT, but when readily available with experienced operators, its relative low cost, lack of radiation exposure, and accessibility in austere conditions make use ideal.
CT offers more detailed imaging and diagnosis of other causes of abdominal pain but also delivers
ionizing radiation. Magnetic resonance imaging presents similar advantages to CT but is more
expensive and cumbersome, so it is reserved for patients where ultrasound would be complicated
and radiation contraindicated, such as pregnant patients. The standard of care for treatment of
appendicitis in the United States remains early surgery. However, Europeans have demonstrated
success in an "antibiotics first" nonsurgical approach for selected patients. Small studies in
the United States have shown this to be feasible and cost-effective.[3] In austere conditions, the
"antibiotics first" approach may prove to be a viable option to balance risk mitigation, resource
utilization, and cost management, particularly when surgery is not readily accessible.

When appendicitis is suspected, it is important to place an IV line and assess vital signs.
Other life-threatening causes of abdominal pain must be excluded, particularly ectopic pregnancy in female patients of childbearing age. Serial abdominal exams must be continued to assess for changes in patient condition. Complete blood count and electrolytes should be obtained.
An ultrasound of the RLQ or CT scan of the abdomen and pelvis should be obtained to confirm
diagnosis, rule out perforation or abscess, and evaluate other causes of abdominal pain.

In this case, the RLQ ultrasound demonstrated appendicitis without perforation (evidenced
by free peritoneal fluid) or abscess. This patient was a candidate for "antibiotics first" treatment
(Table 66.1).[4] Antibiotic regimens should cover aerobes and anaerobes based on local resistance

Table 66.1 Common Features of Randomized Clinical Trials
of "Antibiotics First" Regimens

Patient factors	Consenting adult patient
	Not pregnant
	Not immunocompromised
	Not utilizing specified implantable devices
Imaging factors	No abscess
	No perforation
Clinical factors	No disseminated peritonitis
	No abscess
	Able to receive intravenous antibiotics in hospital for 48 hours
	Able to have serial abdominal reassessment every 6–12 hours
	Able to achieve pain control
	Able to tolerate food orally prior to hospital discharge
	Able to take 7 days of home oral antibiotics

Source: Adapted from Flum DR. Acute appendicitis—appendectomy or the "antibiotics
first" strategy. *N Engl J Med.* 2015;372(20):1937–1943.

patterns and include 1 to 3 days of parenteral antibiotics followed by 7 to 10 days of oral antibiotics. While such regimens have shown promise, one study described a short-term failure requiring surgery in approximately 12% of enrolled patients within 7 days.[5] Meta-analyses of randomized controlled trials revealed failure rates of up to 35% within 1 year, with many of these patients requiring surgery.[6,7] Further, when surgery was required among the "antibiotics first" groups in meta-analyses, peritonitis was more frequent in those who were initially treated nonoperatively.[6]

In the setting of acute appendicitis, care must be taken to assess for signs of sepsis or disseminated peritonitis and consideration of available surgical resources as well as potential adverse outcomes related to potential for future need for surgery must be weighed against potential for early discharge and return to normal activity, decreased hospital costs, and other factors influencing the possibility of nonsurgical management in consultation with acute care surgery.

REFERENCES

1. Rezak A, Abbas HMA, Ajemian MS, Dudrick SJ, Kwasnik EM. Decreased use of computed tomography with a modified clinical scoring system in diagnosis of pediatric acute appendicitis. *Arch Surg*. 2011;146(1):64–67.
2. Farahnak M, Talaei-Khoei M, Gorouhi F, Jalali A, Gorouhi F. The Alvarado score and antibiotics therapy as a corporate protocol versus conventional clinical management: randomized controlled pilot study of approach to acute appendicitis. *Am J Emerg Med*. 2007;25(7):850–852.
3. Talan DA, Krishnadasan A, Amii R, et al. Antibiotics-first versus surgery for appendicitis: a US pilot randomized controlled trial allowing outpatient antibiotic management. *Ann Emerg Med*. 2017;70(1):1–11.
4. Flum DR. Acute appendicitis—appendectomy or the "antibiotics first" strategy. *N Engl J Med*. 2015;372(20):1937–1943.
5. Di Saverio S, Sibilio A, Giorgini E, et al. The NOTA Study (Non Operative Treatment for Acute Appendicitis). *Ann Surg*. 2014;260(1):109–117.
6. Podda M, Cillara N, Di Saverio S, et al. Antibiotics-first strategy for uncomplicated acute appendicitis in adults is associated with increased rates of peritonitis at surgery: a systematic review with meta-analysis of randomized controlled trials comparing appendectomy and non-operative management with antibiotics. *Surg*. 2017;15(5):303–314.
7. Eriksson S, Granstrom L. Randomized controlled trial of appendicectomy versus antibiotic therapy for acute appendicitis. *Br J Surg*. 1995;82(2):166–169.
8. DeKoning E. Acute appendicitis. In: Tintinalli JE, Stapczynski J, Ma O, Yealy DM, Meckler GD, Cline DM, eds. *Tintinalli's Emergency Medicine: A Comprehensive Study Guide*. 8th ed. New York, NY: McGraw-Hill; 2016.

CHAPTER 67

HEAT STROKE

ALEXANDER BERK

SETTING

Emergency Department

CHIEF COMPLAINT

Altered Mental Status

HISTORY

A 25-year-old male who is brought by emergency medical services (EMS) to the emergency department after collapsing during a training run. The patient was wearing a Kevlar vest and gas mask during his run. The patient was taken to the base clinic where cooling measures with fans were begun, and EMS was activated. EMS states that upon arrival, he had a Glasgow Coma Scale (GCS) of 7 (E1V2M4). No other history is available at this time. The patient was transported to the emergency department, receiving 600 mL of lactated Ringer's solution en route. The patient's altered mental status prevents any further history.

Past medical, social, and family history is unknown.

PHYSICAL EXAMINATION

Vital signs: HR 140, BP 105/46, RR 28, SpO$_2$ 98% on room air, temp. 41.7°C (107.1°F), temp. 108.0°F rectal.

Examination reveals a well-developed, well-nourished male in severe distress. Examination of his head and neck is normal, revealing no jugular venous distension, evidence of trauma or deformity. He is tachypneic, and his lungs are clear bilaterally with good air movement. His cardiac rate is tachycardic but regular; no murmurs, rubs, or gallops are appreciated. His abdomen is soft, nontender, and nondistended. He has no lower extremity edema with good peripheral pulses. Neurologic examination reveals that he is moving all extremities, but obtunded, with GCS 6 (E1V1M4). Skin is dry, pale, and hot to the touch.

DIFFERENTIAL DIAGNOSIS

1. Meningitis
2. Heat stroke
3. Head trauma/C-spine injury
4. Seizure
5. Serotonin syndrome

TESTS

Chemistry panel: sodium 138 mmol/L, potassium 6.1 mmol/L, chloride 104 mmol/L, CO$_2$ 23 mmol/L, glucose 205 mg/dL, blood urea nitrogen 30 mg/dL, creatine 1.9 mg/dL, calcium 10/1 mg/dL.

Complete blood count: white blood cell count 10.6 K/uL (56% polymorphonuclear leukocytes [PMN], 32% lymphocytes [LYM]), hemoglobin 17.6 g/dL, hematocrit 52.2%, platelets 242 K/uL normal, troponin I 0.56 ng/mL, lactic acid 4.5 mmol/L, creatine kinase, total 582 units/L.

Lumbar puncture: white blood cell count 0, red blood cell count 2, glucose 98, protein 26.0.

Urine and serum tox screen: negative.

Electrocardiogram: sinus tachycardia rate of 129, normal intervals. Normal axis. ST segment elevation 1 to 2 mm through the anterior/lateral precordial leads. No reciprocal changes. No ectopy.

Chest X-ray: no focal infiltrates or consolidations. No overt pulmonary edema. Normal chest.

Computed tomography (CT) head without contrast: no acute infarctions, intracranial hemorrhages or mass lesions.

CT cervical spine without contrast: negative CT of the cervical spine.

CLINICAL COURSE

Based on history and arrival vital signs, a second IV was established. The patient was placed on high-flow oxygen and a cardiac monitor. Active cooling measures were started, including ice packs, spray bottles and fan, and a cooling blanket. Two liters of cooled normal saline were infused. Due to his depressed GCS, he was intubated for airway protection. After intubation, an orogastric tube was placed, and an ice water lavage was started. The patient's head CT and C-spine CT ruled out trauma, and a lumbar puncture was performed that ruled out meningitis. Cooling measures were discontinued when core temperature reached 102.2°F (39°C). At that point, the patient was noted to respond to simple commands such as eye opening. The patient was then admitted to the intensive care unit. He was successfully extubated after one day in the intensive care unit. With copious IV fluids, his metabolic derangement resolved. He was seen by cardiology for his elevated troponin and electrocardiogram changes and was determined to have demand myocardial ischemia, with no evidence of vaso-occlusive coronary artery disease. The patient improved and walked out of the hospital on his own 2 days after admission.

KEY MANAGEMENT STEPS

1. Consider heat stroke in the differential diagnosis of a patient with hyperthermia and altered mental status. Rule out infectious causes as well.
2. Obtain serum chemistry (including electrolytes and creatinine), total creatine kinase, troponin I, lactate level, and chest X-ray in a patient with suspected heat stroke.
3. Intubate for airway protection if needed.
4. Initiate early active cooling measures with ice packs, water and fans, and cooling blankets. Consider more aggressive internal cooling with cooled IV fluids and ice water lavage. Do not overshoot, target goal of 39°C (102.2°F).[1]
5. Appropriate early consultation with Intensivists to help in management.

DEBRIEF

This patient had altered mental status caused by exertional heat stroke. Exertional heat stroke usually occurs in younger patients who perform high-intensity activities in a hot environment. Typically, patients present with a temperature >41°C (105.8°F) and altered mental status. Although anhidrosis or lack of sweating is commonly seen, some patients will present diaphoretic. Providers must maintain a high index of suspicion for these cases.

The differential diagnosis for patients who are hyperthermic and altered is very broad. Evaluation must be focused equally on ruling out infectious, metabolic, and toxicologic causes as it is in evaluating the overall effect on the patient's organ systems. Workup typically includes serum chemistry, lactate, liver function tests, CBC, total creatine kinase urinalysis, toxicology screen, and cerebrospinal fluid evaluation. Radiologic studies should be considered to evaluate for infection, trauma, and pulmonary edema.

When exertional heat stroke is suspected, it is important to aggressively cool the patient with the goal of not overshooting a target of 39°C (102.2°F). Rectal temperatures are considered the most accurate. Antipyretics have not shown any benefit in heat stroke. Cooling should be initiated in the prehospital setting and continued in the hospital. Remove clothing, place ice packs in axillae and groin, spray with water, and use fans for evaporative heat loss. IV access should be obtained and cooled IV fluids infused. Supplemental oxygen should be given to awake patients as needed, and those unable to protect their airway should be intubated. Place the patient on a cardiac monitor in case of dysrhythmia. Consider other cooling methods that include cold water immersion, cold humidified oxygen, cooling blankets and gastric (via orogastric/nasogastric tube), rectal (via rectal tube), thoracic (via chest tubes), and peritoneal (via peritoneal catheter) ice water lavage.[2]

Provide aggressive fluid support for cases of rhabdomyolysis with careful monitoring for fluid overload state. Correct significant electrolyte abnormalities including assisting clearance of potassium if severely hyperkalemic. Initiate broad spectrum antibiotics for all altered hyperthermic patients until infectious causes are ruled out.

All heat stroke patients should be admitted to a monitored setting for 1 to 2 days.

REFERENCES

1. Smith JE. Cooling methods used in the treatment of exertional heat illness. *Br J Sports Med.* 2005;39(8):503–507; discussion 507.
2. O'Connor JP. Simple and effective method to lower body core temperatures of hyperthermic patients. *Am J Emerg Med.* 2017;35(6):881–884.

FURTHER READING

Lovecchio, F. Heat emergencies. In: Tintinalli J, et al., ed. *Tintinalli's Emergency Medicine: A Comprehensive Study Guide.* 8th ed. New York, McGraw-Hill, 2016: 1365–1370.

Pryor RR, Bennett BL, O'Connor FG, et al. Medical evaluation for exposure extremes: heat. *Wilderness Environ Med.* 2015;26(Suppl 4):S69–S75.

Sylvester JE, et al. Exertional heat stroke and American football: what the team physician needs to know. *Am J Orthop.* 2016;45(6):340–348.

CHAPTER 68

FACIAL DISFIGURATION

DOUGLAS HOFSTETTER, ANDREA AUSTIN, AND RYAN MAVES

SETTING

Military Humanitarian Medical Mission, Peruvian Amazon

CHIEF COMPLAINT

Facial Disfiguration

HISTORY

A 65-year-old woman presents to a humanitarian medical mission clinic in the Peruvian Amazon with severe facial disfiguration. She states that the disfiguration started around 4 years ago as gradual swelling and nose pain. She also complains of nasal stuffiness and several episodes of epistaxis. There are no associated fevers, chills, anorexia, abdominal pain, lethargy, or other skin complaints. She was in her normal state of health prior to noting the skin lesion and did not seek care until now due to poor access to medical care.

  She denies any significant past medical history and surgical history.
  She is not aware of any significant family history of health problems.
  She does not take any medications. She has no drug allergies.

She denies smoking, alcohol, and illicit drug use. She has lived in the area her entire life and spends her time working at home or tending her family's crops in the nearby fields. She has not traveled outside of the region recently.

PHYSICAL EXAMINATION

Vital signs: HR 80, BP 138/91, RR 15, SpO_2 99% on room air, temp. 37.4°C.

Examination reveals an elderly female in no acute distress. Her head is normocephalic and atraumatic, and her neck is supple and nontender. Her eyes are without jaundice, injection, or discharge. Examination of her nose shows deep ulcerations on the inferior and middle turbinates of her right naris with partial destruction of the nasal septum; her left naris is normal. Her orophyanyx is clear, moist, and without any evident ulcerations. Her lungs are clear bilaterally with good air movement. Her heart rate is normal and without murmurs, rubs, or gallops. Her abdomen is soft, nontender, nondistended, and without any hepatosplenomegaly. Her extremities are normal and have strong peripheral pulses. Her skin exam shows a large, disfiguring ulcerative facial lesion with heaped borders and scant serosanguinous discharge as depicted in Figure 68.1. She is alert and oriented, and her neurological exam is normal.

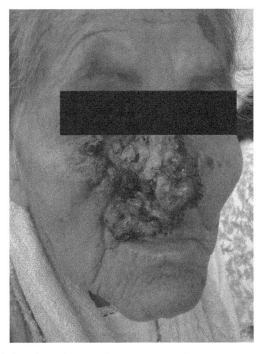

FIGURE 68.1 Leishmanial skin ulceration seen in cutaneous and mucocutaneous leishmaniasis.

Courtesy of Dr. Ryan Maves.

DIFFERENTIAL DIAGNOSIS

1. Staphylococcal infection
2. Squamous cell carcinoma/basal cell carcinoma
3. Leprosy
4. Histoplasmosis
5. Mucocutaneous leishmaniasis
6. Paracoccidioidmycosis
7. Yaws
8. Sporotrichosis
9. Blastomycosis
10. Cutaneous tuberculosis
11. Sarcoidosis
12. Mucormycosis

TESTS

None available.

CLINICAL COURSE

Given the chronic and disfiguring nature of the patient's facial ulcerations, nasal mucosa involvement, and nasal septum destruction, the patient was transferred to a regional referral center for management of suspected mucocutaneous leishmaniasis. Intravenous amphotericin B deoxycholate was initiated, and she underwent surgical debridement of the cutaneous and mucosal lesions. Smears prepared from clean-based cutaneous ulcer scrapings revealed leishmanial amastigotes, confirming the initial diagnosis. DNA polymerase chain reaction (PCR) done on the scrapings would later identify *L. braziliensis* as the species of *Leishmania* involved.

KEY MANAGEMENT STEPS

1. Recognize the skin and mucosal findings typically seen in cutaneous and mucocutaneous leishmaniasis.
2. Understand the different presentations of *Leishmania* infections.
3. Understand the different diagnosis and treatment options for leishmaniasis.

DEBRIEF

In this case, an elderly Peruvian female presented with an impressive area of chronic skin and mucosal ulceration. The appearance of the lesions and the Peruvian Amazon location all suggest mucocutaneous leishmaniasis as the probable diagnosis. This high pretest probability was confirmed via ulcer scrapings and DNA PCR.

Leishmaniasis is a vector-borne protozoan disease caused by over 20 species of intracellular parasites within the *Leishmania* genus. Human populations in developing areas in Latin America, Africa, and Asia bear the brunt of the disease burden.[1] It is estimated that over 12 million people are affected globally with 200,000 to 300,000 deaths reported annually.[2] US cases have been reported and are often linked to travel through endemic area, military operations, and immigrants.[3] Disease transmission occurs through the bite of infected female sandflies.[4]

Depending on the host's immune response and the infecting *Leishmania* species, clinical leishmaniasis can manifest as a cutaneous, mucocutaneous, or visceral disease. Overlap between the categories is common, as are asymptomatic infections. In cutaneous leishmaniasis, patients present with an array of skin findings at the site of inoculation that range from painless papules and nodules to deep, mutilating ulcerations. In mucocutaneous leishmaniasis, destruction of the mucosal tissue and underlying cartilaginous structures ensues, leading to impressive disfiguration.[5] If infected phagocytes continue to spread through the reticuloendothelial system, leishmaniasis can manifest in a life-threatening systemic form called visceral leishmaniasis. Death usually occurs within 2 years if untreated, often from infection, severe anemia, or hemorrhage.[2,6]

A variety of parasitological and immunological techniques are available for the diagnosis of leishmaniasis. For cutaneous leishmaniasis, microscopic examination of skin/ulcer scrapings, aspirates, and biopsies, cultures or DNA PCR may be utilized.[3,7,8] Diagnosis of mucocutaneous leishmaniasis is complicated by the paucity of parasites in affected mucosal tissue; DNA PCR is preferred.[9,10] For visceral leishmaniasis, microscopic visualization of amastigotes in splenic or bone marrow aspirates is required.[11,12]

Given the genetic variability between *Leishmania* species, their geographical distribution, and variability in immune responses between human hosts, developing treatment recommendations for leishmaniasis is challenging. Many cases of cutaneous leishmaniasis resolve on their own. With milder forms of cutaneous leishmaniasis, local therapies such as thermotherapy, cryotherapy, paromomycin ointment, and local infiltrations with pentavalent antimonials are viable options. Oral and parenteral therapy is reserved for more complicated cases and those who have progressed to mucocutaneous or visceral leishmaniasis, with options including azole drugs, antimonials, and amphotericin B formulations.[13,14] Given the complexity of these treatment options, any suspected case of leishmaniasis warrants consultation with an infectious disease specialist.

REFERENCES

1. Parasites-Leishmaniasis. Centers for Disease Control and Prevention. January 10, 2013. https://www.cdc.gov/parasites/leishmaniasis/epi.html.
2. Leishmaniasis. World Health Organization. April 2017. http://www.who.int/mediacentre/factsheets/fs375/en/
3. Kevric I, Cappel MA, Keeling JH. New world and old world leishmanial infections: a practical review. *Dermatol Clin.* 2015;33(3)597–593.
4. Bates PA. Transmission of Leishmania metacyclic promastigotes by phlebotomine sand flies. *Int J Parasitol.* 2007;37(10):1097–1106.
5. Lupi O, Bartlett BL, Haugen RN, et al. Tropical dermatology: tropical diseases caused by protozoa. *J Am Acad Dermatol.* 2009;60(6):897–925.

6. Magill AJ. Leishmania species: visceral (Kala-Azar), cutaneous, and mucosal leishmaniasis. In: Bennett JE, Dolin R, Blaser MJ, eds. *Mandell, Douglas, and Bennett's Principles and Practice of Infectious Diseases*. 8th ed. Philadelphia, PA: Elsevier Saunders; 2014: 3091–3107.

7. Weigle KA, de Dávalos M, Heredia P, Molineros R, Saravia NG, D'Alessandro A. Diagnosis of cutaneous and mucocutaneous leishmaniasis in Colombia: a comparison of seven methods. *Am J Trop Med Hyg*. 1987;36(3):489–496.

8. de Almeida ME, Steurer FJ, Koru O, Herwaldt BL, Pieniazek NJ, da Silva AJ. Identification of Leishmania spp. by molecular amplification and DNA sequencing analysis of a fragment of rRNA internal transcribed spacer 2. *J Clin Microbiol*. 2011;49(9):3143–3149.

9. Magill AJ. Cutaneous leishmaniasis in the returning traveler. *Infect Dis Clin N Am*. 2005;19(1):241–266.

10. Scope A, Trau H, Anders G, Barzilai A, Confino Y, Schwartz E. Experience with New World cutaneous leishmaniasis in travelers. *J Am Acad Dermatol*. 2003;49(4):672–678.

11. Sarker CB, Alam KS, Jamal MF, et al. Sensitivity of splenic and bone marrow aspirate study for diagnosis of kala-azar. *Mymensingh Med J*. 2004;13(2):130–133.

12. Thakur CP. A comparison of intercostal and abdominal routes of splenic aspiration and bone marrow aspiration in the diagnosis of visceral leishmaniasis. *Trans R Soc Trop Med Hyg*. 1997;91(6):668–670.

13. Monge-Maillo B, Lopez-Velez R. Therapeutic options for old world cutaneous leishmaniasis and new world cutaneous and mucocutaneous leishmaniasis. *Drugs*. 2013;73(17):1889–1920.

14. Amato VS, Tuon FF, Siqueira AM, Nicodemo AC, Neto VA. Treatment of mucosal leishmaniasis in Latin America: systematic review. *Am J Trop Med Hyg*. 2007;77(2):266–274.

FEBRILE ILLNESS

DOUGLAS HOFSTETTER, ANDREA AUSTIN, AND RYAN MAVES

SETTING

Emergency Medical Facility—Camp Lemonnier, Djibouti

CHIEF COMPLAINT

Fever

HISTORY

A 20-year-old male Marine presents with 1 day of fever and body aches. The fever has been persistent since onset and has not improved with oral acetaminophen or ibuprofen. The highest temperature was 39°C earlier in the morning. He also reports episodic chills and sweats, persistent malaise, diffuse body aches, a diffuse headache, and 1 day of nonbloody diarrhea. He denies cough, vomiting, and abdominal pain. Prior to his illness, the patient was in his normal state of health. He has been stationed at Camp Lemonnier for 3 months now and has done several training exercises in the rural areas nearby. He received his hepatitis A, hepatitis B, and meningococcal vaccines during boot camp, along with typhoid and yellow fever vaccines prior to deployment. His seasonal influenza vaccine is up to date.

He denies any significant past medical and surgical history.

He denies family history of bleeding disorders and hematological diseases.

He takes 100 mg of oral doxycycline each day for malaria prophylaxis. He missed several doses around 3 weeks ago after failing to pack enough medication for a multiday field exercise. He has no known food or drug allergies.

He denies smoking, alcohol, or illicit drug use.

PHYSICAL EXAMINATION

Vital signs: HR 105, BP 125/83, RR 20, SpO$_2$ 99% on room air, temp. 38.3°C.

Examination reveals a well-built yet fatigued male Marine in mild distress. Examination of his head and neck is normal and reveals no cervical adenopathy. His eyes show conjunctival pallor without scleral icterus. His orophyanyx is clear, moist, and without tonsillar hypertrophy or petechiae. His lungs are clear bilaterally with good air movement. His heart rate is mildly tachycardic but regular and without murmurs, rubs, or gallops. His abdomen is soft, nontender, and nondistended. He has a palpable spleen tip with deep inspiration. His extremities are normal and have strong peripheral pulses. His skin is without jaundice, petechiae, or bruising. He is alert and oriented, and his neurological exam is normal.

DIFFERENTIAL DIAGNOSIS

1. Influenza
2. Infectious mononucleosis
3. Sepsis, bacteremia
4. Malaria
5. Meningitis
6. Dengue fever
7. West Nile virus
8. Zika virus
9. Chikungunya
10. Leptospirosis
11. Yellow fever
12. Typhoid
13. Rickettsial infections
14. Acute schistosomiasis
15. Acute HIV infection

TESTS

Complete blood count: hemoglobin 10.3, hematocrit 32.4%, and a normal mean corpuscular volume. Normal white blood cell count. Platelets 160.

Chemistries: normal sodium, potassium, chloride, and bicarbonate. Blood urea nitrogen 24 and creatinine 1.3. Normal glucose, calcium, magnesium, and phosphate.

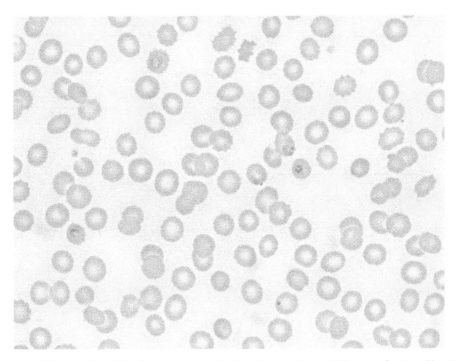

FIGURE 69.1 Thin peripheral blood smear prepared with a Giemsa stain at 100× magnification. Note the ring-shaped immature trophozoites of *Plasmodium falciparum* inside several erythrocytes. The presence of multiple ring forms is typical of *P. falciparum* infections.

Liver function tests: aspartate aminotransferase 75 and alanine aminotransferase 97. Normal alkaline phosphatase, total bilirubin, and albumin.

Coagulation panel: normal prothrombin time, partial thromboplastin time, and international normalized ratio.

Urinalysis: trace ketones but otherwise normal.

Heterophile antibody test: negative.

Rapid influenza antigen swab: negative.

Peripheral blood smear (thin; Giemsa-stained; 100× magnification): Figures 69.1 and 69.2.

CLINICAL COURSE

Based on the patient's presenting symptoms, East African duty station, and brief lapse in antimalarial prophylaxis, a rapid immunochromograph assay for malaria was initially performed on the patient's blood. The rapid diagnostic test was positive for *P. falciparum*, 1 of 5 species of *Plasmodium* protozoa that causes malaria in humans. For confirmation, thick and thin peripheral blood smears were prepared with a Giemsa stain. Microscopic review of the thin smear showed ring-shaped trophozoites residing within the cytoplasm of multiple red blood cells (Figure 69.1). The morphology of these trophozoites was consistent with *P. falciparum,* thus confirming the diagnosis. The patient was admitted to the medical ward for close observation and antimalarial therapy. He completed a 3-day course of oral artemether/lumefantrine and did well following discharge.

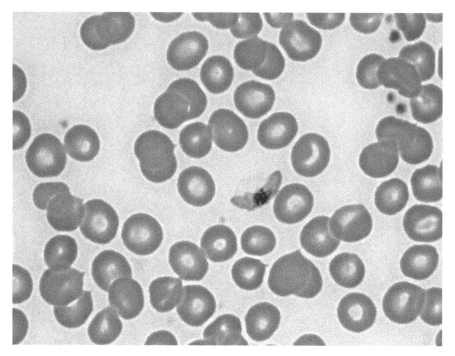

FIGURE 69.2 Thin peripheral blood smear prepared with a Giemsa stain at 100× magnification. The distinctive banana-shaped gametocytes of *Plasmodium falciparum* are pathognomonic when seen in human blood.

KEY MANAGEMENT STEPS

1. Consider zoonotic diseases while evaluating a fever in a foreign country.
2. Diagnose malaria by obtaining thick and thin peripheral blood smears.
3. Differentiate uncomplicated from severe malaria.
4. Understand the different treatment and prophylaxis options for malaria.

DEBRIEF

Malaria is a potentially life-threatening infection caused by several protozoa in the *Plasmodium* genus. There are 4 species that routinely infect humans: *P. falciparum, P. ovale, P. vivax,* and *P. malariae.*[1,2,3]

Malaria is transmitted through the bite of a female *Anopheles* mosquito, which serves as the definitive host and vector of the disease. In *P. vivax* and *P. ovale*, merozoites can enter a dormant phase in the liver and cause relapses of malaria weeks to months after the initial inoculation.[1,2,3] Malaria is normally found in warm, tropical climates. In 2015, the World Health Organization reported over 212 million new cases of malaria with 429,000 deaths.[4]

In uncomplicated malaria, signs and symptoms are often nonspecific. Due to the ongoing hemolysis, patients classically present with fevers followed by a characteristic paroxysm of chills, high fevers, and malaise.[6] Fevers are initially irregular but if untreated, they can adopt regular cycles of 48 to 72 hours depending on the species of *Plasmodium*.[6] Other associated symptoms include headaches, nausea, vomiting, diarrhea, abdominal pain, and myalgias. Physical exam can reveal jaundice and hepatosplenomegaly, with laboratory testing showing a mild anemia.[1,2,5,7]

Uncomplicated malaria can rapidly progress to severe malaria if untreated, especially with *P. falciparum*.[7] Patients with severe malaria can have respiratory distress, intractable vomiting, and prostration.[5,7] Cerebral malaria with neurological symptoms such as seizures and altered mentation can be seen in children and nonimmune adults.[8]

The gold standard for the diagnosis of malaria is light microscopy of Giemsa-stained peripheral blood smears.[9] Thick smears are used to screen a large sample of blood for *Plasmodium*. The thin smear is used to identify the *Plasmodium* species. Both smears can also be used to quantify parasitemia, which is important for estimating disease prognosis.[10,11]

Pharmacotherapy depends on the suspected *Plasmodium* species, the local patterns of drug susceptibility, and the clinical status of the patient. Treatment options include chloroquine, atovaqone/proguanil, or artemether/lumefantrine. Primaquine phosphate may also be required. The Centers for Disease Control has detailed recommendations and an infectious disease specialist should be consulted if providers are inexperienced with malaria treatment.[12] Chemoprophylaxis is recommended for all individuals traveling to regions with endemic malaria.[13]

REFERENCES

1. White NJ, Pukrittayakamee S, Hien TT, Faiz MA, Mokuolu OA, Dondorp AM. Malaria. *Lancet.* 2014;383(9918):723–735.
2. Kantele A, Jokiranta TS. Review of cases with the emerging fifth human malaria parasite. *Clin Infect Dis.* 2011;52(11):1356–1362.
3. White NJ. Malaria. In: Farrar J, Hotez P, Junghanss T, Kang G, Lalloo D, White, N, eds. *Manson's Tropical Diseases.* 23rd ed. Philadelphia, PA: Elsevier-Saunders; 2014: 532–600.
4. World malaria report 2016. World Health Organization 2016. http://www.who.int/malaria/publications/world-malaria-report-2016/report/en/
5. Topical Medicine and International Health. Severe malaria. *Trop Med Int Health.* 2014;19(Suppl 1):7–131.
6. Singh B, Daneshvar C. Human infections and detection of plasmodium knowlesi. *Clin Microbiol Rev.* 2013;26(2):165–184.
7. Miller LH, Baruch DI, Marsh K, Doumbo OK. The pathogenic basis of malaria. *Nature.* 2002;415(6872:)673–679.
8. Newton CR, Chokwe T, Schellenberg JA, et al. Coma scales for children with severe falciparum malaria. *Trans R Soc Trop Med Hyg.* 1997;91(2)161–165.
9. Milne LM, Kyi MS, Chiodini PL, Warhurst DC. Accuracy of routine laboratory diagnosis of malaria in the United Kingdom. *J Clin Pathol.* 1994;47(8):740–742.
10. Fairhurst RM, Wellems TE. Malaria (*Plasmodium* species). In: Bennett JE, Raphael D, Martin JB. *Mandell, Douglas, and Bennett's Principles and Practice of Infectious Diseases.* London, UK: Elsevier-Saunders; 2015: 3070–3090.
11. Division of Parasitic Disease and Malaria. Blood specimens—microscopic evaluation. Centers for Disease Control and Prevention. November 11, 2016. https://www.cdc.gov/dpdx/diagnosticprocedures/blood/microexam.html
12. Treatment of Malaria (Guidelines for Clinicians). Centers for Disease Control and Prevention. July 2013. https://www.cdc.gov/malaria/resources/pdf/clinicalguidance.pdf.
13. Hill DR, Ericsson CD, Pearson RD, et al. The practice of travel medicine: guidelines by the Infectious Diseases Society of America. *Clin Infect Dis.* 2006;43(12):1499–1539.

EXTREMITY SWELLING AND ALTERED MENTAL STATUS

DENISE WHITFIELD

SETTING

Austere Environment

CHIEF COMPLAINT

Altered Mental Status

HISTORY

A 38-year-old male was performing military field operations in South America with his unit. The unit medic was called to evaluate him for altered mental status. Unit members report that the patient was in his usual state of health when he slipped and fell backwards into forest shrubbery. He immediately complained of pain to the left arm. Shortly after, he developed nausea, oral numbness, and lightheadedness, stating he felt faint. A puncture wound was noted on his left upper extremity. His unit medic splinted his affected extremity, began administration of intravenous fluids, and made immediate arrangements for transport to the nearest hospital for further care. During transport, the patient became acutely confused, only oriented to person.

He has no significant past medical history.

He is a smoker, no history of elicit substance use, or recent alcohol.

He has no family history of stroke, intracranial hemorrhage, cardiovascular, or neurologic disease.

PHYSICAL EXAMINATION

Vital signs: HR 134, BP 88/30, RR 28, SpO_2 98% on room air, temp. 37.1°C.

Examination reveals a well-developed, well-nourished male with a Glasgow Coma Scale of 14 (E4V4M6). He appears confused. Head, eye, ear, nose, and throat examination is normal. His lungs are clear bilaterally with good air movement. He is tachycardic; no murmurs, rubs, or gallops are appreciated. His abdomen is soft, nontender and nondistended. Puncture wounds are noted on the medial aspect of his left upper extremity with surrounding edema. He has good peripheral pulses. His extremities are warm and well-perfused. Neurologic examination reveals that he is oriented to person only, with grossly normal strength. Sensation to light touch in the left upper extremity is diminished. Gait and coordination cannot be assessed.

DIFFERENTIAL DIAGNOSIS

1. Snake envenomation
2. Arthropod envenomation
3. Chemical agent exposure
4. Heat-related injury and dehydration
5. Sepsis

TESTS

Upon arrival to the hospital:

Complete blood count: hemoglobin 15.2, hematocrit 45.3, white blood cells 11.2, platelets 98. Normal sodium, potassium, chloride, bicarbonate, blood urea nitrogen, and glucose. Creatinine is slightly elevated to 1.4.

Urinalysis: hemoglobinuria.

Prothrombin time 18.7 seconds, partial thromboplastin time 52.2 seconds, fibrinogen 97 mg/dL.

Chest X-ray: normal cardiac silhouette, clear lungs. No acute abnormality.

Initial puncture wound: Figure 70.1.

CLINICAL COURSE

The patient arrived at a local hospital within 1 hour of symptom onset. He was admitted to the intensive care unit. His mental status remained unchanged on arrival. Notable swelling and ecchymosis developed in the affected upper extremity en route to the hospital. Based on history,

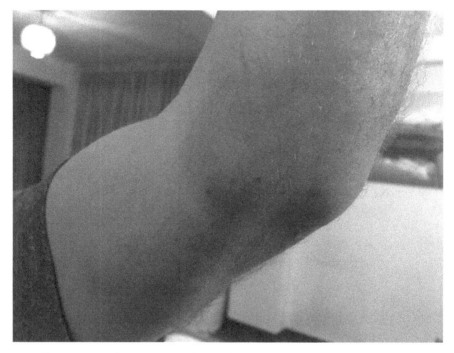

FIGURE 70.1 Puncture wounds consistent with snake bite noted on initial physical examination of a suspected snake bite patient.

Photo courtesy of James Jones, PhD, PA-C.

the patient was placed on a cardiac monitor, and intravenous fluid administration continued. He required vasopressor support for worsening hypotension. The clinical team administered a polyvalent snake antivenom. After the initial dose of antivenom, edema symptoms of the affected extremity improved (as demonstrated by sequential limb circumference measurements), and his hypotension resolved. His mental status returned to baseline. However, his coagulopathy worsened, and his platelet count decreased to a minimum value of 30×10^3 per mm^3. A second dose of antivenom was administered. The patient's coagulopathy improved, and platelet count began to trend upward. His thrombocytopenia and improving coagulopathy were monitored to resolution as an outpatient.

KEY MANAGEMENT STEPS

1. Treatment for snake envenomation in the field requires transporting the patient immediately to the nearest hospital facility with treatment capabilities for evaluation and definitive management.
2. Injured extremities should be immobilized.
3. In the setting of snake envenomation, antivenom is indicated for systemic symptoms (hemostatic abnormalities, hypotension/shock, mental status changes, neurotoxic symptoms) and spreading local swelling.[2,3]
4. Appropriate early consultation with a toxicologist or local expert, based on presentation, can help to guide clinical management.

DEBRIEF

This patient was experiencing local and systemic symptoms from a venomous crotaline snake bite. Snake bites remain a significant global health problem in many tropical and sub-tropical countries causing an estimated 100,000 deaths each year worldwide.[1]

Snake venoms are complex and species specific, containing hundreds of peptides and polypeptides that act as cytotoxins, proteolytic enzymes, and cell-signaling ligands.[3] The particular composition of the inoculating venom determines patient symptoms. In many cases, the venomous snake fails to inoculate during the bite, resulting in a "dry bite." When inoculation occurs, the inoculating venom may work by a variety of mechanisms—cell lysis, capillary leak, hematologic coagulopathy, and/or inhibition of presynaptic and postsynaptic signaling—to cause symptoms.[3]

Snakebite diagnosis is made by the presence of fang marks and correlation with clinical history and presentation. Patients may present with a combination of local, hematologic, neurologic, and systemic symptoms depending on the species of snake.

Worldwide, venomous snakes belong to 4 groups: Elapidae, Crotalinae, Hydrophidae, and Colubridae. In the Americas, native venomous snakes are of the Crotalinae or the Eladpidae groups. The crotaline snake species are also known as "pit vipers."

Envenomations from crotaline species are typically associated with localized pain, swelling, and progressive ecchymosis at the bite site. Local symptoms are mediated by cytotoxic mechanisms that result in cellular damage and an inflammatory response causing swelling, erythema, and pain. Ecchymosis, bullae, and necrosis may develop over time. Early systemic symptoms may include nausea and vomiting, oral paresthesia, tachycardia, or muscle fasciculation. Systemic symptoms may progress to tachycardia, tachypnea, hypotension, and altered mental status.[3,4] Snake venoms may induce abnormalities in the clotting cascade and platelet function systemically as well. Thrombocytopenia, elevated prothrombin time, and hypofibrinogenemia may result.[4]

Elapid envenomation is characterized by predominantly neurotoxic symptoms. There may be few or no local symptoms. Neurotoxic symptoms may include tremor, salivation, acute muscular paralysis, and seizure. Death results from respiratory paralysis. Symptoms may be delayed for several hours.[3,4] Neurotoxic symptoms are the sequelae of the pre- or postsynaptic effects of snake venom on acetylcholine signaling at the neuromuscular junction.[5] Acute neuromuscular paralysis may present as ptosis and ophthalmoplegia early on but can progress to dysarthria, dysphagia, fixed miosis, and acute respiratory failure.

Field Care:

- Safely remove the patient from the snake's striking range.
- Immobilize the affected extremity.
- Pressure immobilization is used in particular parts of the world (Australia, New Guinea) where elapid bites are prevalent and may be fatal. Simple immobilization may be preferred in other global regions.[5–7]
- The use of tourniquets and techniques such as bite incision/suction are contraindicated.
- Administer supportive care focusing on managing the airway, breathing, and circulation. Mortality from crotalid envenomation is often related to third spacing, so the best supportive care is intravenous fluids.
- Treating providers should assume that all bites in the field are envenomation (and not dry bites) and arrange immediate transport to the nearest hospital facility with:

o Personnel that can manage snakebites and antivenom administration complications
o Laboratory capability
o Adequate supply or access to appropriate antivenom[6]

Hospital Care:

- Continue supportive care focused on managing airway, breathing, and circulation. Intravenous fluid administration should be continued to manage hypotension. The patient may require vasopressor support.
- Obtain appropriate laboratory studies to evaluate for systemic envenomation in addition to thorough history and physical examination.
- Administer antivenom in patients with clear clinical or laboratory evidence of systemic envenomation.[4]
- Be prepared to treat adverse effects of antivenom administration including hypersensitivity reactions (anaphylaxis, serum sickness).

Avoidance is the best strategy for preventing snakebites. Individuals who are required to operate in venomous snake endemic regions should wear protective clothing and footwear (long pants, long-sleeved shirts, boots). Lighting (flashlights, headlamps) should be used when they are appropriate for operations.

REFERENCES

1. White J. Bites and stings from venomous animals: a global overview. *Ther Drug Monit.* 2000;22:65–68.
2. Gold BS, Dart RC, Barish, RA. Bites of venomous snakes. *N Engl J Med.* 2002;347(5):347–355.
3. Warrell DA. Venomous bites, stings, and poisoning. *Infect Dis Clin N Am.* 2012;26:207–223.
4. Dart RC, White J. Reptile bites. In: Tintinalli JE, ed. *Tintinalli's Emergency Medicine: A Comprehensive Study Guide.* 8th ed. New York, McGraw-Hill; 2015: 1379–1382.
5. Ranawaka UK, Lalloo DG, de Silva JH. Neurotoxicity in snakebite—the limits of our knowledge. *PLoS Negl Trop Dis.* 2013;7(10):e2302.
6. Long N. Approach to snakebite (blog post) Life in the Fast Lane. July 16, 2017. https://lifeinthefastlane.com/tox-library/basics/approach-to-snakebite/
7. Anz AW, Schweppe M, Halvorson J, Bushnell B, Sternberg M, Koman LA. Management of venomous snakebite injury to the extremities. *J Am Acad Orthop Surg.* 2010;18:749–759.

EYE INJURY

MICHAEL MOHSENI

SETTING

Aircraft Carrier

CHIEF COMPLAINT

Eye Pain

HISTORY

A 23-year-old male presents to the ship's medical department with a complaint of bilateral eye pain and decreased vision after being struck in the face by a large piece of flying debris on the flight deck of an aircraft carrier. He was not wearing eye protection. The discomfort is associated with diffuse swelling around the eyes and markedly decreased vision. He denies vomiting, headache, or syncope. His discomfort is worsened with any attempts to move the right eye. His vision difficulty has progressively worsened since the incident.

He has a no significant past medical history.

He denies any alcohol or tobacco use.

He denies any significant family history.

PHYSICAL EXAMINATION

Vital signs: HR 95, BP 140/90, RR 18, SpO$_2$ 99% on room air, temp. 36.4°C.

Examination reveals a well-developed well-nourished male in moderate distress. Examination of his face reveals multiple small lacerations and abrasions, significant soft tissue swelling and ecchymoses surrounding his right eye. Both pupils are teardrop shaped, and there is loss of direct pupillary response and decreased extraocular motility on the right. His visual acuity is noted to be significantly diminished in the both eyes, with inability to read the Snellen chart. There is an abnormal contour noted to the surface of the right globe; Seidel sign is positive in both eyes on fluorescein testing. Additionally, subconjunctival hemorrhage is noted diffusely in the right eye. The remainder of the neurologic examination reveals grossly normal strength and sensation in all extremities and normal gait and coordination.

DIFFERENTIAL DIAGNOSIS

1. Globe rupture
2. Retrobulbar hematoma
3. Traumatic glaucoma
4. Hyphema
5. Orbital blowout fracture with entrapment

TESTS

Complete blood count: normal hemoglobin, hematocrit, white blood cell count and platelets.

Coagulation panel: normal prothrombin time, partial thromboplastin time, and international normalized ratio.

Maxillofacial computed tomography (CT): unavailable on aircraft carrier.

Radiographs of the orbits: Figure 71.1.

CLINICAL COURSE

Based on the presentation, the patient was placed in an upright position, taking care to avoid any unnecessary manipulation of the eyes. Tetanus immunization status was confirmed. Antiemetics were provided to offset any potential retching, which would increase intraocular pressure. Prophylactic antibiotics were administered. Tonometry was deferred given the appearance of the eye. A protective eye cover was placed to protect both eyes. Ophthalmology was consulted by phone, and medevac was arranged.

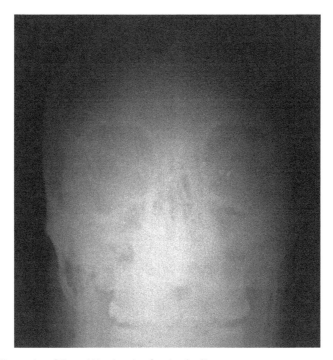

FIGURE 71.1. Radiographs of the orbits showing foreign bodies.

KEY MANAGEMENT STEPS

1. Avoid any unnecessary manipulation of the globe (including tonometry) to prevent any extrusion of intraocular contents.
2. Obtain appropriate imaging to rule out concomitant bony injury or intracranial trauma.
3. Provide analgesia and antiemetics to prevent Valsalva maneuvers that may worsen globe rupture.
4. A protective rigid eye shield should be utilized to prevent any additional injury; eye patches are contraindicated.
5. Provide prophylactic antibiotics to help prevent endophthalmitis.
6. Ensure tetanus immune status.

DEBRIEF

This patient was experiencing eye pain and vision loss from bilateral traumatic globe rupture, caused by blunt and penetrating force to the eye. Typical symptoms of globe rupture include eye deformity, eye pain, and vision loss, though depending on the clinical suggestion the deformity may not be readily apparent on exam. Radiopaque foreign bodies were noted in both orbits and vision loss and globe deformity were present on the initial evaluation.

Globe rupture occurs when there is a defect in the cornea, sclera, or both structures. Most often globe rupture occurs after direct penetrating trauma; however, if sufficient blunt force is applied to the eye, the intraocular pressure can increase enough to rupture the sclera.

Thorough evaluation for any concomitant intracranial and facial bony injury should be pursued. A high number of globe ruptures are associated with fractures, in particular of the orbital floor. Extraocular motility testing may be decreased in the affected eye because of entrapment or intrinsic globe deformity.

Physical examination findings may reveal decreased vision or frank vision loss, irregular contour of the globe, teardrop pupil, hyphema, or a shallow anterior chamber on slit-lamp exam. The Seidel sign is positive in globe rupture, indicating flow of aqueous humor from the injury site in the fluorescein-stained eye. However, if the globe rupture is obvious, testing for the Seidel sign should be avoided.

Emergency treatment includes supportive measures to prevent worsening of globe rupture or extrusion of intraocular contents. Hence, antiemetics should be provided to prevent Valsalva from vomiting, which could lead to increased intraocular pressures and subsequent loss of aqueous fluid. Analgesia should be provided as needed. A rigid eye shield should be placed and additional manipulation of the eye should be avoided. The patient should be placed in a semi-recumbent position.

Laboratory evaluation should be pursued as the clinical situation dictates in the setting of trauma or anticoagulant use. CT imaging can rule out any additional maxillofacial injuries while confirming globe rupture. CT can reveal globe deformity, scleral disruption, and vitreous hemorrhage in the setting of this diagnosis. CT is often unavailable in operational and remote settings.

In the setting of likely globe injury, emergent consultation with ophthalmology was warranted. Definitive management is surgical repair by the appropriate ophthalmologic specialist.

FURTHER READING

Acerra J, Golden D. Globe rupture. eMedicine. April 13, 2017. http://emedicine.medscape.com/article/798223-overview

Babineau MR, Sanchez LD. Ophthalmologic procedures in the emergency department. *Emerg Med Clin North Am*. 2008;26(1):17–34.

Bhatia K, Sharma R. Eye emergencies. In: Adams JG, Barton ED, Collings JL, DeBlieux PMC, Gisondi MA, Nadel ES, eds. *Emergency Medicine Clinical Essentials*. 2nd ed. Philadelphia, PA: Elsevier Saunders; 2013: 224.

Bord SP, Linden J. Trauma to the globe and orbit. *Emerg Med Clin North Am*. 2008;26(1):97–123.

DYSPNEA AND HEMOPTYSIS AFTER A RIGOROUS, OPEN-WATER SWIM

PATRICK ENGELBERT, JOHN HAGGERTY, AND STEVEN PORTOUW

SETTING

Military Health Clinic, Coronado Island, California

CHIEF COMPLAINT

Dyspnea and Hemoptysis

HISTORY

A 27-year-old military recruit reported dyspnea and cough producing a pink, frothy sputum, which started during a training swim in 17°C (63°F) ocean water; he was in the water for approximately 30 minutes and not wearing a wetsuit. He did not report the symptoms until after the swim during a conditioning run when he performed well below his previous ability and fell behind the rest of his training group. He was evaluated by his training team, found to have an O_2 saturation of 85%, and sent into the base clinic.

At the base clinic, he denied any history of similar symptoms as well as any current chest pain or other symptoms beyond dyspnea, cough, and fatigue from his efforts during the swim and run. Specifically, he denied recent illness, dyspnea, or cough before the swim.

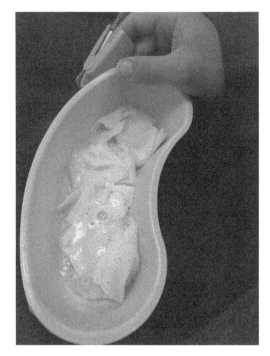

FIGURE 72.1 Characteristic pink, frothy sputum seen with SIPE.

He denied any previous medical, surgical, or significant family medical history.

PHYSICAL EXAMINATION

Vital signs: HR 71, BP 138/67, RR 24, SpO_2 87% on room air, temp. 36.4°C.

On exam, he was observed to have a frequent cough with pink, frothy sputum (Figure 72.1) and conversational dyspnea but was otherwise not in distress. His head and neck exam was normal including without evidence of jugular venous distension. Pulmonary auscultation revealed bibasilar rales. His cardiac exam was normal and without appreciable murmurs, rubs, or gallops. He had no extremity edema and had strong peripheral pulses in all extremities. There were no focal neurologic deficits appreciated.

DIFFERENTIAL DIAGNOSIS

1. Swimming-induced pulmonary edema (SIPE)
2. Congestive heart failure
3. Pulmonary embolism
4. Pneumonia
5. Tuberculosis

TESTS

Chest X-rays: Figure 72.2A.

CLINICAL COURSE

He was passively warmed, administered supplemental O_2 at 2 L/min via nasal cannula and observed in clinic. After 2 to 3 hours of observation, his O_2 saturation on room air was measured at 95%. He reported significant improvement in his dyspnea and decreased frequency of cough.

He was pulled from training with no further treatment other than rest. After 48 hours, he reported resolution of his symptoms except minor dyspnea when going up stairs. A follow-up chest X-ray showed significant radiographic improvement (Figure 72.2B). A gradual increase in activity was initiated until he was performing at previous levels of intensity, first on land and then in water. Two weeks later he was cleared as medically able to return to training.

KEY MANAGEMENT STEPS

1. SIPE should be considered in a patient with dyspnea, hemoptysis, rales, and hypoxia following vigorous exercise during cold-water immersion.
2. Laboratory values are not helpful in the diagnosis of SIPE unless being used to rule out alternative diagnoses.
3. Treatment is primarily supportive with the most important treatment being removal from immersion and exercise.
4. Rapid resolution of symptoms is typically expected.

DEBRIEF

The patient was experiencing shortness of breath, hemoptysis, and hypoxia from SIPE, a condition often associated with rigorous open-water swims such as seen in this case.

The underlying pathophysiology is not fully understood, but it has been proposed that SIPE likely occurs from the effects caused by immersion, particularly in cold water, in conjunction with vigorous exertion. This can lead to central shunting of blood, in part due to peripheral vasoconstriction, with a subsequent increase in preload, cardiac output, and afterload, which contributes to increased pulmonary capillary pressures. This increase in pulmonary capillary pressure may lead to capillary fracture and ultimately the development of pulmonary edema and hemoptysis.[1] There is also thought that over-hydration may play a role in the development of SIPE.[2]

Presenting signs and symptoms of SIPE typically include shortness of breath, hemoptysis, hypoxia, and rales occurring while performing, or immediately after performing, a rigorous cold-water swim. Chest x-ray may be consistent with pulmonary edema. No particular labs confirm the diagnosis of SIPE, including brain natriuretic peptide (BNP).[3]

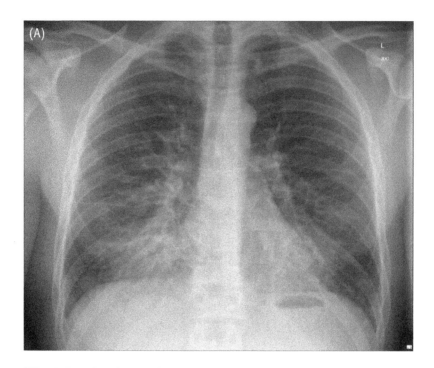

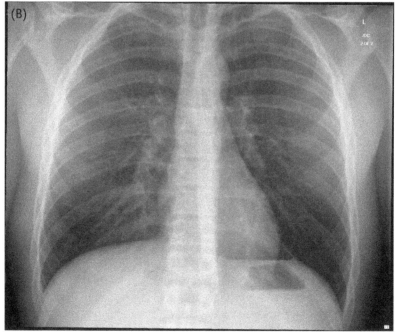

FIGURE 72.2 (A) Initial chest X-ray that revealed patchy consolidations of the hila, right middle, and left lower lobe, along with fluid with the minor fissure. (B) Chest X-ray 48 hours after initial presentation with near resolution of abnormal findings.

Treatment is predominately supportive and includes removal from immersion and exertional activities with placement into a warm, dry environment. Typically, the recovery is quick once the patient is removed from the offending environment. Inhaled beta$_2$-agonists and supplemental oxygen may further hasten the recovery process. Diuretics are typically not indicated.[1] Sildenafil has been evaluated as a way to reduce pulmonary vascular pressures and potentially reduce the risk for SIPE.[4] This prophylactic treatment, however, likely requires additional research and is not a treatment currently employed by US Navy medical teams.

If evaluated in the emergency department, patients with SIPE can often be discharged after oxygen saturations have returned to baseline without the need for supplemental oxygenation. Prognosis of SIPE is good with complete resolution of symptoms typically seen within 72 hours.[3]

REFERENCES

1. Lund KL, Mahon RT, Tanen DA, Bakhda S. Swimming-induced pulmonary edema. *Ann Emerg Med*. 2003;41(2):251–256.
2. Yoder JA, Viera AJ. Management of swimming-induced pulmonary edema. *Am Fam Physician*. 2004;69(5):1046–1049.
3. Shearer D, Mahon R. Brain natriuretic peptide levels in six Basic Underwater Demolitions/ SEAL recruits presenting with swimming induced pulmonary edema (SIPE). *J Spec Oper Med*. 2009;9(3):44–50.
4. Moon RE, Martina SD, Peacher FD, et al. Swimming-induced pulmonary edema: pathophysiology and risk reduction with sildenafil. *Circulation*. 2016;133(10):988–996.

CHAPTER 73

PENETRATING CHEST TRAUMA

KATHERINE BIGGS

SETTING

Military Aid Station in a Combat Zone, Surgical Capability

CHIEF COMPLAINT

Hit by a Rocket-Propelled Grenade (RPG)

HISTORY

A 25-year-old male presents to the military aid station after being hit by an RPG while on patrol. He was walking along the road when he was hit in the chest. He denies loss of consciousness. He has trouble breathing and can only speak in one-word answers. He is having chest pain and abdominal pain. Injury occurred 20 minutes ago.

He denies a past medical history, tonsillectomy as a child.

He denies smoking and drinks occasionally.

Family history includes hypertension.

PHYSICAL EXAMINATION

Vital signs: HR 120, BP 91/54, RR 25, SpO_2 93% on room air, temp. 36.9°C.

Examination reveals a well-developed, well-nourished male in acute distress. He is able to speak in one-word answers. There is no blood coming from oropharynx. There are two approximately 3 cm circular wounds on his left anterior chest and right flank that are actively bleeding. There is unequal chest rise on the left with no breath sounds. His trachea is midline. Pulses are intact in all four extremities. Pupils are 3 mm, equal, round, and reactive. He is able to move all extremities. Abdomen is tender.

1. Open pneumothorax
2. Tension pneumothorax
3. Hemothorax
4. Cardiac tamponade
5. Liver laceration
6. Bowel perforation
7. Tracheobronchial injury
8. Pulmonary contusion
9. Rib fractures

TESTS

Extended focused assessment with sonography for trauma (eFAST) exam: absent lung slide on left, no fluid around heart, free fluid in Morrison's pouch.

Chest X-ray: left-sided moderate pneumothorax with hemothorax.

Complete blood count: normal hemoglobin, hematocrit, white blood cell count, and platelets.

Basic metabolic panel: normal sodium, potassium, chloride, bicarbonate, blood urea nitrogen, creatinine, and glucose.

CLINICAL COURSE

The patient presented as a penetrating chest and abdominal trauma. During the primary survey the airway was determined to be patent. He had a sucking chest wound to the left anterior chest and, an Asherman chest seal was placed (Figure 73.1). During the assessment, ancillary staff placed the patient on 2 L nasal cannula, established a second large-bore intravenous (IV) and started IV fluid. eFAST showed free fluid in Morrison's pouch. After the secondary assessment was completed, a left-sided tube thoracostomy was performed with 200 mL of blood drained. Due to the open pneumothorax and penetrating abdominal trauma, the patient was emergently taken to the operating room for exploration and repair of wounds.

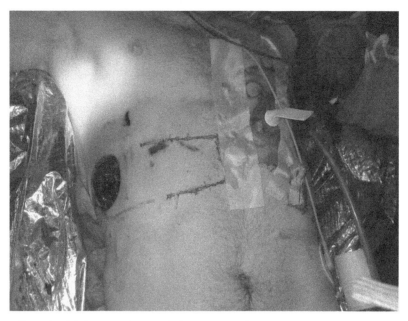

FIGURE 73.1 Example of Asherman chest seal placed on a sucking chest wound on the left anterior chest.

KEY MANAGEMENT STEPS

1. For all trauma evaluations and resuscitations start with a primary survey: airway maintenance with cervical spine protection, breathing and ventilation, circulation with hemorrhage control, disability (neurologic status), and exposure/environment control. This is followed by a secondary survey.
2. With open chest wounds, place a 3-sided occlusive dressing to prevent converting to a tension pneumothorax, ideally in the prehospital setting.
3. Definitive management of open pneumothorax is a chest tube.
4. Penetrating abdominal trauma will likely require laparotomy.

DEBRIEF

Trauma resuscitations, no matter the setting or injuries, should be run the same. An organized primary and secondary survey should be assessed, deviating only for life-saving interventions. This case involves a young male with penetrating chest and abdominal trauma with an open pneumothorax. During a trauma evaluation, simultaneously resuscitate the patient with IV fluids, blood products, and procedures as indicated with frequent reevaluations.

If there are signs of airway obstruction or compromise, the evaluation should be stopped and airway intervention initiated. During the breathing assessment, if there is a sucking chest wound, as this case, a 3-sided occlusive dressing or Asherman chest seal dressing needs to be applied. Ideally, a sterile dressing should be used but any dressing or occlusive material can work to cover the wound, taping on 3 sides. This dressing acts like a valve, allowing air to escape the chest cavity but preventing air from entering. The Asherman chest seal is an improvement on the 3-sided occlusive dressing; it completely covers the wound and has a 1-way valve built in. Both of these dressings are temporary measures but help prevent conversion to tension pneumothorax. If there are signs of a tension pneumothorax (hypotension, jugular venous distension, tracheal deviation), a needle thoracostomy must be performed immediately. This is accomplished by inserting a 5 cm 14 G needle in the second intercostal space at the mid-clavicular line, or in the fifth intercostal space anterior to the mid-axillary line. A rush of air should be heard, indicating the needle made it into the chest cavity, relieving the tension. In large and muscular people or those wearing Kevlar vests, the mid-axillary line approach is better and now the primary recommended location. This approach is more accessible, and the distance to the thoracic cavity is shorter. If the patient has improved with these interventions, continue with the primary survey.

Once the primary and secondary surveys are completed, including eFAST if available, more definitive treatments of the injuries need to be established. Indications for tube thoracostomy include:

- Traumatic pneumothorax (except asymptomatic, apical pneumothorax)
- Moderate to large pneumothorax
- Respiratory symptoms
- Increasing size of pneumothorax despite conservative measures
- Recurrence of pneumothorax after removing initial chest tube
- Need for ventilator (positive pressure) support
- Associated hemothorax
- Bilateral pneumothorax
- Tension pneumothorax

Even a small pneumothorax may require a chest tube if the patient is going to be transported by air to avoid expansion during flight.

This patient also had penetrating abdominal injury with free fluid seen on the eFAST and was taken to the operating room. Indications for laparotomy following penetrating trauma are hemodynamic instability, peritoneal signs, evisceration, diaphragmatic injury, gastrointestinal hemorrhage, implement in situ, and intraperitoneal air.

FURTHER READING

American College of Surgeons. Abdominal and pelvic trauma. In: *Advanced Trauma Life Support Student Course Manual.* 9th ed. Chicago, IL: Second Impression; 2012: 94–121.

American College of Surgeons. Thoracic trauma. In: *Advanced Trauma Life Support Student Course Manual.* 9th ed. Chicago, IL: American College of Surgeons; 2012: 122–147.

Eckstein M, Henderson SO. Thoracic trauma. In: Marx JA, Rosen P, eds. *Rosen's Emergency Medicine: Concepts and Clinical Practice.* 8th ed. Philadelphia, PA: Elsevier/Saunders; 2013: 431–458.

Kirsh TD. Tube thoracostomy. In: Roberts JR, ed. *Roberts and Hedges' Clinical Procedures in Emergency Medicine.* 6th ed. Philadelphia, PA: Elsevier/Saunders; 2014: 175–196.

Platz JJ, Fabricant L, Norotsky M. Thoracic trauma: injuries, evaluation and treatment. *Surg Clin North Am.* 2017;97(4):783–799.

Puskarich MA, Marx JA. Abdominal trauma. In: Marx JA, Rosen P, eds. *Rosen's Emergency Medicine: Concepts and Clinical Practice.* 8th ed. Philadelphia, PA: Elsevier/Saunders; 2013: 459–478.

INDEX

Note: Page numbers followed by *f* or *t* indicate a figure or table.